Parent-Infant Nursing Science: *Paradigms, Phenomena, Methods*

Lorraine O. Walker, R.N., Ed.D., F.A.A.N.
Luci B. Johnson Centennial Professor in Nursing
The University of Texas at Austin
School of Nursing
Austin, Texas

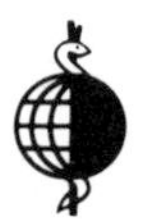

F. A. DAVIS COMPANY • Philadelphia

Printed in the United States of America

Last digit indicates print number: 10 9 8 7 6 5 4 3 2 1

NOTE: As new scientific information becomes available through basic and clinical research, recommended treatments and drug therapies undergo changes. The author(s) and publisher have done everything possible to make this book accurate, up to date, and in accord with accepted standards at the time of publication. The authors, editors, and publisher are not responsible for errors or omissions or for consequences from application of the book, and make no warranty, expressed or implied, in regard to the contents of the book. Any practice described in this book should be applied by the reader in accordance with professional standards of care used in regard to the unique circumstances that may apply in each situation. The reader is advised always to check product information (package inserts) for changes and new information regarding dose and contraindications before administering any drug. Caution is especially urged when using new or infrequently ordered drugs.

Library of Congress Cataloging-in-Publication Data

Walker, Lorraine Olszewski.

Parent-infant nursing science : paradigms, phenomena, methods / Lorraine O. Walker.

p. cm.

Includes bibliographical references and index.

ISBN 0-8036-9028-2 (hardback : alk. paper)

1. Maternity nursing. 2. Maternity nursing—Research. I. Title.

[DNLM: 1. Maternal-Child Nursing—methods. 2. Parent-Child Relations. WY 157.3 W181p]

RG951.W29 1991

610.73'678—dc20

DNLM/DLC

for Library of Congress 91-25136

CIP

This book is dedicated to my parents, Mary Krupnik Olszewski and Clement J. Olszewski, Sr.

Preface

My goal in writing this book was to increase the accessibility of parent-infant nursing research and to organize that research according to the field's emerging paradigms. My motivation to undertake such a project can be traced back to my baccalaureate program at the University of Dayton with Ann Franklin. We students, even in the early 1960s, were constantly confronted with the absence of a body of knowledge upon which to base our nursing practice. During my masters program at Indiana University we were sent out to comb through any available science that might be found to demonstrate the rational basis for nursing practices. Thus, having been well-schooled in the importance of "hunting expeditions" and the exhilaration of a "find," it is only logical that I would do a book like this. Having been gently persuaded by Betty Grossman that parenthood remains one of life's most intriguing mysteries, it was only natural that I should do this book in my specialty field of parent-infant nursing.

As ambitious as my goal was in undertaking this writing, the final product has its limitations and I share these freely with readers so that they not be lulled into thinking that everything is here. First, I worked diligently to locate as much research published by nurses in the parent-infant field as possible. Often, early writings in the field, however, made finding a clear answer to the question, "Is this research?" difficult or impossible. Second, many practice journals did not clearly indicate in the table of contents which articles reported research findings. Finally, a number of nurse investigators reported research findings in book chapters or journals in other disciplines. Both of these posed formidable problems in identification. For the most part this book represents research published in major nursing research journals, clinical nursing journals that designate research articles in the tables of contents, articles cited in major published research reviews, and other sources as these were known to me.

Specifically, the studies covered in this book emphasize the following journals from 1978 to 1989: *Nursing Research, Research in Nursing and Health, Advances in Nursing Science, Journal of Nurse-Midwifery,* and *Maternal-Child Nursing Journal* (ending with volume 18, number 1). *Journal of Obstetric, Gynecologic, and Neonatal Nursing* and *Western Journal of Nurs-*

PART ONE

Specialization and the Nursing Discipline

CHAPTER 1

A Disciplinary Perspective on Parent-Infant Nursing

Knowledge is a key factor in advancing the nursing profession and the practice of nurses. In particular, knowledge generated by nurses about specific populations served by nurses empowers both the profession and its practitioners. Specialized knowledge about populations served by nurses expands our understanding about how to enhance client health and well-being. Specialization—in the area of academic knowledge or practice—is a mark of a maturing profession. According to Hoeffer and Murphy (1984), "Specialization is created primarily by complexity of knowledge and new technologies, attained by advanced education, and maintained by delimiting practice" (p. 8). Thus, in order to specialize, practitioners must have mastered advanced knowledge focused on a specific area of practice.

In this view, nursing specialization is *not* the opposite of holistic care; rather it integrates fundamental nursing values, such as caring, with thorough knowledge of particular populations served by nurses. Knowledge—particularly scientific knowledge—and caring are not incompatible entities. Each represents part of the modes of knowing and experiencing needed in the rich and complex world of nursing practice (Carper, 1978; Kidd & Morrison, 1988).

Further, nursing scholars have advocated that nursing science, rather than the science of other fields, become the basis for nursing specialties (Hoeffer & Murphy, 1984). Increasingly, there is a belief that nursing science is now an emerging reality. That reality is supported by studies such as those by Moody, Wilson, Smyth, Schwartz, Tittle, and Van Cott (1988). In their analysis of scientific nursing literature, Moody et al. identified 720 articles on nursing practice research published between 1977 and 1986 in six nursing research journals. Further, they documented the clinical populations of interest in nursing studies. For example, of the research they reviewed, 12 percent focused on maternal-infant nursing, 8 percent on child health, and 7.4 percent on women's health. Shortly thereafter, Beck's (1989) analytic review of maternal-newborn nursing research from 1977 to 1986 supported the emergence of a distinct field of parent-infant nursing science.

As background to the exposition of parent-infant nursing science, it is helpful to first consider the discipline, the profession, and the practice of nursing. Each aspect of nursing is briefly examined in the next section, and that is followed by development of a perspective for parent-infant nursing as an area of specialization in nursing.

DIMENSIONS OF NURSING

The *discipline* of nursing as an academic field embodies both the current knowledge base of nursing and the scholarly processes through which nursing knowledge is developed. (See Table 1–1 for definitions related to the concept of discipline.) Just as the information used in the practice dimension of nursing is directed at the artful, humane, and effective provision of care to clients, so the knowledge sought within the disciplinary dimension reflects the phenomena of concern to nursing. According to Donaldson and Crowley,

> *Typically, disciplines have evolved as a consequence of a distinct perspective and syntax, which determine what phenomena or abstractions are of interest, in what context such phenomena are to be viewed, what questions are to be raised, what methods of study are to be used, and what canons of evidence and proof are to be required. (1978, p. 114)*

Thus, the discipline is shaped not by discrete technical information but rather by the broad viewpoint, values, and perspective adopted by its theoreticians and researchers (Carveth, 1987). In that regard, Greene defined nursing as "a service discipline that provides care, concern, and comfort to recipients experiencing a broad range of health-illness phenomena through the synergistic combination of its art and science" (1979, p. 63).

The discipline of nursing is especially concerned with describing and explaining phenomena of concern in terms of fundamental processes that endure across time and place. In parent-infant nursing science—an emerging specialty area within the discipline—examples of important phenomena of interest include maternal attachment (Avant, 1979), role attainment (Rubin, 1967), and behavioral organization in infants (Anderson, Raff, Duxbury, & Carroll, 1979).

Table 1–1
DEFINITIONS RELATED TO THE CONCEPT OF DISCIPLINE

Discipline

A defined field of knowledge marked by a community of scholars who are experts in the subject matter and methods of a field, a body of scholarly knowledge which may include one or more paradigms guiding scholarly work and standards which guide the conduct of scholarly inquiry in a field. In essence, a discipline is "characterized by a unique perspective, a distinct way of viewing all phenomena, which ultimately defines the limits and nature of its inquiry." (Donaldson & Crowley, 1978, p. 113.)

Paradigm

A family of related theories which share similar concepts and structural features rooted in a relatively shared set of starting theoretical assumptions (e.g., that the unconscious mind exists; that humans are in constant interaction with the environment) as well as similar criteria of evidence. While individual theories within a paradigm may be tested, the paradigm is not directly tested because of its abstract and evolving nature.

Theory

"An internally consistent group of relational statements (concepts, definitions, and propositions) that represent a systematic view of a phenomenon and which is useful for description, explanation, prediction, and control." (Walker & Avant, 1983, pp. 17–18.)

Phenomenon

An event occurring in reality as opposed to the idea of the event held in mind.

Phenomena of Concern

The key concepts which depict at an abstract level the recurrent kinds of events (i.e., the major types of events) that have been, are currently, or are proposed to be the central focus of a field of study or discipline.

Clinical Phenomena

Concepts which depict at an abstract level the recurrent kinds of events that are the focal concern of a field of professional practice. These may be less abstract than the phenomena of concern to a discipline in that they encompass typical events observed in practice and thus often have defined clinical manifestations (e.g., signs and symptoms) and predictable circumstances when they are likely to occur (etiologies). Often clinical phenomena which represent a problematic state of affairs in terms of patient well being or development are expressed as nursing diagnoses.

Concept

Mental representation of an individual; or mental representation of a class of individuals or events. "Terms" or "words" are used in communication between people to express concepts.

Clinical Concepts

Linguistic labels which capture key or recurrent types of events observed in practice. Clinical "concepts" is partially a misnomer in that clinical terms express linguistically the mental representations, perceptions, or classificatory schemes used by clinicians; concepts are not spoken, but rather they are represented in language.

The *profession* of nursing denotes a skilled occupation the practitioners of which are educated and credentialed to carry out a range of health care services. The requisite professional services are specified by statutory and other regulatory mechanisms. In turn, the members of the profession are recognized by the general public as expert in providing specialized services associated with nursing. In *Nursing: A Social Policy Statement* (American Nurses' Association (1980, p. 7), the relationship of a profession to society is called a social contract.

Development of theory has been an important ingredient in building nursing's autonomy as a profession. In this regard, Chinn and Jacobs note "that theoretical knowledge is a basis of power" (1987, p. 20). In historical perspective, possession of a body of knowledge has repeatedly been used as one of the criteria for assessing the status of nursing as a profession (Bixler & Bixler, 1945, 1959). Theoretical knowledge expressed in nursing science is a necessity for professional status because it provides a firm foundation for the practice of nursing.

The *practice* dimension of nursing of special interest here is the nursing approach to assessing, diagnosing, treating/ameliorating, and evaluating the health care needs of clients. This approach is critical to the American Nurses' Association definition of nursing as "the diagnosis and treatment of human responses to actual and potential health problems" (p. 9). The practice of nursing is more than a set of techniques; it includes consideration of (1) phenomena, (2) theory application, (3) nursing actions, and (4) evaluation of effects of action in relation to phenomena (American Nurses' Association, 1980, p. 9). The multitude of very complex skills, techniques, and information needed to administer care is grounded in nursing science and nursing values.

Application of these skills, techniques, and information is guided by such criteria as standards of practice. A key feature of the practice dimension is recognized patterns of expectable care for clients with specific health problems or health needs, all things being equal. Such patterns can be identified by reading nursing textbooks or interviewing expert nurses. The information needed in practice is aimed at achieving desired client outcomes within the constraints of nursing values, available science, technology, and resources.

There is, of course, no sharp line dividing the practice and disciplinary dimensions of nursing described here. Indeed, much of nurses' research—a key activity within the disciplinary dimension—has been directed at both exploring phenomena and improving practice. For example, Mercer (1986) conducted a study directed at gaining a better understanding of the phenomenon of maternal role attainment over the span of the first year of motherhood. While directed at expanding knowledge of fundamental processes, Mercer's work also has identified factors that lead to impaired parenting. As the nursing discipline expands fundamental knowledge of clinical phenomena, clinical assessment and intervention may be transformed.

The link between the discipline and practice of nursing is well demonstrated in the work of Barnard. Barnard's research (e.g., Bee, Hammond, Eyres, Barnard, & Snyder, 1986) identified predictors of infant development and subsequently led to the development of clinical assessment protocols. Nurses may now receive training in a variety of assessment tools relevant to infants and their environments that emerged from the research.

FOCUS OF THE NURSING DISCIPLINE

What is the focus of the nursing discipline? According to Donaldson and Crowley (1978), three themes have predominated:

---

1. *Concern with principles and laws that govern the life processes, well-being, and optimal functioning of human beings, sick or well. For example, a concern with the discovery of laws that govern health, knowledge of reparative processes, and prevention was manifest in the late nineteenth or early twentieth century in Nightingale's writings and certainly in Rogers' concern with laws and principles governing life processes in the past two decades.*
2. *Concern with the patterning of human behavior in interaction with the environment in critical life situations. As evidence of this theme, Rogers' writings reflect a concern with life rhythms and their relationship to environmental rhythms. Similarly, Johnson's writings in the 1960s focused attention on systems of behavior, pattern-maintenance, and pattern-disruption. The conceptual frames for most nursing curricula today include coping processes, adaptation, and supportive and nonsupportive environments.*
3. *Concern with the processes by which positive changes in health status are affected. Peplau addressed herself to nursing as an interpersonal process, an educative force, whereas; Kreuter as well as Leininger and others addressed the particular type of process of support system seen as nursing's unique contribution (1978, p. 113).*

Subsequently, Fawcett slightly modified and expanded on Donaldson and Crowley's work. Fawcett argued that the "relationships between and among the concepts—person, environment, health, nursing—are elaborated in recurring themes found in the work of nurse scholars since Nightingale." (1984, p. 84). Those themes included the following:

> 1. *The principles and laws that govern the life-process, well-being, and optimal function of human beings, sick or well.*
> 2. *The patterning of human behavior in interaction with the environment in* normal life events *and critical life situations [emphasis added].*
> 3. *The process by which positive changes in health status are effected (1984, p. 85).*

Although these themes are helpful in suggesting broad boundaries of the nursing discipline, they are in need of extensive elaboration to be useful in further identifying nursing phenomena of concern. To be effective, the elaboration should be done by specialists who carve out defined and manageable programs of research and theory development focused at the specialty level. In that regard, clinical specialty areas have a tremendous contribution to make in elaborating the subject matter of the discipline. Development of nursing science within specialty areas is the next step in the development of the nursing discipline. The emphasis on specific populations in specialty areas encourages a steady accretion of knowledge based on research, clinical studies, and theory formulation related to a limited set of phenomena.

SPECIALIZATION AND THE NURSING DISCIPLINE

The relation between specialization in knowledge and practice and the nursing discipline has evolved gradually. The American Nurses' Association (1980) has described specialization in nursing practice as follows:

> *Specialization means a narrowed focus on a part of the whole field of nursing. It entails application of a broad range of theories to selected phenomena within the domain of nursing, in order to secure depth of understanding as a basis for advances in nursing practice. (p. 21)*

Further, graduate education, the route to specialization, "includes in-depth study of theories relevant to the particular area of specialization and faculty-supervised clinical practice" (p. 23).

The concept of specialization as expressed by the American Nurses' Association can be taken one step further today. Specialization for nursing practice requires more than "application of a broad range of theories to selected phenomena" and "in-depth study of theories relevant to the particular area of specialization." It requires mastery of theoretical knowledge about the phenomena within a specific part of the nursing discipline. Thus, specialty practice for nursing has its roots in specialized knowledge within the nursing discipline

In a related vein, Murphy and Hoeffer (1983) have critiqued the American Nurses' Association statement about specialization. They assert that it is based on

> *the belief that nursing is primarily an applied science. Thus, it emphasizes the* application *of a broad range of theories borrowed from other disciplines to understand subsets of phenomena, rather than the* generation *of nursing theories or the* adaptation *of borrowed theories and concepts for nursing practice. (p. 34)*

They proposed instead that "nursing specialties can best contribute to nursing science by generating and testing middle-range or limited-scope theories" (pp. 34–35) relevant to practice concerns within specialty areas. Consistent with this theme, Walker (1989) proposed a revised definition of specialization in nursing as

> *an intensive focus on the health and developmental processes, needs, and experiences of an identifiable population served by nurses. It entails developing, testing, and revising middle-range or limited-scope theories within the discipline of nursing in order to secure depth of understanding as a basis for advances in nursing practice and nursing science. (p. 16)*

If in-depth, specialized knowledge is required for specialty practice, then the development of the discipline must logically precede the development of specialty practice. That, of course, has not been the chronological sequence in nursing. Nursing specialization has often been based on advances in *medical science* and technology rather than on advances in *nursing science* and nursing innovations. However, as nursing science grows, the source of innovations in practice can increasingly be expected to come from the nursing-specialty science rather than other disciplines.

PARENT-INFANT NURSING SCIENCE

Parent-infant nursing is a specialty area that is developing a rich and bountiful literature within the nursing discipline (see reviews by Mercer,

1985a, 1985b; Barnard & Blackburn, 1985; Barnard & Neal, 1977; Barnard, 1983; Lederman, 1984, 1986; McBride, 1984). This literature constitutes the basis for an identifiable specialty within the nursing discipline and serves as an emerging foundation for specialty nursing practice.

Pregnancy, birth, and postpartum serve as "marker events" in both the practice and knowledge base for parent-infant nursing. These marker events are important, however, for all the scientific and professional disciplines that study reproduction and parenting. Thus, they are not necessarily the primary subject matter of parent-infant nursing.

If pregnancy, childbirth, and postpartum are not the primary subject matter of parent-infant nursing, then what is? This book is premised on the belief that the concepts, theories, and paradigms used to construct coherent accounts of human experiences related to reproduction and parenting are that subject matter. The subject matter of parent-infant nursing includes, but is not limited to, the following:

1. Stress and coping processes in the reproductive and parenting cycles, including the influence of social support and personal and social resources on those processes
2. Mastery of the transition to parenthood, including role and relational aspects, and transitions in health conditioned by reproduction and parenting
3. Patterns of health behaviors and health status during pregnancy, childbirth, early parenting, and infancy
4. Human interaction with special emphasis on that between parent and infant
5. Human development with special emphasis on the developing infant

Running through each of these phenomena of concern to parent-infant nursing is the larger concern of fostering health and development. Indeed, two of the defining attributes of parent-infant nursing may be a focus on health and a focus on development. In that regard, the American Nurses' Association states: "The phenomena with which maternal and child nurses are concerned independently are the observable responses of women, children, and families to actual or potential *health* or *developmental* problems" [emphasis added] (1983, p. 3).

Thus, parent-infant nursing concerns itself specifically with the health status and health behaviors, parental role development, stress and coping, and person-environment interactions of parents and infants. More broadly, parent-infant nursing includes concepts and theories that blend health and developmental perspectives or that at a minimum have implications for health and development of parents and infants. Further, viewed within the context of the recurring themes of nursing (Donaldson & Crowley, 1978), parent-infant nursing concerns reflect population-specific elaborations of nursing's metaparadigm. Table 1–2 presents examples of that elaboration in parent-infant nursing science.

Table 1–2
EXAMPLES OF ELABORATIONS OF THE NURSING METAPARADIGM IN PARENT-INFANT NURSING SCIENCE*

THEMES AND CONCEPTS IN NURSING METAPARADIGM			
Parent-infant concerns	Principles and laws that govern the life-process, well-being, and optimal functioning (person and health)	Patterning of human behavior in interaction with the environment (person, environment, and health)	Processes by which positive changes in health status are effected (person, health, environment, and nursing)
Stress and coping	—	Descriptive and predictive theories related to the effects of stress, coping, and social support during pregnancy, early parenting, and infancy	Practice theories aimed at stress management, coping, and support mobilization
Parental role	Descriptive and predictive theories related to parental role development	—	Practice theories aimed at enhancing parental role performance, cognitions, and attitudes
Health behaviors and health status	Descriptive and predictive theories related to parental and infant health	—	Practice theories aimed at risk reduction and health promotion in parents and infants
Human interaction	—	Descriptive and predictive theories of behavioral organization and interaction during infancy	Practice theories aimed at facilitating behavioral organization and parent-infant interaction
Human development	—	Descriptive and predictive theories of early development in the context of the environment	Practice theories aimed at enhancing infant development within the context of the parenting environment

Note: This table represents ideas derived from Donaldson and Crowley (1978) and Fawcett (1984).

EXISTING PARADIGMS WITHIN PARENT-INFANT NURSING SCIENCE

What paradigms are used to study the phenomena of concern to parent-infant nursing science? Choice of paradigm depends on what specific phenomena are under study and how closely phenomena fit with concepts in existing paradigms. For example, childbirth may be viewed from either a *stress-and-coping* paradigm or from a *role attainment* paradigm depending on the circumstances. Similarly, the relation between premature infant and parent may be understood in terms of either parent-infant *interaction* patterns or *health status* of the infant. However, if a preterm infant is being moved from an incubator with scheduled feedings to an open crib and demand feedings, the paradigm of *behavioral organization* may be more useful than a stress paradigm. Thus, multiple paradigms are needed to cover the scope of parent-infant nursing science and thought is needed to apply them suitably. The classification system for parent-infant paradigms and their component phenomena to be used in this book is as follows:

1. Stress, coping, and support
   a. Stress
   b. Coping
   c. Social support
2. Health
   a. Health status
   b. Health behaviors
3. Parental development
   a. Transition to parenthood
   b. Parental role attainment
   c. Attachment
   d. Separation and loss
4. Behavioral interaction and behavioral organization
   a. Behavioral organization in infancy
   b. Behavioral interaction
5. Person-environment interaction and development

The classificatory system presented here was developed through careful review and analysis of nursing research literature dating from 1982 to 1987. *Nursing Research, Research in Nursing and Health,* and *Western Journal of Nursing Research* were examined for all articles that related to parent-infant nursing. A sample of 101 articles was identified as pertinent to parents and infants, and the articles were examined for their phenomena of concern as expressed in the titles, abstracts, research questions, and study variables within articles. Initial categories for classifying articles were based on an earlier analysis of emerging research themes done by Walker and Avant (1988). To cross-validate the classificatory system, parent-infant–focused articles appearing in *Maternal Child Nursing Journal* for the same time period as used in the initial analysis were reviewed and classified. Categories in the classificatory system worked well in sorting this second set of articles into conceptual groups.

The classification system presented here represents one way of organizing knowledge, and it is not a proposal for what the desired directions for parent-infant science should be. The paradigms and phenomena of concern in the classificatory system represent an attempt at delineating the directions currently being adopted by nursing scholars in parent-infant nursing. Thus, the aim of this book is to facilitate the future work of scholars in parent-infant nursing science by synthesizing information about the paradigms, phenomena, and methods of the science. The synthesis is not of itself prescriptive.

PARENT-INFANT NURSING SCIENCE AND PRACTICE

Although the disciplinary aspects of parent-infant nursing science have been growing rapidly in the past 5 years, less notice has been directed to the potential that much of this work bears for the future of practice. The discipline has special relevance for practice by virtue of (1) identifying information needed for accurate assessment of pregnant women, their partners, and infants, (2) testing theoretical principles on which to base nursing interventions, and (3) developing methods for evaluating quality of care. A first step in linking the science and the practice is synthesizing nursing research findings and incorporating them in clinical nursing textbooks. A second step will require overcoming several problems: (1) gaps in the scope of nursing intervention research, (2) weak links between phenomena of concern and research-based interventions, and (3) the need to develop the theoretical grounds for existing interventions.

RELATION OF THE FOLLOWING CHAPTERS TO THE STRUCTURE OF PARENT-INFANT NURSING SCIENCE

In Part I, the importance of nursing science in developing nursing specialization was presented. Further, a classification system for parent-infant nursing science based on recurrent phenomena investigated in nursing research was proposed. The system included five major paradigms that capture the bulk of parent-infant nursing science at this time. The remaining sections of this book elaborate on the paradigms and their component phenomena.

In Part II, the stress, coping, and social support paradigm is presented.

Chapter 2 presents an overview of the paradigm using literature from the broad field of stress research. In Chapters 3 to 5 each component of that paradigm is examined specifically in relation to parent-infant nursing science.

The paradigm of health, including both health status and health behaviors, is presented in Part III. Chapter 6 focuses on an overview of alternative models of health in nursing and in the larger field of health research. In Chapters 7 and 8, parent-infant nursing science relating to health status and health behaviors is presented.

In Part IV the family of related theories comprising the parental development paradigm is presented. Chapter 9 provides an overview of alternative views of approaching the study of parental development and relational ties. In Chapters 10 to 15, transitions, role attainment, attachment, and loss are examined in the context of parent-infant nursing science. The voluminous research on role attainment across the antepartal, intrapartal, and postpartal periods is presented in Chapters 11 to 13.

Table 1–3
REVIEWS CITING PARENT-INFANT NURSING SCIENCE LITERATURE

Review	Dates for Literature Search	Topic
Barnard & Neal (1977)	1952–1975	Maternal-child nursing
Mercer (1985b)	1956–1982	Teenage pregnancy
Barnard (1983)	1977–1981	Children under 5 yr
Mercer (1985a)	1973–1983	Obstetrical nursing
Barnard & Blackburn (1985)	Not stated	Newborn infant
McBride (1987a)	Not stated	Women's mental health
McBride (1987b)	Not stated	Nursing and child development
McBride (1985)	Not stated	Women's health
McBride (1984)	To July-Aug. 1982	Parenting
Lederman (1984)	Not stated	Anxiety/fears in pregnancy related to maternal health
Lederman (1986)	Not stated	Anxiety/fears as related to delivery and infant outcomes

In Part V the paradigm of behavioral organization and behavioral interaction is presented. In Chapter 16 the paradigm is introduced by using literature from both nursing and human development, particularly during the period of infancy. Chapters 17 and 18 relate behavioral organization and behavioral interaction specifically to parent-infant nursing science.

In Part VI the paradigm of person-environment as it relates to development is presented. Chapter 19 contains an overview of the paradigm based on theorizing from the field of human development, particularly early childhood. In Chapter 20 the components of the paradigm (person, environment, and development) are examined within parent-infant nursing science.

Gathering the body of research and theoretical literature comprising parent-infant nursing science was immensely facilitated by the review articles cited in Table 1-3. In addition, hand searches were made of all major nursing research journals and selected clinical journals from 1978 to 1989. Potentially missing from the parent-infant nursing literature cited in this book is research published as chapters of books or other sources which are not regularly cataloged in information retrieval systems. Also potentially missing is parent-infant nursing research published in nonnursing research journals, which are not readily identifiable. Locating parent-infant nursing science literature would be greatly facilitated if nurse researchers would publish in nursing journals some key pieces exemplifying their work.

REFERENCES

American Nurses' Association. (1980). *Nursing: A social policy statement.* Kansas City, MO: American Nurses' Association.

American Nurses' Association. (1983). *Standard for maternal and child health nursing practice.* Kansas City, MO: American Nurses' Association.

Anderson, G. C., Raff, B., Duxbury, M., & Carroll, P. (Eds.). (1979). *Newborn behavioral organization: Nursing research and implications.* New York: Liss. March of Dimes Birth Defects Foundation. *Birth Defects: Original Article Series, 15*(7), 1-228.

Avant, K. (1979). Nursing diagnosis: Maternal attachment. *Advances in Nursing Science, 2*(1), 45-55.

Barnard, K. E. (1983). Nursing research related to infants and young children. *Annual Review of Nursing Research, 1,* 3-25.

Barnard, K. E., & Blackburn, S. (1985). Making a case for the ecologic niche of the newborn. *NAACOG invitational research conference. Birth Defects: Original Article Series, 21*(3), 71-88.

Barnard, K. E., & Neal, M. V. (1977). Maternal-child nursing research. *Nursing Research, 26,* 193-200.

Beck, C. T. (1989). Maternal-newborn nursing research published from 1977 to 1986. *Western Journal of Nursing Research, 11,* 621-626.

Bee, H. L., Hammond, M. A., Eyres, S. J., Barnard, K. E., & Snyder, C. (1986). The impact of parental life change on the early development of children. *Research in Nursing and Health, 9,* 65-74.

Bixler, G., & Bixler, R. W. (1945). The professional status of nursing. *American Journal of Nursing, 45,* 730-735.

Bixler, G., & Bixler, R. W. (1959). The professional status of nursing. *American Journal of Nursing, 59,* 1142-1147.

Carper, B. A. (1978). Fundamental patterns of

knowing in nursing. *Advances in Nursing Science, 1*(1), 13-23.

Carveth, J. A. (1987). Conceptual models in nurse-midwifery. *Journal of Nurse-Midwifery, 32*(1), 20-25.

Chinn, P. L., & Jacobs, M. K. (1987). *Theory and nursing—A systematic approach* (2nd ed.). St. Louis: Mosby.

Donaldson, S. K., & Crowley, D. M. (1978). The discipline of nursing. *Nursing Outlook, 26*(2), 113-120.

Fawcett, J. (1984). The metaparadigm of nursing: Present status and future refinements. *Image, 16,* 84-87.

Greene, J. A. (1979). Science, nursing and nursing science: A conceptual analysis. *Advances in Nursing Science, 2*(1), 57-64.

Hoeffer, B., & Murphy, S. A. (1984). *Issues in professional nursing practice:* Vol. 2. *Specialization in nursing practice.* Kansas City, MO: American Nurses' Association.

Kidd, P., & Morrison, E. F. (1988). The progression of knowledge in nursing: A search for meaning. *Image, 20,* 222-224.

Lederman, R. P. (1984). Anxiety and conflict in pregnancy: Relationship to maternal health status. *Annual Review of Nursing Research, 2,* 27-61.

Lederman, R. P. (1986). Maternal anxiety in pregnancy: Relationship to fetal and newborn health status. *Annual Review of Nursing Research, 4,* 3-19.

McBride, A. B. (1984). The experience of being a parent. *Annual Review of Nursing Research, 2,* 63-81.

McBride, A. B. (1985). Women's health: Research for the future. *NAACOG invitational research conference. Birth Defects: Original Article Series, 21*(3), 17-28.

McBride, A. B. (1987a). Developing a women's mental health research agenda. *Image, 19,* 4-8.

McBride, A. B. (1987b). *The National Center for Nursing Research: Social Policy Report.* Washington, D.C.: Society for Research in Child Development.

Mercer, R. T. (1985a). Obstetric nursing research: Past, present, and future. *NAACOG invitational research conference. Birth Defects: Original Article Series, 21*(3), 29-70.

Mercer, R. T. (1985b). Teenage pregnancy as a community problem. *Annual Review of Nursing Research, 3,* 49-76.

Mercer, R. T. (1986). *First-time motherhood: Experiences from teens to forties.* New York: Springer.

Moody, L. E., Wilson, M. E., Smyth, K., Schwartz, R., Tittle, M., & Van Cott, M. L. (1988). Analysis of a decade of nursing practice research: 1977-1986. *Nursing Research, 37,* 374-379.

Murphy, S. A., & Hoeffer, B. (1983). Role of the specialties in nursing science. *Advances in Nursing Science, 5*(4), 31-39.

Rubin, R. (1967). Attainment of the maternal role: 1. Processes. *Nursing Research, 16,* 237-245.

Walker, L. O. (1989, June). Conceptual bases for the organization and advancement of nursing knowledge: Clinical content. *Proceedings for the 1989 National Forum on Doctoral Education in Nursing.* Indianapolis: Indiana University.

Walker, L. O., & Avant, K. C. (1983). *Strategies for theory construction in nursing.* Norwalk, CT: Appleton-Century-Crofts.

Walker, L. O., & Avant, K. C. (1988). *Strategies for theory construction in nursing* (2nd ed.). Norwalk, CT: Appleton & Lange.

READINGS

Doheny, M. O., & Cook, C. B. (1982). *The discipline of nursing: An introduction.* Bowie, MD: Brady.

PART TWO

Stress, Coping, and Social Support

CHAPTER 2

The Paradigm of Stress, Coping, and Social Support

OVERVIEW

The stress, coping, and social support pardadigm is of interest to nursing for several reasons. First, providing support to patients has been a long-standing nursing principle of practice. Second, a growing body of research literature indicates that, under conditions of stress, social support may protect persons from adverse effects on their health. Third, clinical wisdom indicates that even when facing a common stressor, people cope differently. Despite the simplicity of these reasons, the paradigm of stress, coping, and social support is anything but a simple one. [*Note:* Although stress is often measured in relation to health outcomes, the concept of health is examined in a separate chapter to more fully explore its meanings and relationships (Chapter 6).]

To study the paradigm of stress, coping, and social support is a bit like entering a city that does not have a clearly defined downtown. Instead of a sharply zoned area where business and shopping are concentrated, multiple sites are scattered throughout. Some sites are connected by expressways; others are more remote to major connecting transportation links. Always there are multiple pathways from one site to another, some more desirable than others. Sites often exist in competition with each other because they duplicate the services provided elsewhere. There is no clear answer to the question: Where is the downtown area? It is everywhere.

The paradigm of stress, coping, and social support is as complex as the city described above. To portray it with less complexity would simply be incorrect. Briefly, stress, coping, and social support have been concepts explored independently of each other. They have also been concepts linked together loosely in broad conceptual frameworks, as well as in more concrete models guiding research. The concepts of stress, coping, and support do not have generally accepted individual meanings; instead, they have multiple definitions depending on the theoretical perspective adopted. Finally, the concepts have been applied to almost every facet of health and illness. Indeed, it may be misleading to speak of the stress-coping-support paradigm because stress, coping, and support have been approached in so many different ways. At the same time, however, it is premature to declare one approach as either the best or as insignificant for fear that such a claim may later be proved wrong. Thus, Laux and Vossel conclude: "There is no single paradigm in stress and coping research and certainly no one on which all authors in the field agree" (1982, p. 203). However, the term "paradigm" as used in this book (Chapter 1) refers to a family of related theories, not one unified theory. Thus, it seems reasonable to use the term "paradigm" when referring to the concept of stress and its associated concepts: coping and social support.

KEY CONCEPTS AND RELATIONSHIPS

STRESS

To provide some clarity to the complex status of contemporary approaches to stress as used in parent-infant nursing science, first a broad beginning definition of stress is provided, and then alternative concepts of stress are examined. Because the concept of stress did not originate in nursing literature, looking to the field of stress literature is necessary. Following Cohen, Evans, Stokols, and Krantz (1986), "stress" is used broadly in this book to refer to "the study of situations in which the demands on individuals tax or exceed their adaptive capacities" (p. 3). Further, there are three broad approaches to the theory and measurement of stress: (1) stimulus-oriented, (2) response-oriented, and (3) interactional (Derogatis, 1982; Hobfoll, 1989). These three approaches roughly approximate viewing stress from social, physiological, and psychological perspectives, respectively.

Stimulus-oriented approaches "view stress as a potential residing within the stimulus properties of the organism's environment" (Derogatis, 1982, p. 272). The demands of stimuli (stressors), if excessive, wear down or overload a person's ability to adapt to them, and illness ensues. Stress is understood to comprise the demands or events that challenge a person's adaptive capacities. Tabulating the amount of stressful life events experienced by a person reflects this stimulus-oriented concept of stress (Dohrenwend & Dohrenwend, 1974; 1981). Providing community-wide interventions for anyone undergoing such an event as divorce, a natural disaster, or a major holiday also reflects a stimulus-oriented concept of stress. An individual is seen as more vulnerable under such a circumstance because environmental demands may exceed his or her ability to adapt to or cope with it.

In response-oriented approaches, however, "it is the response of the individual to the events of the environment that is treated as defining the presence of stress" (Derogatis, 1982, p. 272). Emotional dysfunction or the presence of an organ change (Selye, 1982) is an indicator of stress. Stress is thus a response within the individual that might be termed maladaptive. Stress and disease are almost synonymous. Resultant pathology is believed to come about from activation of (1) the sympathetic-adrenal medullary system (SAM) and/or (2) the pituitary-adrenocortical axis (PAC) (Cohen et al., 1986). Excessive activation of SAM results in secretion of catecholamines (epinephrine and norepinephrine) and has been linked to a number of cardiovascular pathologies (see Cohen et al., 1986, pp. 3–4; Schneiderman & McCabe, 1985). Activation of PAC results in the release of corticosteriods and in the general adaptation syndrome described by Selye (1982). Although not all stress is considered distress (Selye, 1982), two aspects of Selye's concept of stress have influenced ideas about how the stress process operates: (1) individuals have a finite reserve for dealing with stressors, and (2) pathological changes can occur as a result of adaptation to a stressor, the adaptive-cost hypothesis (Cohen et al., 1986). [For a fuller discussion of physiological responses to stressors, see Schneiderman and McCabe (1985) and Gunnar (1987).]

In interactional approaches to stress, processes engaged by the individual regulate whether a response to an event occurs and, if so, what the nature of the response will be. The work of Lazarus and Folkman (1984) exemplifies this concept of stress. In that work, cognitive appraisal is the central mediator between a potentially stressful event and a person's response to it. A person's assessment of the available resources and options influences the appraisal of an event for potential benefits, harms, or threats. In the interactional approach, stress is the relationship between a person and the environment. The meaning and gravity of stressors are related to the appraisals made of them. In turn, coping with a stressor is influenced by the cognitive appraisal made of it and the alternatives available to the person in a given environment.

Because scientific fields do not remain static, but continue to change as new data and theories are proposed, the three concepts of stress have been influenced by one other. Thus, stimulus-oriented stress researchers have increasingly attempted to incorporate mediators or moderators into theoretical models of stress (Gore, 1981; Cutrona & Troutman, 1986). Also, the concept of stressful events has been expanded beyond that of single-occurrence, dramatic events to include chronic stressors (Pearlin, Menaghan, Lieberman, & Mullan, 1981) and hassles of daily living (Kanner,

Coyne, Schaefer, & Lazarus, 1981). In turn, research and theoretical models using an interactional concept of stress are expanding to identify environmental resources, for example, social support, and other factors that lead individuals to appraise similar stressors differently and thus have different responses to those stressors (Yarcheski & Mahon, 1986; Heller & Swindle, 1983). Because of this paradigm blending, this author has found it useful to use more specific terminology when referring to the various aspects of stress. *Stressor* or *stressful event* is used to refer to an occurrence of a situation with potential for being appraised as taxing available capacities. *Stress appraisal* denotes a judgment that a situation is threatening, harmful, or challenging to an individual at a specific time. *Stress response* refers to psychological and/or physiological arousal following appraisal of a situation as exceeding available capacities. Finally, *stressor effects* or *stress effects* is used to denote the damaging effects of a stress response on parenting behaviors or health status.

COPING

Like stress, "coping" is a term with diverse meanings linked loosely to different concepts of stress. Broadly, coping is effort undertaken by an individual to manage either the stressor itself or its effects. Although the parallel between concepts of stress and concepts of coping is not a direct one in each case, there is enough parallelism to warrant making the connection. In stimulus-oriented approaches to stress, the emphasis is on coping with the stressful event or its environmental consequences. In response-oriented approaches to stress, organ pathology or dysfunction is often seen as an outcome of the cost of coping with a stressor. Thus, coping may lead to disease even after a stressor is no longer present and, in a sense, coping may precede stress. In interactional approaches to stress, coping may be directed at dealing with either the events appraised as stressful or the emotional, cognitive, or physical consequence of the appraisal itself (Holroyd & Lazarus, 1982).

There is no widespread agreement on what constitutes successful coping (Lazarus, 1980, pp. 53, 63–64). Haan (1982) differentiates between coping, an adaptive response, and defense, a maladaptive response. Moreover, some authors have focused on coping resources (somewhat enduring personal and environmental factors) and others on coping processes (strategies undertaken by a person or family to deal with a situation [Moos & Billings, 1982; Gore, 1985]). Included among coping resources are ego development, self-efficacy, cognitive styles, and problem-solving ability; in turn, coping processes include responses aimed at (1) defining the meaning of a situation (appraisal-focused coping), (2) altering a situation so that it is no longer a source of stress (problem-focused coping), and (3) managing emotions brought about by a situation seen as stressful (emotion-focused coping) (Moos & Billings, 1982).

The distinction between problem-focused coping and emotion-focused coping has been extensively explicated and studied by R. S. Lazarus (e.g., Folkman & Lazarus, 1985). Determining suitability of different coping strategies (e.g., problem-focused vs. emotion-focused) for different types of situations has motivated a good deal of research. To date, no single coping strategy has been shown to be adaptive in all situations (Folkman, 1984). Instead, Folkman proposes that a match is needed between appraisal and reality:

> *A time-honored principle of effective coping is to know when to appraise a situation as uncontrollable and hence abandon efforts directed at altering that situation . . . and turn to emotion-focused processes in order to tolerate or accept the situation (1984, p. 849).*

Holroyd and Lazarus (1982, pp. 26–27) have elaborated on the potential pathways by which coping with a stressful situation may affect health: (1) Coping strategies may influence health by affecting how often and how long neuroendocrine stress responses occur. (2) As a secondary gain, illness itself may become a stable coping response. (3) Coping behaviors selected may be ones that are injurious to health, for example, smoking or drug use. (4) Choice of coping strategies may directly affect an existing health problem, for example, taking needed medication as directed. In a related vein, Cohen et al. (1986), blending both an interactional and a physiological response model of stress, have linked coping to adaptive costs. Even when coping has been successful, that is, "the stressor has been neutralized by an apparently adjustive coping strategy," three secondary effects of coping may occur: (1) cumulative fatigue effects, (2) overgeneralization of a coping strategy, and (3) coping side effects (p. 8). Rigorous testing of each of these proposed mechanisms is needed. To date, preliminary evidence supports the overgeneralization hypothesis (Cohen et al, 1986, p. 236).

SOCIAL SUPPORT

Whereas the concept of coping has focused on efforts made by an individual in relation to a stressful situation, the concept of social support emphasizes the environment available to the individual. In its broadest form, social support is defined as "the resources provided by other persons" (Cohen & Syme, 1985, p. 4). Reviews of research evidence support the conclusion that social support is related to (1) vulnerability to mental distress (Kessler & McLeod, 1985) and (2) mortality and morbidity caused by physical illness (Berkman, 1985). The pathways by which social support effects its influence are less clear. Most broadly, social support may act directly to promote health regardless of persons' levels of stress, that is, the direct-effect hypothesis or social support may exhibit its influence primarily in the presence of stress by protecting persons from the effects of stress, that is, the buffering hypothesis (Cohen & Syme, 1985, pp. 6–7). These potential pathways have been outlined by Gore (1981) and are shown in Figure 2–1.

In the figure, arrows 1(a) and 1(b) represent buffering effects by which social support influences the relation between two variables (between objective stress and subjective stress or between subjective stress and strains), rather than affect the variables directly. Arrows 2 and 3 represent direct and reciprocal effects of social support and the stress variables. Not shown in the diagram, but also a potential pathway for direct effects, is an arrow connecting social support and subjective stress.

Despite repeated findings that social support is an important influence on health, particularly in times of stress, the concept of support is anything but a simple one. In this regard House and Kahn have stated:

> *The research appeal of social support . . . is based neither on the specificity of the concept nor on the emergence of some uniquely successful empirical measure. Rather, like the related concept of stress, social support has attracted researchers and stimulated research across the biomedical, behavioral, and social sciences because of its integrative promise and intuitive appeal. (1985, p.84)*

In an effort to clarify the concept of social support, House and Kahn (1985, p. 85) delineated three aspects of support (Figure 2–2): (1) Social support refers to the functional content of social relationships as these fulfill needs for information, instrumental aid, or emotional regard. (2) Social integration/isolation refers to the presence and amount of social relationships. (3) Social network refers to the structural properties of a person's social relationships, for example, density and homogeneity.

A related concept is social competence, that is, the ability to attract and maintain social relationships. All aspects of the overall social support construct might be expected to be interrelated, but each represents a distinct dimension of social relationships. [*Note:* For a readable introduction to the literature on social support, see Mitchell and Trickett (1980). For reviews of social support done from a nursing perspective, see Dimond and Jones (1983) and Cronenwett (1983).]

INTERRELATIONSHIPS AMONG STRESS, COPING, AND SOCIAL SUPPORT

There is, of course, no single accepted theoretical integration of the relationships among the concepts of stress, coping, and social support.

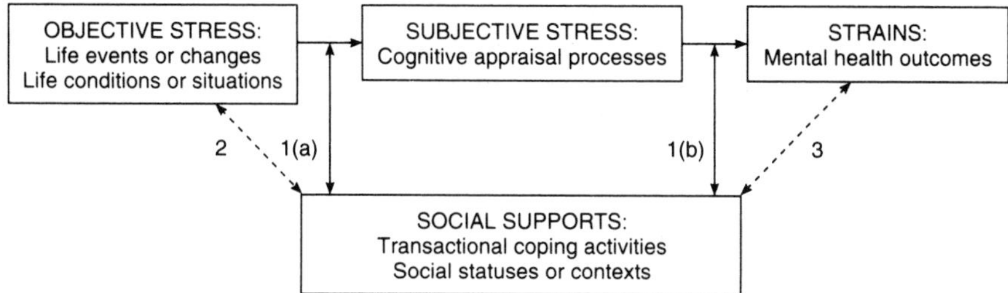

Figure 2–1
Functions of social support in stress processes. (From *Stressful Life Events and Their Contexts*, edited by Barbara S. Dohrenwend and Bruce P. Dohrenwend. Copyright © 1981, Neale Watson Academic Publications, Inc.; copyright © 1984, Rutgers University, The State University. Printed with permission of Rutgers University Press.)

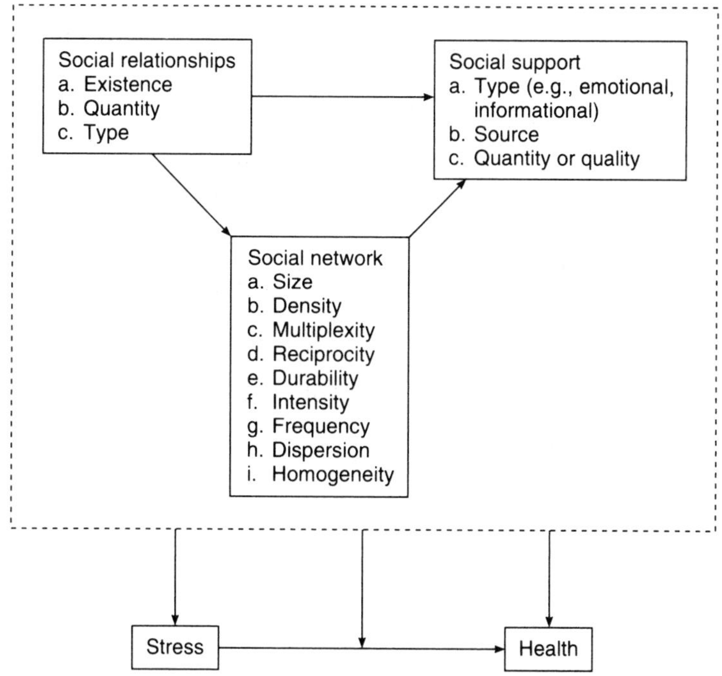

Figure 2–2
Components of social support. (From *Social Support and Health* (p. 86) by S. Cohen and S.L. Syme, 1985 Florida: Academic Press. Copyright 1985 by Academic Press. Reprinted by permission.)

Indeed, as the nature of the stressor varies from acute stresses to chronic ones, it may well be that different types of support are needed (Kessler and McLeod, 1985). There also remains the issue of the competing hypotheses as to whether (1) social support is related to health status only at high levels of stress (buffering hypothesis); (2) social support has a positive influence on health regardless of the presence of stress (direct or main effects hypothesis) or (3) both (1) and (2) may hold true but under different circumstances (see review by Kessler & McLeod, 1985). Similarly, a meta-analysis of coping strategies suggests that different types of coping may be needed for different types of stressors (Suls & Fletcher, 1985). Thus, Suls and Fletcher state:[11] [Strategies] involving *avoidant* tactics are effective in reducing pain, stress, and anxiety in some cases, whereas nonavoidant strategies appear to be more effective in others" (1985, p. 250).

Another matter clouding the theoretical integration of stress, coping, and social support is the relatively independent research traditions surrounding social support and coping (Gore, 1985). Social support has been the preoccupation of demographic, epidemiological, and sociological studies, whereas the construct of coping has been investigated in primarily psychological studies. Because the research of disciplines is typically published in distinct, specialized journals, it is not surprising that two or more disciplines may independently study similar phenomena.

Fortunately, some scholars have been interested in bridging the intrapersonal focus of coping and the interpersonal focus of social support (Gore, 1985; Heller & Swindle, 1983). For example, Heller and Swindle have proposed a model linking components of social support with coping and stressful events (Figure 2–3). In that model the following are distinguished as separate components of the overall social support construct: Social competence in accessing social resources, social connections (network), perceptions of being supported, and support seeking as a coping behavior. In addition to stressful events, personal characteristics and social connections influence the dimensions of appraisal, including perceived social support. Appraisal, in turn, influences coping behaviors, one of which may be support seeking. Tenets of the Heller-Swindle model include the following: (1) The components of support are not static, but developmental. (2) Individuals are not simply the passive recipients of support, but may influence the type of support they receive. (3) Individuals may use a variety of coping strategies, not only social support.

METHODOLOGY

Methods used in stress, coping, and social support research are closely tied to the overall type of conceptual approach taken to stress (stimulus-oriented, response-oriented, or interactional). Ideally, research methods should follow from the guiding conceptual scheme, not the reverse. Thus, it is important to give careful consideration to the phenome-

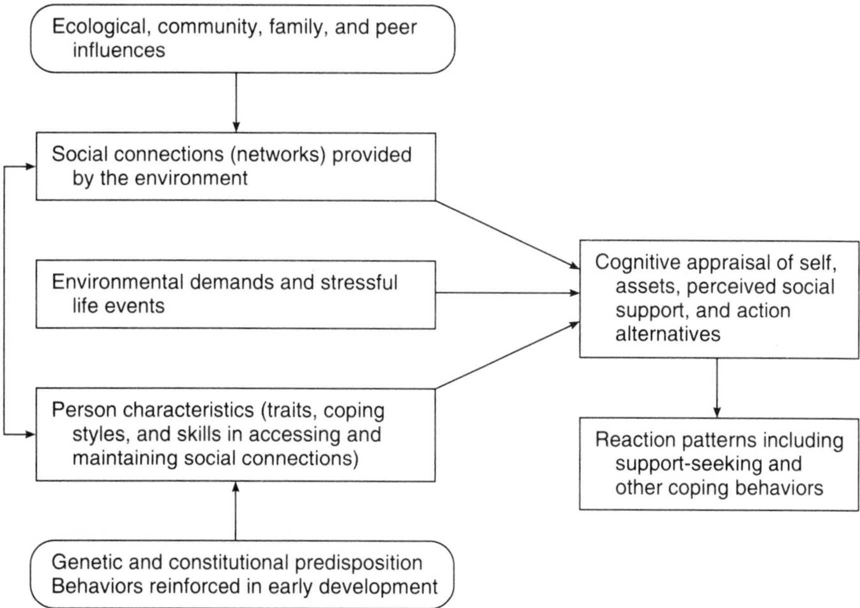

Figure 2–3
A model of stress, social support, and coping. (Reprinted with permission from *Preventive Psychology.* Heller and Swindle: "Social networks, perceived social support, and coping with stress." Copyright 1983, Pergamon Press PLC).

non of interest prior to selecting a particular stress paradigm and its accompanying research methods.

Stimulus-oriented approaches to stress have relied heavily on survey research methods, such as interviews and questionnaires. By using cross-sectional or panel designs, data are typically analyzed by relating stress and illness indicators to a variety of demographic characteristics of survey respondents (e.g., Verbrugge, 1983). Thus, the existing evidence for beneficial effects of social support are largely correlational in nature and thereby make causal inferences tenuous. Limitations of correlational research methods must be acknowledged, but they should not hold back the next logical steps in stress research. To the contrary, Cohen and Syme propose that "significant advances in the understanding of support-health relationships will occur only if future studies focus on the *process* by which support is linked to well-being instead of on determining merely whether a link exists" (1985, p. 15).

Both prospective longitudinal studies and experimental studies that provide differing levels of social support would aid in clarifying questions about the processes by which stress, coping, and social support influence health or adaptive outcomes. Because threats to internal validity are problematic in correlational designs (those in which the independent variable is not manipulated by the investigator), it is important to use data analytic procedures that provide checks for threats (Dooley, 1985). See Table 2-1 for a summary of statistical methods that provide some control of validity threats in correlational research designs. Further consideration of special methodological issues in measuring buffering effects may be found in Heller and Swindle (1983, pp. 100–101), Thoits (1982), LaRocco (1983), and Dooley (1985, p. 120).

Psychometric issues of reliability and validity must be carefully considered in selecting indicators of stress, coping, and social support. Of all psychometric issues, the demonstration of construct validity is often the one neglected. Strong evidence of construct validity should include attention to both the *convergent* and the *discriminant* validity of measures (Campbell & Fiske, 1959). That is, a measure of a construct should correlate more highly with other measures of that same construct than with measures of other constructs. Excellent reviews of tools and issues related to measuring stress, coping, and social support are available in Derogatis (1982); Dohrenwend, Dohrenwend, Dodson, and Shrout (1984); Lazarus, DeLongis, Folkman, and Gruen (1985); Barrera (1986); House and Kahn (1985); Hyman (1988); Payne and Jones (1987); and Cohen (1987).

Response-oriented approaches to stress have largely relied on presence of pathology as a stress index. Because morbidity is related to age (Verbrugge, 1983), many stress-related disorders, such as coronary artery disease, may not be suitable indices of stress in adults of childbearing age. A number of obstetric complications have been linked to stress, however, and they might be useful indicators of stress effects (see reviews by Lederman, 1984, 1986). Although it is important to tap the phenomenological dimensions of stress when using interactional approaches, Cohen and Syme caution that "Symptom measures cannot be viewed as proxies for direct measures of clinical pathology" (1985, p. 8). This caution is especially important in response-oriented approaches to stress and measurement of such outcomes as depression (Davis & Jensen, 1988).

Interactional approaches to stress, coping, and social support require thoughtful and intricate research designs. These designs may involve questionnaires or interviews; in any case, it is important that the information gathered will capture the unfolding of the stress process. This may require carefully prepared questionnaire or interview items to elicit all relevant contextual and subjective aspects of the appraisal of, the coping with, and the consequences of an encounter with a stressful situation. It is also likely that thorough study of a stressful encounter will necessitate repeated measurement of key variables through (1) prospective, short-term longitudinal designs (e.g., Folkman & Lazarus, 1985) or (2) designs involving continuous monitoring techniques (e.g., Bandura, Taylor, Williams, Mefford, & Barchas, 1985). In addition, because different stressors may necessitate different forms of support and coping, both correlational (Kessler & McLeod, 1985) and interventive (Gore, 1985) studies will be more informative if they focus on specific stressors.

Table 2–1
SUMMARY OF CORRELATIONAL METHODS

Method	Purpose	Technique	Requirements and Limitations
Cross-lag panel correlation	To determine causal predominance	Sequence of tests of equality of pairs of correlations	Panel data; no test of buffering; low power; assumes synchronicity, stationarity, and equal stabilities
Longitudinal path analysis	To estimate direct and indirect effects, including reciprocal lagged relations in panel data; buffering	Estimation of standardized regression or path coefficients in equations determined by theory	No estimation of simultaneous reciprocity; requires errorless independent variables, no serial correlation of residuals of lagged variables, and no spuriousness
Two-stage least-squares analysis	To estimate reciprocal relations without lag	Regression equations for each simultaneous reciprocal path based on instrumental variables	Availability of instrumental variables, errorless control variables, and no spuriousness
Causal analysis with latent variables	To estimate structural equations, including buffering with errorless latent variables; simultaneous reciprocity possible if model is identified	Maximum likelihood estimates of coefficients and overall model fit statistics	Each latent variable needs multiple indicators; based on strong normality of distribution assumptions and no spuriousness
Logit analysis	Causal analysis when dependent variable is dichotomous; includes buffering	Log-linear analysis when all variables are categorical and logistic regression when some independent variables are continuous	Large sample size necessary; no simultaneous reciprocity

Source: D. Dooley, Causal inference in the study of social support. In S. Cohen & S. L. Syme (Eds.), *Social Support and Health,* Orlando, FL: Academic Press, 1985, p. 122.

Finally, issues related to parental gender should be considered. In a spirit of egalitarianism, it has become customary to speak of "parenting" and to consider mothers and fathers, generically, as "parents." Although the ideology underlying this language is commendable, it does not always serve the science of nursing well in that it presupposes common processes for men and women. Whether women and men as parents display similar patterns to stressors during pregnancy and postnatal period is of special interest to parent-infant nurses. Indeed, evidence of gender differences in response to stressors is growing but is still incomplete (Barnett, Biener, & Baruch, 1987). Research reviews support the conclusion that in achievement-oriented situations men may be more reactive to stress on some variables, such as plasma and urinary epinephrine, than women (Polefrone & Manuck, 1987). Findings of gender differences for other neuroendocrine substances either show no differences, for example, norepinephrine, or inconsistent differences across studies, for example, cortisol. Findings for cardiovascular responses to stress also show inconsistent gender differences (Polefrone & Manuck, 1987). In contract, by psychological measures women have been shown to experience more emotional distress, particularly depressive symptoms, in response to crises in their social network than men (Wethington, McLeod, & Kessler, 1987). This difference is partly explained by the wider social networks to which women are responsive compared to men: "Women seem to cast a wider net of concern and so are affected emotionally not only by the well-being of their immediate family but also by lives of those to whom they may be less intimately related" (Wethington, McLeod, & Kessler, 1987, p. 150).

The accrued evidence of some gender differences in response to stressors warrants attention in studies of stress during pregnancy and early parenting. When possible, it would advance the state of parent-infant nursing science (1) if future research would include both mothers and fathers in research studies and (2) if analysis of data specifically would focus on detecting gender differences in addition to testing the main hypotheses. There may be some phenomena for which a common model applies to both mothers and fathers, but there will also be those for which distinct gender models fit the data more correctly. Differentiating between the two circumstances is important in understanding the full complexity of the early parenting experience.

REFERENCES

Bandura, A., Taylor, C. B., Williams, S. L., Mefford, I. N., & Barchas, J. D. (1985). Catecholamine secretion as a function of perceived coping self-efficacy. *Journal of Consulting and Clinical Psychology, 53,* 406–414.

Barnett, R. C., Biener, L., & Baruch, G. K. (1987). *Gender and stress.* New York: Free Press.

Barrera, M. (1986). Distinctions between social support concepts, measures, and models. *American Journal of Community Psychology, 14,* 413–445.

Berkman, L. F. (1985). The relationship of social networks and social support to morbidity and mortality. In S. Cohen & S. L. Syme (Eds.), *Social support and health* (pp. 241-262). New York: Academic Press.

Campbell, D. T., & Fiske, D. W. (1959). Convergent and discriminant validation by the multitrait-multimethod matrix. *Psychological Bulletin, 56,* 81-105.

Cohen, F. (1987). Measurement of coping. In S. V. Kasl & C. L. Cooper (Eds.), *Stress and health: Issues in research methodology* (pp. 283-305). New York: Wiley.

Cohen, S., Evans, G. W., Stokols, D., & Krantz, D. S. (1986). *Behavior, health, and environmental stress.* New York: Plenum.

Cohen, S., & Syme, S. L. (1985). Issues in the study and application of social support. In S. Cohen & S. L. Syme (Eds.), *Social support and health* (pp. 3-22). New York: Academic Press.

Cronenwett, L. R. (1983). When and how people help: Theoretical issues and evidence. In P. L. Chinn (Ed.), *Advances in nursing theory development* (pp. 251-270). Rockville, MD: Aspen.

Cutrona, C. E., & Troutman, B. R. (1986). Social support, infant temperament, and parenting self-efficacy: A mediational model of postpartum depression. *Child Development, 57,* 1507-1518.

Davis, T., & Jensen, L. (1988). Identifying depression in medical patients. *Image, 20,* 191-195.

Derogatis, L. R. (1982). Self-report measures of stress. In L. Goldberger & S. Breznitz (Eds.), *Handbook of stress* (pp. 270-294). New York: Free Press.

Dimond, M., & Jones, S. L. (1983). Social support: A review and theoretical integration. In P. L. Chinn (Ed.), *Advances in nursing theory development* (pp. 235-249). Rockville, MD: Aspen.

Dohrenwend, B. S., & Dohrenwend, B. P. (Eds.). (1974). *Stressful life events: Their nature and effects.* New York: Wiley.

Dohrenwend, B. S., & Dohrenwend, B. P. (Eds.). (1981). *Stressful life events and their contexts.* New York: Prodist.

Dohrenwend, B. S., Dohrenwend, B. P., Dodson, M., & Shrout, P. E. (1984). Symptoms, hassles, social supports, and life events: Problem of confounded measures. *Journal of Abnormal Psychology, 93,* 222-230.

Dooley, D. (1985). Causal inference in the study of social support. In S. Cohen & S. L. Syme (Eds.), *Social support and health* (pp. 109-125). New York: Academic Press.

Folkman, S. (1984). Personal control and stress and coping processes: A theoretical analysis. *Journal of Personality and Social Psychology, 46,* 839-852.

Folkman, S., & Lazarus, R. (1985). If it changes it must be a process: Study of emotion and coping during three stages of a college examination. *Journal of Personality and Social Psychology, 48,* 150-170.

Gore, S. (1981). Stress-buffering functions of social supports: An appraisal and clarification of research methods. In B. S. Dohrenwend & B. P. Dohrenwend (Eds.), *Stressful life events and their contexts* (pp. 202-222). New York: Prodist.

Gore, S. (1985). Social support and styles of coping with stress. In S. Cohen & S. L. Syme (Eds.), *Social support and health* (pp. 263-278). New York: Academic Press.

Gunnar, M. R. (1987). Psychobiological studies of stress and coping: An introduction. *Child Development, 58,* 1403-1407.

Haan, N. (1982). The assessment of coping, defense and stress. In L. Goldberger & S. Breznitz (Eds.), *Handbook of stress* (pp. 254-269). New York: Free Press.

Heller, K., & Swindle, R. W. (1983). Social networks, perceived social support, and coping with stress. In R. D. Felner, L. A. Jason, J. N. Moritsugu, & S. S. Farber (Eds.), *Preventive psychology* (pp. 87-103). Elmsford, NY: Pergamon.

Hobfoll, S. E. (1989). Conservation of resources: A new attempt at conceptualizing stress. *American Psychologist, 44,* 513-524.

Holroyd, K. A., & Lazarus, R. S. (1982). Stress, coping and somatic adaptation. In L. Goldberger & S. Breznitz (Eds.), *Handbook of stress* (pp. 21-34). New York: Free Press.

House, J. S., & Kahn, R. L. (1985). Measurers and concepts of social support. In S. Cohen & S. L. Syme (Eds.), *Social support and health* (pp. 83-108). New York: Academic Press.

Hyman, R. B. (1988). Measures of stress and related constructs: A guide for research and clinical practice. *Scholarly Inquiry for Nursing Practice,* 2(1), 5-66.

Kanner, A. D., Coyne, J. C., Schaefer, C., & Lazarus, R. S. (1981). Comparison of two modes of stress measurement: Daily hassles and uplifts versus major life events. *Journal of Behavioral Medicine.* 4(1), 1-39.

Kessler, R. C., & McLeod, J. D. (1985). Social support and mental health in community samples. In S. Cohen & S. L. Syme (Eds.), *Social support and health* (pp. 219-240). New York: Academic Press.

LaRocco, J. M. (1983). Comment: Theoretical distinctions between causal and interaction effects of social support. *Journal of Health and Social Behavior, 24,* 91-92.

Laux, L., & Vossel, G. (1982). Paradigms in stress research: Laboratory versus field and traits versus processes. In L. Goldberger & S. Breznitz (Eds.), *Handbook of stress* (pp. 203-211). New York: Free Press.

Lazarus, R. S. (1980). The stress and coping paradigm. In L. A. Bond & J. C. Rosen (Eds.), *Competence and coping during adulthood* (pp. 28-74). Hanover, NH: University Press of New England.

Lazarus, R. S., DeLongis, A., Folkman, S., & Gruen, R. (1985). Stress and adaptational outcomes. *American Psychologist, 40,* 770-779,.

Lazarus, R. S., & Folkman, S. (1984). *Stress, appraisal, and coping.* New York: Springer.

Lederman, R. P. (1984). Anxiety and conflict in pregnancy: Relationship to maternal health status. *Annual Review of Nursing Research, 2,* 27-61.

Lederman, R. P. (1986). Maternal anxiety in pregnancy: Relationship to fetal and newborn health status. *Annual Review of Nursing Research, 4,* 3-19.

Mitchell, R. E., & Trickett, E. J. (1980). Social networks as mediators of social support: An analysis of the effects and determinants of social networks. *Community Mental Health Journal, 16,* 27-44.

Moos, R. H., & Billings, A. G. (1982). Conceptualizing and measuring coping resources and processes. In L. Goldberger & S. Breznitz (Eds.), *Handbook of stress* (pp. 211-230). New York: Free Press.

Payne, R. L., & Jones, J. G. (1987). Measurement and methodological issues in social support. In S. V. Kasl & C. L. Cooper (Eds.), *Stress and health: Issues in research methodology* (pp. 167-205). New York: Wiley.

Pearlin, L. I., Menaghan, E. G., Lieberman, M.A., & Mullan, J. T. (1981). The stress process. *Journal of Health and Social Behavior, 22,* 337-356.

Polefrone, J. M., & Manuck, S. B. (1987). Gender differences in cardiovascular and neuroendocrine responses to stress. In R. C. Barnett, L. Biener, & G. K. Baruch (Eds.), *Gender and stress* (pp. 13-38). New York: Free Press.

Schneiderman, N., & McCabe, P. M. (1985). Biobehavioral responses to stressors. In T. M. Field, P. M. McCabe, & N. Schneiderman (Eds.), *Stress and coping* (pp. 13-61). Hillsdale, NJ: Erlbaum.

Selye, H. (1982). History and present status of the stress concept. In L. Goldberger & S. Breznitz (Eds.), *Handbook of stress* (pp. 7-17). New York: Free Press.

Suls, J., & Fletcher, B. (1985). The relative efficacy of avoidant and nonavoidant coping strategies: A meta-analysis. *Health Psychology, 4,* 249-288.

Thoits, P. A. (1982). Conceptual, methodological, and theoretical problems in studying social support as a buffer against life stress. *Journal of Health and Social Behavior, 23,* 145-159.

Verbrugge, L. M. (1983). Multiple roles and physical health of women and men. *Journal of Health and Social Behavior, 24,* 16-30.

Wethington, E., McLeod, J. D., & Kessler, R. C. (1987). The importance of life events for explaining sex differences in psychological distress. In R. C. Barnett, L. Biener, & G. K. Baruch (Eds.), *Gender and stress* (pp. 144-156). New York: Free Press.

Yarcheski, A., & Mahon, N. E. (1986). Perceived stress and symptom patterns in early adolescents: The role of mediating variables. *Research in Nursing and Health, 9,* 289-297.

CHAPTER 3

Parent-Infant Nursing Research on Stress

DEFINITIONS AND DESCRIPTIONS OF STRESS

DEFINING STRESS IN PARENT-INFANT NURSING

For the most part, nursing investigations of stress in pregnancy and early parenting have simply adopted an approach to the stress concept (stimulus-oriented, response-oriented, or interactional) but have devoted little attention to conceptual definitions of the concept. Instead, definitions of stress have been made implicitly through selection of operational definitions of the stress concept. Several studies are noteworthy, however, in their efforts to define stress within the context of pregnancy and parenting. Mercer, May, Ferketich, and DeJoseph, for example, defined antepartum stress as "a complication of pregnancy or at-risk condition (pregnancy risk) and negatively perceived life events" (1986, p. 339). In a study of stressors in antepartum hospitalization, White and Ritchie (1984) adopted Cox's definition of stress: "An imbalance between the perceived demand and the person's perception of his ability to meet the demand" (1978, p. 18). In a related definition, Glazer (1989) defined stressors as "stimuli that are characterized by threat and that tax or exceed resources of the system" (p. 50).

Are pregnancy and early parenting in and of themselves stressful events or crises? This issue has been addressed in nonnursing literature in debates about the appropriateness of calling parenthood a crisis or a "normal crisis." Among others, Rossi (1968) called for dropping the concept of normal crisis and instead speaking directly "of the transition to and impact of parenthood" (p. 28). Thus, there is some basis for separating normative changes associated with parenthood from stressful events that tax or exceed those normative changes.

In nursing, positions vary as to the exact relationship between stress and pregnancy. (See Table 3–1 for statements illustrative of prevailing positions.) At the heart of the issue is the suitability of the stress paradigm for understanding pregnancy and early parenting under "normal circumstances."

To study normal pregnancy and early parenting from the standpoint of a stress paradigm runs the risk of stretching the paradigm beyond its scientific utility. That is, a theoretical approach that can be applied everywhere loses its precision and specificity. For that reason, the position adopted here is that the stress paradigm is most usefully applied to circumstances that are marked by atypical risk or adverse outcome. Such circumstances may occur during pregnancy, childbirth, early parenthood, or infancy. Modal concerns and needs of new parents—those typically experienced by parents—are considered to be outside the stress context and to be a part

Table 3–1
DESCRIPTIONS OF STRESS RELATED TO PREGNANCY AND EARLY PARENTING

"Certain kinds of stress prove most disruptive to women during pregnancy. Four categories have been identified: (1) any adverse event the woman perceives as having the potential to damage her fetus; (2) any defect or conflict in the woman's support system, particularly involving mother or mate; (3) the woman's perception that she is poorly prepared, inexperienced, or otherwise inadequate to assume the maternal role; and (4) any maternal condition the woman believes might be worsened by the pregnancy." (Stern, Tilden, & Maxwell, 1980, pp. 70–71)

"Stress is essentially the rate of wear and tear caused by adjustment in everyday life. It is often the stress of . . . life adjustments under difficult circumstances that causes a change in normal coping behavior." (Robbins, 1981, p. 219)

"Although the amount of experienced disequilibrium varies considerably among expectant parents, research and clinical observation suggest that a first pregnancy is at least somewhat stressful." (Brown, 1986, p. 72)

"It seems universally true that women experience pregnancy as a psychological crisis." (Kuhn, 1982, p. 96)

"Stress results not from a particular life event per se but from the individual's perception of that event and of his or her ability to control and deal with the event." (Mercer & Ferketich, 1988, p. 26)

"Theorists agree that for most persons pregnancy is a maturational crisis." (White & Ritchie, 1984, p. 48)

"Although pregnancy itself is considered to constitute a stressful experience, it is not uniformly stressful among women or for the same woman at different times in her life." (Norbeck & Tilden, 1983, p. 33)

"Birth of a child and the advent of parenthood inevitably bring about change and stress in the lives of family members." (Brooten et al., 1988, p. 213)

of normative processes associated with the transition to parenting (Chapter 10) and parental role attainment (Chapters 11 to 13). That position is not meant to deny that certain parents experience the normative changes of pregnancy and parenting as stressful (e.g., Tilden, 1984). The position adopted here is based primarily on conceptual distinctions.

There is an additional reason for viewing normative aspects of pregnancy and parenthood as generally outside the stress paradigm. Stimulus-oriented approaches to stress have typically focused on major identifiable events, often of an unpredictable and irreversible nature. The approach does not fit easily with the role preparation and rehearsal and positive anticipation that can precede parenthood. By contrast, labor more easily conforms to a stress paradigm. Still, there is not a consensus on the matter of stress and its suitability to normative events. For example, Pridham, Egan, Chang, and Hansen (1986) have reported day-to-day stressors in the lives of new mothers.

To distribute content on normative changes, the author generally chose to place the research literature on concerns and needs related to the parenting role in the chapters on role attainment or the chapter on health behaviors, depending on focus. Research literature explicitly using stress terminology to describe pregnancy or the parenting role was placed in this chapter.

MODELS AND FRAMEWORKS FOR STUDYING STRESS

To better understand stressors that affect childbearing families, Avant (1988) proposed a classification system for studying those stressors. Using Bronfenbrenner's (1979) model of the ecology of human development, Avant identified four systems from which stressors may emanate: The microsystem of the family, the mesosystem (several systems within which the family directly participates), the exosystem (external systems that influence the family), and the macrosystem (the highest level of system usually comprising the culture and the national level). Although Avant states that nurses work primarily with childbearing families at the microsystem and mesosystem levels, her analysis provides a rich template for organizing nursing research on stressors that influence childbearing families.

Although a number of studies in parent-infant nursing have tested the relations of life event stress to health or parenting outcomes, the most clearly expressed model of variable relations is found in the work of Mercer et al. (1986). Their theoretical model for studying the effect of antepartum stress provides hypotheses for research on pathways between stressful events and health and family outcomes. See Figure 3–1 for a diagram expressing the proposed pathways linking antepartum stress and health outcomes. (Partial tests of this model are reported in Chapter 5.)

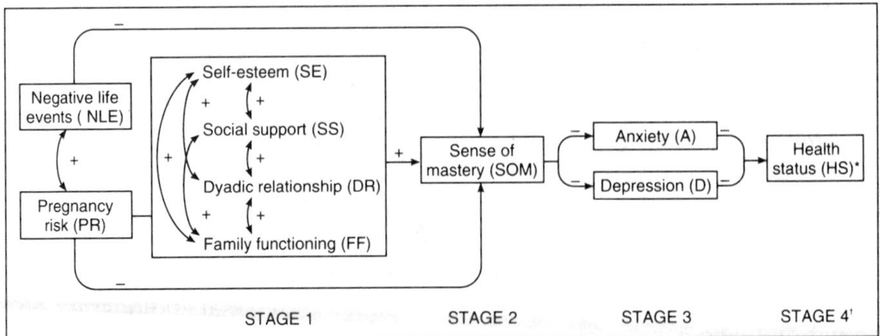

*A model may be tested for mothers, fathers, and infants.
†Stages represent the temporal ordering of variables, i.e., Stage 1 variables predict Stage 2 variables, which predict Stage 3 variables, which predict the outcome variable HS. In the proposed longitudinal model, HS will be predicted at Stages 5, 6, 7, and 8, i.e., birth, 1, 4, and 8 months postpartum.

Figure 3–1
Effect of antepartum stress on health status. (Copyright 1986, American Journal of Nursing Company. Reprinted from *Nursing Research*, Nov/Dec, 1986, *35*(6), p. 340. Used with permission. All rights reserved.)

MEASUREMENT

GENERAL STRATEGIES

A wide variety of strategies are available for measuring stress. Many of the strategies follow from one of the broad approaches to stress (stimulus-oriented, response-oriented, or interactional) identified in Chapter 2. For general reviews of tools and methods for measuring stress, see Derogatis (1982), Everly and Rosenfeld (1981), and Hyman (1988).

Stimulus-oriented approaches to measuring stress include (1) self-report measures such as questionnaires to tabulate the occurrence of stressful events in parents' lives and (2) presence of a specific stressor, such as high-risk pregnancy or preterm birth.

Response-oriented approaches to stress usually focus on negative health outcomes theorized to be the end stage of the stress process. Thus, this approach includes presence of physical or mental pathology, emotional distress indexed by depression, anxiety, or somatic complaints, and obstetric or neonatal complications.

Interactional approaches to stress focus on either the appraisal or perception of events as stressful. Self-report methods typically are employed to capture appraisal or perceptions of stress. Because appraisal influences the extent and type of arousal that may follow, measures of emotional state and some physiologic indicators (e.g., cardiovascular and neuroendocrine responses) also have a place in interactional approaches to stress.

SPECIFIC TOOLS

Parent-infant nursing studies have included a wide variety of approaches to measuring stress. The most predominant tools used for measuring stress have been questionnaires, particularly those focused on cumulative life events. Other measurement methods include behavioral rating scales, health diaries, levels of plasma cortisol and catecholamines, oxygen tension (in infants), and pain scales. Specific tools relevant to stress research in parent-infant nursing are summarized in Table 3–2. Also indicated in Table 3–2 are parent-infant research studies in which those tools have been used. In addition, several tools suitable for parent-infant studies were identified in research with other populations, and they also are included. (*Note:* Because response-oriented approaches to stress typically involve measurement of a health state or outcome, as a rule those measures are not presented in this chapter. They are included in Chapter 7, on health status.)

Pain or discomfort associated with childbirth has been a stressor of particular interest to parent-infant nurse researchers. Investigators have focused on both the measurement of pain and the simulation of clinical pain. To aid investigators in selecting suitable pain measures, McGuire (1984) has presented an analysis of self-report scales, physiological/behavioral measures, and multidimensional measures of clinical pain. The measurement measures are summarized in Table 3–3.

Finally, three parent-infant methodological studies of pain are of note. Franck (1986) has conducted a pilot study to develop a quantitative method for measuring pain responses in infants by using photogrammetric techniques. In a study of pain during labor, Geden, Beck, Brouder, and O'Connell (1983) explored the similarity of four laboratory pain stimuli to pain associated with the transitional stage of labor. The Forgione-Barber pain stimulator was identified as the stimulus of choice for analogue research of labor pain. In another study of labor pain, Lowe and Roberts (1988) tested the convergence of self-reported pain in labor with postpartum recall of labor pain. Some discrepancies between women's reports of pain measured in labor and postpartum recall of that pain were identified. Specifically, postpartum pain reports for early labor were lower and reports of transitional labor were higher than those measured in labor.

SUMMARY OF NURSING RESEARCH

SCOPE OF STRESS RESEARCH

Stress research in parent-infant nursing science encompasses three broad categories: Descriptive, relational/predictive, and interventive. Parent-infant research studies falling in those three broad categories are presented in Table 3–4.

Table 3–2
MEASURES/TOOLS FOR THE CONCEPT OF STRESS

Tool	Source Described in	Studies Using Tool
	LIFE EVENTS QUESTIONNAIRES	
Life Experiences Survey: Sixty-item questionnaire of life events and impact; 1984 version has 82 items	Sarason, Johnson, & Siegel (1978) Norbeck (1984) (revised version)	Norbeck & Tilden (1983) Brandt (1984) Mercer & Ferketich (1988) Mercer (1986) Tilden (1983) Tilden (1984) Curry (1987) Norbeck & Anderson (1989a) Becker (1987) Booth, Barnard, Mitchell, & Spieker, (1987) Booth et al. (1989) Norbeck & Anderson (1989b) Ferketich & Mercer (1989) Mercer, Hackley, & Bostrom (1983) Mercer, Ferketich, DeJoseph, May, & Sollid (1988a) Mercer et al. (1988b)
Social Readjustment Rating Scale: Forty-two-item life events scale (related scales: Schedule of Recent Experiences; Recent Life Changes Questionnaire)	Holmes & Rahe (1967)	White & Dawson (1981) Lenz et al. (1986) Bee et al. (1986) Nuckolls, Cassel, & Kaplan (1972) Woods (1985) Kirgis et al. (1977) Dooher (1980) Riesch (1984) Bee et al. (1982) Mitchell, Bee, Hammond, & Barnard (1985)

Review of Life Experiences: Brief life events scale	Hurst, Jenkins, & Rose (1978)	Miles (1985)
Stress Amount Checklist: Twelve-item scale of stressful events common to pregnancy	Brown (1986)	Brown (1986)
Adolescent Life Change Event Scale: Five-point scale for adolescents	Robbins (1981)	Robbins (1981) Thomas & Groer (1986) Yarcheski & Mahon (1986)
Family Inventory of Life Events & Changes: Seventy-one-item family life event scale	McCubbin, Patterson, & Wilson (1981)	Sund & Ostwald (1985)
OTHER STRESS SCALES AND INTERVIEWS		
Parenting Stress Index: One hundred twenty-item questionnaire with three subscales: Child domain, parent domain, life stress	CPPC Tests 4 Conant Square Brandon, VT 05733	Abidin (1982) Mash & Johnston (1983) Dormire, Strauss, & Clarke (1989)
Difficult Life Circumstances Scale: Twenty-eight-item scale of chronic, current family stressors	Booth et al. (1989)	Booth et al. (1989)
Ireton Personal Inventory: Scale to survey worries and concerns	Ireton (1980)	Clinton (1986)
Parental Experiences Interview: Interview guide related to monitoring infant apnea	Nuttall (1988)	Nuttall (1988)

Table 3–2
MEASURES/TOOLS FOR THE CONCEPT OF STRESS *(Continued)*

Tool	Source Described in	Studies Using Tool
	OTHER STRESS SCALES AND INTERVIEWS	
Feelings about Pregnancy Questionnaire: Tool for number and intensity of stressors	Glazer (1989)	Glazer (1989)
Changes in Toddler Behavior: Interview guide for changes after birth of sibling	Kayiatos et al. (1984)	Kayiatos et al. (1984)
Perceived Stress Scale: Fourteen-item scale for global stress	Cohen, Kamarck, & Mermelstein (1983)	Walker (1989a, 1989b)
Hassles Scale: One hundred seventeen-item list of daily hassles	Kanner, Coyne, Schaefer, & Lazarus (1981)	Murphy (1986)
Antepartum Hospital Stress Inventory: Forty-seven-item scale of stressors	White & Ritchie (1984)	White & Ritchie (1984)
Behavior Cues Index: Observer ratings of stress behavioral cues	Hegyvary & Chammings (1975)	Barsevick & Llewellyn (1982)
Stress Rating Scale: Observer ratings of stress in labor	R. Lederman et al. (1985)	R. Lederman et al. (1985)
Labor Anxiety Inventory: Sixteen-item self-report scale	R. Lederman et al. (1985)	R. Lederman et al. (1985)
State Anxiety Inventory: Twenty-item scale for state anxiety (some studies also include trait subscale)	Spielberger, Gorsuch, Lushene, Vagg, & Jacobs (1983)	Glazer (1989) Kemp & Hatmaker (1989) Mercer & Ferketich (1988) Albrecht & Rankin (1989)
Morse Pain Stimulus Scale: Thirty-six items of paired pain comparisons	Morse & Park (1988)	Morse & Park (1988)

BIOPHYSICAL STRESS INDICATORS		
Plasma cortisol and catecholamines	—	R. Lederman et al. (1985) R. Lederman et al. (1979) R. Lederman et al. (1977) E. Lederman et al. (1981) R. Lederman et al. (1978)
Urinary catecholamines	—	Kemp & Hatmaker (1989)
Oxygen tension	Norris et al. (1982)	Norris et al. (1982)
PAIN MAGNITUDE AND RELATED INDICATORS		
McGill Pain Questionnaire: Twenty-item pain questionnaire	Melzack (1983)	Lowe (1987) Keller & Bzdek (1986) Geden et al. (1983) Lowe & Roberts (1988) Lowe (1989)
"Pain thermometer": Single descriptive scale for subjective rating of pain	Chaves & Barber (1974)	Geden et al. (1986) Manderino & Bzdek (1984)
Pain-o-meter: Hard plastic gauge for pain intensity	Gaston-Johansson et al. (1988)	Gaston-Johansson et al. (1988) Fridh et al. (1988)
Visual Analogue Scale: Ten-centimeter line for pain intensity	Gaston-Johansson et al. (1988)	Gaston-Johansson et al. (1988)
EVENT DIARIES		
Health diary: Daily log of experiences	Pridham et al. (1986) Killien & Brown (1987)	Pridham et al. (1986) Pridham et al. (1982) Killien & Brown (1987)

Note: Measures of stressor effects can be found in Table 7–1.

Table 3–3
COMPARISON OF PAIN INSTRUMENTS

Instrument	Dimension(s) Measured	Reliability / Validity	Type of Pain Best Suited for	Ease of Understanding	Time Required for Explanation and Administration, min	Time Required for Scoring, min
Verbal Descriptor Scale	Intensity	Good / Probable	Clinical: Acute, Chronic, Progressive	Very easy	<5	0
Visual Analogue Scale	Intensity	Good / Probable	Clinical: Acute, Chronic, Progressive	Easy to difficult depending on sample	<5	<2
Chambers-Price Pain Rating Scale	Intensity Anxiety Attention paid to pain Physiologic parameters	Probable / Questionable	Clinical: Acute	Moderately easy	5–15	<5
Johnson's Two-Component Scales	Physical intensity Emotional distress	Unclear / Unclear	Experimental and probably clinical	Moderately easy	<5	<2
McGill Pain Questionnaire	Location Sensation Affective aspects Evaluation Intensity Pattern	Good / Good	Clinical: Acute, Chronic, Progressive	Moderately easy to very difficult	15–30	5–10
Card sort method	Sensation Affective aspects Evaluation Intensity	Probable / Probable	Clinical: Acute	Moderately easy to difficult	10–20	5–10

Source: D. B. McGuire. The measurement of clinical pain. *Nursing Research, 33,* p. 155.

Table 3–4
STRESS RESEARCH IN PREGNANCY AND EARLY PARENTING*

DESCRIPTIVE

Stressors Identified

Glazer (1989), expectant fathers
J. W. Griffith (1983a, 1983b), women 25 to 65 years of age
Kayiatos et al. (1984), toddler siblings
Killien & Brown (1987), hassles of adult women
Nuttall (1988), mothers of apnea-monitored infants
Pridham et al. (1982, 1986), new mothers
White & Ritchie (1984), hospitalized pregnant women

Stress Patterns and Experiences

Blackburn & Lowen (1986), premature birth
Dean (1986), monitoring apneic infant
Kuhn (1982), unwed adolescent pregnancy
Leonard (1981), depressive response to twins
Loos & Julius (1989), hospitalization during pregnancy
Lovell & Fiorino (1979), oppression of institution of motherhood
Steren et al. (1980), culturally induced stress
Tentoni & High (1980), cultural attitudes

Differences in Stress Patterns

Becker (1987), adolescent vs. adult mothers
S. Griffith (1976), mothers vs. fathers
Kemp & Hatmaker (1989), low- vs. high-risk pregnant women
Mercer & Fertekich (1988), high-risk (hospitalized) vs. low-risk pregnancy; mothers vs. fathers
Robbins (1981), pregnant vs. nonpregnant adolescents
Schroeder-Zwelling & Hock (1986), diabetic vs. nondiabetic mothers
Tilden (1984), single vs. partnered women
White & Dawson (1981), parents of low-, moderate-, and high-risk infants
Zigrossi & Riga-Ziegler (1986), gestational vs. chronic diabetes

RELATIONSHIPS AMONG VARIABLES/PREDICTIVE MODELS

Life Events as Predictors

Becker (1987)
Bee et al. (1986)
Brandt (1984)
Brown (1986)
Downs (1977)
Ferketich & Mercer (1989)
Kirgis et al. (1977)
Lenz et al. (1986)
Mercer & Ferketich (1988)
Mercer et al. (1988a)
Norbeck & Anderson (1989a)
Norbeck & Anderson (1989b)

Table 3–4
STRESS RESEARCH IN PREGNANCY AND EARLY PARENTING* *(Continued)*

RELATIONSHIPS AMONG VARIABLES/PREDICTIVE MODELS
Norbeck & Tilden (1983)
Nuckolls et al. (1972)
Sund & Ostwald (1985)
Tilden (1983)
Relationships among Psychological and Physiological Stress Measures
E. Lederman et al. (1981)
R. Lederman et al. (1977)
R. Lederman et al. (1978)
R. Lederman et al. (1979)
R. Lederman et al. (1985)
Pain Experience in Childbirth
Cahill (1989)
Fridh et al. (1988)
Gaston-Johansson et al. (1988)
Lowe (1987)
Lowe (1989)
Morse & Park (1988)
Relationships with Specific Stressors and Stress Contexts
Maternal expectations (Fishbein, 1984)
Maternal employment, infant difficultness (Walker, 1989a, 1989b)
Routine nursing care procedures (Norris et al. 1982)
High-risk birth (Lamm, 1983)
War environment (Zahr et al. 1988)
INTERVENTION TO PREVENT OR REDUCE STRESS†
Cagan & Meier (1983), discharge-planning tool
Consolvo (1986), care-by-parent unit
Wilford & Andrews (1986), sibling classes

*Concerns and needs of parents are included in the chapters on role attainment.
†Interventions aimed at teaching coping skills are not included here; see the chapter on coping. Interventions aimed at teaching parenting skills are presented in the chapters on role attainment.

Descriptive research includes studies that identify specific stressors and stress patterns common during pregnancy and early parenting, the experiences of parents facing specific stress events, such as premature birth, and, finally, differences in stress between subgroups based on gender, age, and marital status, among others.

Aimed at explicating the relations among sets of variables, relational/predictive research includes studies about the effects of life events and other forms of stressful events on parenting and health status, relations between psychological and physiological stress measures, biophysical and psychosocial factors affecting the pain experience in labor, expectations as predictors of stress, and the relation of stressful events to physiological and behavioral responses of infants.

Intervention research covers investigations of the efficacy of nursing interventions to prevent or reduce stress. This category comprises the area with the fewest studies related to stress.

DESCRIPTIVE RESEARCH

Stressors among Women of Childbearing Age

J. Griffith (1983a) surveyed 579 women, ages 25 to 65 years, about stressors, coping patterns, and physical and emotional symptoms. Among respondents, 63 percent were married. Stressors were identified by a disparity between level of importance and satisfaction of 22 life-goal items. For women in the primary childrearing age group, 25 to 34 years, stressors occurred in the following areas: Personal time (32 percent), physical health (26 percent), personal success (12 percent), love relationships (8 percent), social relationships (1 percent), and parent-child relationships (0 percent). By contrast, parent-child relationships were stressors for 6 percent of women in the 45 to 54 age group. In the physical health category, the two most frequent foci of stress were exercise and nutrition for women from 25 to 54 years of age. Findings relative to coping patterns and stress responses (symptoms) reported by Griffith (1983b) are summarized in Chapters 4 and 7, respectively. In a related study, Killien & Brown (1987) identified hassles (daily stresses) experienced by women in four different role configurations (e.g., married working mother, homemaker). The overall occurrence of hassles did not differ for the four role configurations, and hassles related to the self was the most frequently occurring category for three of the four role patterns.

Stressors among New Mothers

Identification of stressors specific to new mothers of well infants has been reported by Pridham, Hansen, Bradley, and Heighway (1982) and Pridham et al. (1986). Using daily logs, new mothers (N = 62) reported the stressors and supports they experienced during the first 90 days of their infants' lives. Through content analysis, occurrence of stressors and supports were tabulated for seven major categories: (1) self, (2) responsibilities and tasks, (3) resources, (4) activities and plans, (5) behavior of self and other, (6) conditions, and (7) events.

Stressors and supports were also classified according to whether they were social or nonsocial (existential) in nature (Pridham et al., 1986). During the first 15 days, stressors in the self category were most frequent. Thereafter, stressors in the category of responsibilities and tasks were most frequent. Overall totals of stressors and supports were approximately equivalent for the 90-day period. Both nonsocial stressors and supports exceeded social ones for the overall 90-day period. Overall frequency of stressors and supports decreased during the 90 days, but the level of three stressors remained fairly constant: Responsibilities and tasks, conditions, and events. Overall, there was a positive relationship between the frequencies of stressors and supports.

Responses of Fathers and Siblings

In a study of stressors and anxiety in 108 expectant fathers, Glazer (1989) reported that the four most frequent specific stressors were concern about whether the baby would be healthy and normal, partner's pain in childbirth, baby's condition at birth, and unexpected events during childbirth. Overall, the areas of childbirth, finances, and baby were most frequently identified as sources of stress. Mean state anxiety levels were not high; expectant fathers on average had lower state anxiety than male high school or college students. Levels of stressors and state anxiety were related to fathers' age, income, and education. Stressor levels were also related to fathers' weight gain.

To determine mothers' concerns about sibling rivalry, Kayiatos, Adams, and Gilman (1984) conducted telephone interviews of 29 mothers of toddlers at 3 to 6 weeks after birth of a sibling. Ninety-three percent of the mothers reported regressive behavior in toddlers. Changes in toddler behavior occurred in general behavior (e.g., tantrums, use of security items), eating, toileting, and sleep habits. Regressive changes in general behavior was the area about which mothers most frequently expressed concern.

Stress of Hospitalization and Apnea Monitoring

White and Ritchie (1984) studied stressors associated with hospitalization of 61 pregnant women with at-risk conditions. Highest levels of stress were associated with separation from home and family and disturbing emotions. Next came stress associated with changing family circumstances, health concerns, and changing self-image. Lowest levels of stress were associated with communications with health professionals and the hospital environment. In women hospitalized more than 2 weeks (n = 12), overall stress levels increased significantly from those initially experienced.

In a related study of 11 women hospitalized for complications of pregnancy, Loos and Julius (1989) reported similar findings. In particular, their phenomenological method revealed experiences of loneliness, boredom, and powerlessness.

Dean (1986) described stress patterns experienced by 20 mothers of infants being monitored for apnea. By using qualitative methods for data analysis of open-ended interviews, five dimensions of mothers' experiences were identified: (1) constant watchfulness, (2) struggles with leaving the baby, (3) limitations imposed by monitoring, (4) changes in relating to other children, and (5) concerns about terminating monitoring.

In a still larger sample (N = 74), Nuttall (1988) conducted interviews of women whose infants had had home apnea monitoring. To identify types of upsets mothers experienced related to monitoring, interviews were content-analyzed. Nine types of upsets were identified: Fear, lack of credibility, problems with the monitor, disrupted family life, emotional effects, lack of support, concerns for the infant, unresolved problems, and unhelpfulness of health professionals.

Stress Associated with Preterm Birth

By use of a convenience sample, Blackburn and Lowen (1986) conducted a survey of reactions of parents and grandparents to premature birth. Both parents and grandparents reported high levels of anxiety. In addition, both mothers and fathers reported high levels of fear, lack of control, and helplessness. Mothers were regarded by the researchers as most needy, and one third received less emotional support than needed. The primary concern of grandparents was concern about the infant's parents. For parents, concerns focused on coping with the situation, strain, and finances. Grandparents identified less concern for the infant's survival and more concern about the infant's future intellectual development than parents.

Stress and Mental Health of Mothers

Kuhn (1982) examined the role of stress in a pregnant adolescent who developed postpartum psychosis. By use of case study methodology, prenatal, intrapartal, and postpartal stresses were described as related to pregnancy, adolescence, and unwed parenthood. In a related vein, Leonard (1981) reported on the occurrence of depression in three mothers of twins. By using case study methods, depression was linked to stress in parental, marital, and personal roles.

Cultural Expectations and Beliefs as Stressors

Three studies examined the role of cultural expectations and beliefs as a source of stress. Lovell and Fiorino (1979) studied stress in the mothering role stemming from institutionalized myths about motherhood. Occurrence of stress was linked to four concepts: (10) nonmotivating pain, (2) a sense of powerless, (3) good mother/bad mother conformity, and (4) an external source of identity. Clinical validation with 26 mothers supported the presence of the four concepts in myths about motherhood. In a related vein, Tentoni and High (1980) identified three negative changes experienced by pregnant women, for example, changes in body proportions. These were theorized to lead to loss of self-esteem and subsequent depression. Finally, by using field research methods, Stern, Tilden, and Maxwell (1980) investigated stress stemming from interactions between Philippino-American families and Western health professionals. Western obstetric care was stressful to pregnant women raised with non-Western models of childbearing. Stress stemmed from three sources: (1) cultural beliefs and practices, (2) interpersonal style, and (3) language barriers.

Group Differences in Stress

A number of studies compared differing subpopulations of parents by using various measures of stress. The small number of subjects sampled in many of those studies warrants caution in extrapolating the findings. In a comparison of 23 adolescent and 22 adult mothers of infants, Becker (1987) found no significant differences in life change events during pregnancy. Similarly, Robbins (1981) found no differences in life events when comparing pregnant and nonpregnant adolescents.

In a large sample of expectant parents aged 18 and above, Mercer and Ferketich (1988) found no differences in life events experienced by expectant mothers compared to fathers. However, women with high-risk pregnancies reported more negative life events than women with low-risk pregnancies. Also comparing stress levels in women with low-risk and high-risk pregnancies, Kemp and Hatmaker (1989) reported the two groups did not differ in state anxiety or urinary norepinephrine levels. Women with high-risk pregnancies did have higher urinary epinephrine levels.

White and Dawson (1981) explored differences in life events associated with parental gender as well as infant-risk status. Using data from 99 families, White and Dawson found no significant differences in life events when comparing mothers and fathers, nor was level of infant-risk status associated with significant differences in parents' reported life events.

In a study of expectant parents, S. Griffith (1976) examined the subjects' interpersonal needs. Although data were not tested statistically, the investigator identified differences between husbands and wives related to meeting interpersonal needs as a potential source of stress. Tilden (1984) compared pregnant women on life event stress and found that those who were single ($n = 25$) had significantly higher life event stress than those who were partnered ($n = 116$).

Combining both gestational and chronic diabetic pregnant women into one group ($n = 20$), Schroeder-Zwelling and Hock (1986) reported no differences between them and a nondiabetic comparison group ($n = 20$) on an anxiety indicator of stress. However, Zigrossi and Riga-Ziegler (1986) concluded that pregnant women with gestational diabetes (n = 20) found their medical regimens more stressful than those with chronic diabetes (n = 18); however, this conclusion was drawn without benefit of statistical testing.

RELATIONAL AND PREDICTIVE RESEARCH

Impact of Life Events on Parenting and Family Functioning

A number of studies have investigated the relationship of life-event stress to developmental, parenting, and health outcomes. Becker (1987) found life events related to some aspects of mothers' assessment of infant behavior. In a longitudinal study from birth to age 4, Bee et al. (1986) reported modest correlations between life event changes and later child developmental outcomes. The relation between life event changes and development was most pronounced if mothers were low in both resources and social support. Brandt (1984) failed to find direct relations between stress and parenting, that is, maternal discipline. Instead, there was a trend for the stress and support interaction to predict parenting. In a study of family stress, Sund and Ostwald (1985) found life events to be related to life-style variables as well as to parental age and number of children.

In a major study (N = 593) of expectant parents, Mercer, Ferketich, DeJoseph, May, and Sollid (1988a) tested a theoretical model of the effects of prenatal stress on family functioning. Contrary to expectation, the model had low explanatory power for both women with high-risk pregnancies and their partners, as well as for women with low-risk pregnancies and their partners. The model for women with high-risk pregnancies was respecified with the following outcomes: Sense of mastery, trait anxiety, and relationship with own father as a child predicted significant amounts of variance in women's reports of family functioning. Distinct respecified models were also provided for women with low-risk pregnancies and the partners of both groups of women.

Impact of Life Events on Health Status

The largest number of nursing studies of life events have focused on the relation between stress and health-illness status. Stressful events have been linked to neonatal pathology (Downs, 1977), as well as to health status (Brown, 1986) and depression and state anxiety among expectant parents (Mercer & Ferketich, 1988). In a more elaborate test of the relation between stress and health, Kirgis, Woolsey, and Sullivan (1977) examined psychosocial factors in pregnant women (n = 51) that in association with physical factors may predict neonatal outcomes, specifically infant Apgar scores. Maternal life-event stress was correlated significantly with Apgar scores. Further, in multiple regression analysis with nine predictors, an interaction variable (stress in past 6 months and number of past pregnancy complications) was most highly correlated with Apgar scores. However, in a triethnic sample of 208 low-risk pregnant women, Norbeck and Anderson (1989b) found no significant relation between life event stress and pregnancy complications. Further, in a multivariate causal model of fathers' health status (pregnancy through 8 months postpartum), Ferketich and Mercer (1989) reported no direct health-status effects of negative life events or pregnancy risk, but there were some indirect effects for both predictors.

Nuckolls, Cassel, and Kaplan (1972) demonstrated that stressful events in and of themselves may not always lead to pathology. Their research showed that life events did not predict pregnancy outcomes directly. Rather, life events were associated with pregnancy outcomes only when events were high but psychosocial assets were low, that is, the interaction effect of stress and resources in relation to health outcomes. Several studies have specifically tested both the direct effects of stress on health outcomes and the interaction effects. Lenz, Parks, Jenkins, and Jarett (1986) studied the relation of life events to illness among mothers of 6-month-old infants. Although life events added significantly to the prediction of illness, the interaction of life events and support did not. Similarly, Tilden (1983) found that life events directly predicted emotional disequilibrium in pregnancy and that the interaction of life events and support resources was not statistically significant. In still another study, Norbeck and Tilden (1983) used a prospective design to control for prior medical problems as well as social factors. Both emotional disequilibrium and overall pregnancy complications were predicted by prior life events, but their interaction with social support was not predictive of either outcome. However, when gestational, labor, and infant complications were separately considered, each was predicted by the interaction of life events during pregnancy and tangible support. The latter finding is consistent with the stress-buffering hypothesis (Chapter 2). Finally, Norbeck and Anderson (1989a) examined the effects of life events on state anxiety in healthy, low-income women (N = 190) during the second and third trimester of pregnancy. In cross-sectional and longitudinal analyses, life events predicted state anxiety. In two of three analyses, the interactions of life events and social support were significant: Women with high stress and low support had the highest mean anxiety.

Pain Experiences in Childbirth

To understand the experience of pain in childbirth, several related studies have compared subgroups of women and occasionally their partners in relation to labor-pain magnitude. In a comparison of pain during labor, Lowe (1987) found that *primiparas* and *multiparas* did not differ in overall pain (main effects) during labor. A significant statistical interaction was reported; it indicated that primiparas may have more pain in early labor and less pain in second-stage labor than multiparas.

Gaston-Johansson, Fridh, and Turner-Norvell (1988) further described the pain experience across successive phases of labor among Swedish women. Overall, the sensory component of pain (assessed by such words as "sharp" and "cramping") exceeded the affective component of pain during labor (assessed by such words as "terrifying" and "dreadful"). However, for primiparas the affective component exceeded the sensory one at 8 to 10 cm of cervical dilitation. At most points in labor, primiparas reported more sensory and affective pain than multiparas. They also used more pain medication than multiparas.

In a further exploration of factors associated with pain in childbirth, Fridh, Kopare, Gaston-Johansson, and Norvell (1988) reported that both the number of children and the maternal age were negatively correlated with pain in labor. For primiparas, both emotional variables and history of trouble with menstrual pain correlated with pain in labor. For multiparas, history of trouble with menstrual pain, but not emotional variables, correlated with pain in labor.

In still another study of variables affecting the pain experience in active labor, Lowe (1989) tested the explanatory power of nine variables, both physiological and psychosocial. Three variables explained significant amounts of variance in labor pain: Confidence in ability to handle labor, preparation for childbirth, and frequency of uterine contractions.

The choice of birth setting on perceptions of labor pain was the focus of a study by Morse and Park (1988). To test cognitive methods that parents use to bolster decisions made about birth setting, the investigators compared parents electing home birth versus hospital birth. As predicted, home birth parents rated pain in childbirth as significantly lower than hospital birth parents.

In a study of the relation between beta-endorphin levels and pain, Cahill (1989) reported that pregnant women had significantly higher plasma levels of beta-endorphins than nonpregnant women. During actual labor, however, no association between pain levels and plasma beta-endorphin levels was found.

Relations between Psychological and Physiological Measures of Stress and Childbirth

Relations between psychological and physiological measures of stress have been studied within the context of pregnancy and labor. R. Lederman, McCann, Work, and Huber (1977) reported that plasma catecholamines of primigravidas rose during labor compared to third-trimester concentrations. However, the latter were similar to concentrations for normal, nonpregnant subjects. Elsewhere, R. Lederman, E. Lederman, Work, and

McCann (1978) reported evidence of relations in phase 2 labor between plasma epinephrine and self-reported anxiety, uterine contractile activity (Montevideo units), and progress in labor. Although plasma cortisol was unrelated to epinephrine levels, cortisol was related to anxiety and uterine contractility. In phase 3 labor, epinephrine was negatively related to duration of labor.

Additionally, R. Lederman et al. (1979) reported relations between psychological factors in pregnancy, for example, conflict about accepting the pregnancy, and labor variables such as plasma epinephrine and progress in labor. In examining fetal-newborn health status, E. Lederman, R. Lederman, Work, and McCann (1981) reported that both anxiety in labor and plasma epinephrine were related to fetal heart rate pattern in active-phase labor. Also, prenatal conflict about acceptance of pregnancy was inversely related to 5-minute Apgar scores. Among multigravid women, R. Lederman et al. (1985) found evidence that duration of labor (from 3 to 6 cm) was related to plasma epinephrine and norephinephrine levels; longer labors were associated with higher catecholamines. In turn, several measures of patient anxiety were related to catecholamine levels. Further, fetal heart rate patterns at 7 to 10 cm of cervical dilitation were related to earlier levels of epinephrine and anxiety.

Expectations as Predictors of Stress

Fishbein (1984) explored the role of expectations as a source of stress for expectant fathers. As predicted, if expectant couples did not share congruent expectations of the fathers' involvement in child care, fathers had a higher state of anxiety ($r = 0.24$). Lamm (1983) investigated the impact of a previous high-risk birth on mothers' dyadic adjustment; mothers of infants with severe respiratory distress syndrome evidenced significant inverse relations between the number of previous preterm births and dyadic adjustment.

Stress of Maternal Employment and Infant Difficultness

Using maternal employment and infant difficultness as stressor variables, Walker (1989b) proposed a stress-process model in which perceived stress mediated the effects of stressors on the maternal role. In addition, health-promotive life-style was proposed to buffer the maternal role from stress effects. The mediating role of perceived stress was supported for both stressors. Health-promotive life-style did not demonstrate buffering effects; instead, it was related directly to the maternal role. In a longitudinal retesting of the stress-process model (Walker, 1989a), earlier results were replicated when maternal employment, but not infant difficultness, served as the stressor.

Infant Responses to Stressful Events

Focusing on stress in infants, Norris, Campbell, and Brenkert (1982) examined the relations of three nursing procedures (suctioning, repositioning, and conducting a heel-stick) to transcutaneous oxygen tension in premature infants. Decrease in transcutaneous oxygen was greatest during suctioning, followed by repositioning. Changes associated with heel-sticks were not statistically significant.

In a study of the effects of prenatal stress on neonatal behavior, Zahr, Khoury, and Nugent (1988) compared two groups of Lebanese newborns living in a war environment: One living in a dangerous part of Beirut in which daily shelling and gunfire occurred and a second group living in a relatively safe part of Beirut. Both groups of infants were healthy, full-term infants weighing more than 2500 g at birth. Of seven variables compared, infants differed on two: Habituation and range of infant state. Infants living in the more dangerous area performed better than those in the safer region. The researchers hypothesized that differences may be a function of adaptation to auditory stimuli associated with gunfire and shelling (cf. Barnard et al., 1985, p. 252).

Intervention Research

Using a nonequivalent control-group design, Cagan and Meier (1983) evaluated the impact of a discharge-planning tool with parents of high-risk infants. The tool was aimed at standardizing teaching given to parents in preparation for home care of their infants. The intended purpose of the tool was to minimize the crisis parents underwent following discharge of their infants from the hospital. A visiting nurse from the nursery administered a follow-up questionnaire in the home setting to compare the routine-teaching group with the planning-tool group. Focused on how well parents felt nurses prepared them for home care, the follow-up questionnaire showed that parents in the planning-tool group felt more prepared. In a similar study, Consolvo (1986) used a one-group, pretest-posttest group design to evaluate the effectiveness of a care-by-parent unit to prepare mothers for assuming the home care of their infants being released from the intensive care unit. Maternal anxiety was significantly reduced in one of four questionnaire scenarios in which mothers were asked to respond to illness of a child.

In another study, Wilford and Andrews (1986) evaluated the effectiveness of sibling preparation classes for preschoolers in reducing stress after birth of a sibling. Nonequivalent groups were used: One group received sibling preparation classes and the other did not. The sibling preparation class lasted about 2 hours; its content was focused on family changes with a new baby. Slides, book reading, and holding a doll were used. After birth of infants, sibling groups were compared on child behavior. No significant differences were found between preschool siblings who received preparation classes and those who did not.

Future Research Directions

Although the nursing literature on stress in pregnancy and early parenting is impressive in amount, future work would benefit from more careful consideration of the conceptual approach to stress that is adopted and the selection of measurement methods to attain consistency with the approach taken. Sorting out the conceptual distinctions between stressful events, chronic strains, stress appraisal, stress response, and stress effects should be considered in future nursing research on stress (Chapter 2).

Also evident is a need to more precisely and deliberately trace the pathways by which stress leads to negative outcomes. Two tasks in particular must be addressed by investigators. First, future studies should be based on thoughtful proposals about modes by which stressful experiences may leave their imprint upon parenting and health status (Hyman & Woog, 1982). Second, in future work, investigators should carefully build on advances in knowledge and methods coming forth from other investigators whose work closely parallels their own. This building is emerging in the areas of life event stress and prediction of childbirth pain.

In sum, future research should be done with an eye to two issues: (1) Is there a clear match between the stress concept as defined at the theoretical level and the operational procedures selected for its measurement? (2) Does the proposed research clarify the manner by which stress experiences lead to negative health, developmental, or parenting outcomes? The model testing reported by Mercer et al. (1988a) and Walker (1989a, 1989b) provides some tests of proposed stress pathways, but further research in this area is clearly needed.

Although descriptive and predictive research has shown that stress is related to developmental and health outcomes, little progress has been made in systematically developing and testing nursing interventions to prevent or reduce stress for parents and infants. Information on the nature and patterning of stress in a variety of circumstances during pregnancy and early parenting is available. Comparative data also exist to aid in identifying client groups likely to experience higher levels of stress. In addition, relational/predictive models that link various stressors to health and other adaptive outcomes have been tested. However, nursing interventions specifically aimed at preventing or reducing cumulative or specific sources of stress or preventing or reducing stress appraisal or arousal triggered by stressful events are few in number. To be truly preventive, such interventions would not be aimed at managing (coping with) the emotions and problems precipitated by stressful events. Instead, their aim would be to interrupt the early phases of the stress process so that stress appraisal and arousal would not occur. That represents a new and challenging area of research in parent-infant nursing science in need of attention.

REFERENCES

Abidin, R. R. (1982). Parenting stress and the utilization of pediatric services. *Children's Health Care, 11*(2), 70–73.

Albrechts, S. A., & Rankin, M. (1989). Anxiety levels, health behaviors, and support systems of pregnant women. *Maternal-Child Nursing Journal, 18,* 49–60.

Avant, K. C. (1988). Stress on the childbearing family. *Journal of Obstetric, Gynecologic, and Neonatal Nursing, 17,* 179–185.

Barnard, K. E., Hammond, M., Mitchell, S. K., Booth, C. L., Spietz, A., Snyder, C., & Elsas, T. (1985). Caring for high-risk infants and their families. In M. Green (Ed.), *The psychosocial aspects of the family* (pp. 245–266). Lexington, MA: Heath.

Barsevic, A., & Llewellyn, J. (1982). A comparison of the anxiety-reducing potential of two techniques of bathing. *Nursing Research, 31,* 22–27.

Becker, P. T. (1987). Sensitivity to infant development and behavior: A comparison of adolescent and adult single mothers. *Research in Nursing and Health, 10,* 119–127.

Bee, H. L., Barnard, K. E., Eyres, S. J., Gray, C. A., Hammond, M. A., Spietz, A. L., Snyder, C., & Clark, B. (1982). Prediction of IQ and language skill from perinatal status, child performance, family characteristics, and mother-infant interaction. *Child Development, 53,* 1134–1156.

Bee, H. L., Hammond, M. A., Eyres, S. J., Barnard, K. E., & Snyder, C. (1986). The impact of parental life change on the early development of children. *Research in Nursing and Health, 9,* 65–74.

Blackburn, S., & Lowen, L. (1986). Impact of an infant's premature birth on the grandparents and parents. *Journal of Obstetric, Gynecologic, and Neonatal Nursing, 14,* 173–178.

Booth, C. L., Barnard, K. E., Mitchell, S. K., & Spieker, S. J., (1987). Successful intervention with multi-problem mothers: Effects on the mother-infant relationship. *Infant Mental Health Journal, 8,* 288–306.

Booth, C. L., Mitchell, S. K., Barnard, K. E., & Spieker, S. J. (1989). Development of maternal social skills in multiproblem families: Effects on the mother-child relationship. *Developmental Psychology, 25,* 403–412.

Brandt, P. A. (1984). Stress-buffering effects of social support on maternal discipline. *Nursing Research, 33,* 229–234.

Bronfenbrenner, U. (1979). *The ecology of human development: Experiments by nature and design.* Cambridge, MA: Harvard University Press.

Brooten, D., Gennaro, S., Brown, L. P., Butts, P., Gibbons, A. L., Bakewell-Sachs, S., & Kumar, S. P. (1988). Anxiety, depression, and hostility in mothers of preterm infants. *Nursing Research, 37,* 213–216.

Brown, M. A. (1986). Social support, stress, and health: A comparison of expectant mothers and fathers. *Nursing Research, 35,* 72–76.

Cagan, J., & Meier, P. (1983). Evaluation of a discharge planning tool for use with families of high-risk infants. *Journal of Obstetric, Gynecologic, and Neonatal Nursing, 12,* 275–281.

Cahill, C. A. (1989). Beta-endorphin levels during pregnancy and labor: A role in pain modulation. *Nursing Research, 38,* 200–203.

Chaves, J., & Barber, T. X. (1974). Cognitive strategies, experimental modeling, and expectations in the attenuation of pain. *Journal of Abnormal Psychology, 83,* 356–363.

Clinton, J. F. (1986). Expectant fathers at risk for couvade. *Nursing Research, 35,* 290–295.

Cohen, S., Kamarck, T., & Mermelstein, R. (1983). A global measure of perceived stress. *Journal of Health and Social Behavior, 24,* 385–396.

Consolvo, C. A. (1986). Relieving parental anxiety in the care-by-parent unit. *Jour-*

nal of Obstetric, Gynecologic, and Neonatal Nursing, 15, 154–159.

Cox, T. (1978). *Stress.* Baltimore: University Park Press.

Curry, M. A. (1987). Maternal behavior of hospitalized pregnant women. *Journal of Psychosomatic Obstetrics and Gynaecology, 7,* 165–182.

Dean, P. G. (1986). Monitoring an apneic infant: Impact on the infant's mother. *Maternal-Child Nursing Journal, 15,* 65–76.

Derogatis, L. R. (1982). Self-report measures of stress. In L. Goldberger & S. Breznitz. (Eds.), *Handbook of stress* (pp. 270–294). New York: Free Press.

Dooher, M. E. (1980). Lamaze method of childbirth. *Nursing Research, 29,* 220–224.

Dormire, S. L., & Strauss, S. S., & Clarke, B. A. (1989). Social support and adaptation to the parent role in first-time adolescent mothers. *Journal of Obstetric, Gynecologic, and Neonatal Nursing, 18,* 327–337.

Downs, F. S. (1977). Maternal stress in primigravidas as a factor in the production of neonatal pathology. In F. S. Downs & M. A. Newman (Eds.), *A source book of nursing research* (2nd ed., pp. 129–139). Philadelphia: F. A. Davis.

Everly, G. S., & Rosenfeld, R. (1981). *The nature and treatment of the stress response.* New York: Plenum.

Ferketich, S. L., & Mercer, R. T. (1989). Men's health status during pregnancy and early fatherhood. *Research in Nursing & Health, 12,* 137–148.

Fishbein, E. G. (1984). Expectant father's stress—due to the mother's expectations? *Journal of Obstetric, Gynecologic, and Neonatal Nursing, 13,* 325–328.

Franck, L. S. (1986). A new method to quantitatively describe pain behavior in infants. *Nursing Research, 35,* 28–31.

Fridh, G., Kopare, T., Gaston-Johansson, F., & Norvell, K. T. (1988). Factors associated with more intense labor pain. *Research in Nursing and Health, 11,* 117–124.

Gaston-Johansson, F., Fridh, G., & Turner-Norvell, K. (1988). Progression of labor pain in primiparas and multiparas. *Nursing Research, 37,* 86–90.

Geden, E., Beck, N., Brouder, G., & O'Connell, E. (1983). Identifying procedural components for analogue research of labor pain. *Nursing Research, 32,* 80–83.

Geden, E., Beck, N. C., Anderson, J. S., Kennish, M. E., & Mueller-Heinze, M. (1986). Effects of cognitive and pharmacologic strategies on analogued labor pain. *Nursing Research, 35,* 301–306.

Glazer, G. (1989). Anxiety and stressors of expectant fathers. *Western Journal of Nursing Research, 11,* 47–59.

Griffith, J. W. (1983a). Women's stressors according to age groups: 1. *Issues in Health Care of Women, 6,* 311–326.

Griffith, J. W. (1983b). Women's stress responses and coping patterns according to age groups: 2. *Issues in Health Care of Women, 6,* 327–340.

Griffith, S. (1976). Pregnancy as an event with crisis potential for marital partners: A study of interpersonal needs. *Journal of Obstetric, Gynecologic, and Neonatal Nursing, 5,* 35–38.

Hegyvary, S. T., & Chammings, P. A. (1975). The hospital setting and patient care outcomes: Part I. *Journal of Nursing Administration, 5*(March–April), 29–32.

Holmes, T., & Rahe, R. (1967). The social readjustment rating scale. *Journal of Psychosomatic Research, 11,* 213–218.

Hurst, M. W., Jenkins, C. D., & Rose, R. M. (1978). The assessment of life change stress: A comparison and methodological study. *Psychosomatic Medicine, 40,* 126–141.

Hyman, R. B. (1988). Measures of stress and related constructs: A guide for research and clinical practice. *Scholarly Inquiry for Nursing Practice, 2*(1), 5–66.

Hyman, R. B. & Woog, P. (1982). Stressful life events and illness onset: A review of crucial variables. *Research in Nursing and Health, 5,* 155–163.

Ireton, H. R. (1980). A personal inventory. *Journal of Family Practice, 11,* 137–140.

Kanner, A. D., Coyne, J. C., Schaefer, C., & Lazarus, R. S. (1981). Comparison of two modes of stress measurement: Daily hassles and uplifts versus major life events. *Journal of Behavioral Medicine, 4*(1), 1–39.

Kayiatos, R., Adams, J., & Gilman, B. (1984). The arrival of a rival: Maternal perceptions of toddlers' regressive behaviors after the birth of a sibling. *Journal of Nurse-Midwifery, 29,* 205-213.

Keller, E., & Bzdek, V. M. (1986). Effects of therapeutic touch on tension headache pain. *Nursing Research, 35,* 101-106.

Kemp, V. H., & Hatmaker, D. D. (1989). Stress and social support in high-risk pregnancy. *Research in Nursing and Health, 12,* 331-336.

Killien, M., & Brown, M. A. (1987). Work and family roles of women: Sources of stress and coping strategies. *Health Care of Women International, 8*(2-3), 169-184.

Kirgis, C. A., Woolsey, D. B., & Sullivan, J. J. (1977). Predicting infant apgar scores. *Nursing Research, 26,* 439-442.

Kuhn, J. C. (1982). Stress factors preceding postpartum psychosis: A case study of an unwed adolescent. *Maternal-Child Nursing Journal, 11,* 95-108.

Lamm, N. H. (1983). The second high-risk birth: Impact on maternal dyadic adjustment. *Issues in Health Care of Women, 4,* 251-259.

Lederman, E., Lederman, R. P., Work, B. A., & McCann, D. S. (1981). Maternal psychological and physiologic correlates of fetal-newborn health status. *American Journal of Obstetrics and Gynecology, 139,* 956-958.

Lederman, R. P., Lederman, E., Work, B. A., & McCann, D. S. (1978). The relationship of maternal anxiety, plasma catecholamines, and plasma cortisol to progress in labor. *American Journal of Obstetrics and Gynecology, 132,* 495-500.

Lederman, R. P., Lederman, E., Work, B. A., & McCann, D. S. (1979). Relationship of psychological factors in pregnancy to progress in labor. *Nursing Research, 28,* 94-97.

Lederman, R. P., Lederman, E., Work, B., & McCann, D. S. (1985). Anxiety and epinepherine in multiparous women in labor: Relationship to duration of labor and fetal heart rate pattern. *American Journal of Obstetrics and Gynecology, 153,* 870-877.

Lederman, R. P., McCann, D. S., Work, B., & Huber, M. J. (1977). Endogenous plasma epinephrine and nonepinephrine in last-trimester pregnancy and labor. *American Journal of Obstetrics and Gynecology, 129,* 5-8.

Lenz, E. R., Parks, P. L., Jenkins, L. S., & Jarrett, G. E. (1986). Life change and instrumental support as predictors of illness in mothers of 6-month-olds. *Research in Nursing and Health, 9,* 17-24.

Leonard, L. G. (1981). Postpartum depression and mothers of infant twins. *Maternal-Child Nursing Journal, 10,* 99-109.

Loos, C., & Julius, L. (1989). The client's view of hospitalization during pregnancy. *Journal of Obstetric, Gynecologic, and Neonatal Nursing, 18,* 52-56.

Lovell, M. C., & Fiorino, D. L. (1979). Combating myth: A conceptual framework for analyzing the stress of motherhood. *Advances in Nursing Science, 1*(4), 75-84.

Lowe, N. K. (1987). Parity and pain during parturition. *Journal of Obstetric, Gynecologic, and Neonatal Nursing, 16,* 340-346.

Lowe, N. K. (1989). Explaining the pain of active labor: The importance of maternal confidence. *Research in Nursing and Health, 12,* 237-245.

Lowe, N. K., & Roberts, J. E. (1988). The convergence of between in-labor report and postpartum recall of parturition pain. *Research in Nursing and Health, 11,* 11-21.

Manderino, M. A., & Bzdek, V. M. (1984). Effects of modeling and information on reactions to pain: A childbirth-preparation analogue. *Nursing Research, 33,* 9-14.

Mash, E. J., & Johnston, C. (1983). Parental perceptions of child behavior problems, parenting self-esteem, and mothers' reported stress in younger and older hyperactive and normal children. *Journal of Consulting and Clinical Psychology, 51*(1), 86-99.

McCubbin, H. I., Patterson, J. M., & Wilson, L. R. (1981). Assessing family stress: Family inventory of life events and changes (FILE). In H. I. McCubbin, & J. M. Patterson (Eds.), *Family stress: Resources and coping* (pp. 21-39). St. Paul: University of Minnesota.

McGuire, C. B. (1984). The measurement of clinical pain. *Nursing Research, 33,* 152-156.

Melzack, R. (1983). The McGill pain questionnaire. In R. Melzack (Ed.), *Pain Measure-*

ment and assessment. New York: Raven Press.

Mercer, R. T. (1986). Predictors of maternal role attainment at one year postbirth. *Western Journal of Nursing Research, 8,* 9–25.

Mercer, R. T., & Ferketich, S. L. (1988). Stress and social support as predictors of anxiety and depression during pregnancy. *Advances in Nursing Science, 10*(2), 26–39.

Mercer, R. T., Ferketich, S. L, DeJoseph, J., May, K. A., & Sollid, D. (1988a). Effect of stress on family functioning during pregnancy. *Nursing Research, 37,* 268–275.

Mercer, R. T., Ferketich, S., May, K., DeJoseph, J., & Sollid, D. (1988b). Further exploration of maternal and paternal fetal attachment. *Research in Nursing & Health, 11,* 83–95.

Mercer, R. T., Hackley, K. C., & Bostrom, A. G. (1983). Relationship of psychosocial and perinatal variables to perception of childbirth. *Nursing Research, 32,* 202–207.

Mercer, R. T., May, K. A., Ferketich, S., & DeJoseph, J. (1986). Theoretical models for studying the effect of antepartum stress on the family. *Nursing Research, 35,* 339–346.

Miles, M. S. (1985). Emotional symptoms and physical health in bereaved parents. *Nursing Research, 34,* 76–81.

Mitchell, S. K., Bee, H. L., Hammond, M. A., & Barnard, K. E. (1985). Prediction of school and behavior problems in children followed from birth to age eight. In W. K. Frankenburg, R. N. Emde, & J. W. Sullivan (Eds.), *Early identification of children at risk* (pp. 117–132). New York: Plenum.

Morse, J. M., & Park, C. (1988). Home birth and hospital deliveries: A comparison of the perceived painfulness of parturition. *Research in Nursing and Health, 11,* 175–181.

Murphy, S. A. (1986). Status of natural disaster victims' health and recovery 1 and 3 years later. *Research in Nursing and Health, 9,* 331–340.

Norbeck, J. S. (1984). Modification of life event questionnaires for use with female respondents. *Research in Nursing and Health, 7,* 61–71.

Norbeck, J. S., & Anderson, N. J. (1989a). Life stress, social support, and anxiety in mid- and late-pregnancy among low income women. *Research in Nursing and Health, 12,* 281–287.

Norbeck, J. S., & Anderson, N. J. (1989b). Psychosocial predictors of pregnancy outcomes in low-income black, hispanic, and white women. *Nursing Research, 38,* 204–209.

Norbeck, J. S., & Tilden, V. P. (1983). Life stress, social support, and emotional disequilibrium in complications of pregnancy: A prospective, multivariate study. *Journal of Health and Social Behavior, 24*(March), 30–46.

Norris, S., Campbell, L. A., & Brenkert, S. (1982). Nursing procedures and alterations in transcutaneous oxygen tension in premature infants. *Nursing Research, 31,* 330–336.

Nuckolls, K. B., Cassel, J., & Kaplan, B. (1972). Psychosocial assets, life crisis, and the prognosis of pregnancy. *American Journal of Epidemiology, 95,* 431–441.

Nuttall, P. (1988). Maternal responses to home apnea monitoring of infants. *Nursing Research, 37,* 354–357.

Pridham, K. F., Egan, K. B., Chang, A. S., & Hansen, M. R. (1986). Life with a new baby: Stressors, supports, and maternal experience. *Public Health Nursing, 3*(40), 225–239.

Pridham, K. F., Hansen, M. F., Bradley, M. E., & Heighway, S. M. (1982). Issues of concern to mothers of new babies. *Journal of Family Practice, 14,* 1079–1085.

Riesch, S. K. (1984). Occupational commitment and the quality of maternal infant interaction. *Research in Nursing and Health, 6,* 295–503.

Robbins, R. (1981). A study of the relationship between adolescent pregnancy and life-change events. *Issues in Mental Health Nursing, 3,* 219–236.

Rossi, A. S. (1968). Transition to parenthood. *Journal of Marriage and Family, 30*(1), 26–39.

Sarason, I., Johnson, J., & Siegel, J. (1978). Assessing the impact of life changes: Development of the life experiences survey.

Journal of Consulting and Clinical Psychology, 46, 932–946.

Schroeder-Zwelling, E., & Hock, E. (1986). Maternal anxiety and sensitive mothering behavior in diabetic and nondiabetic women. *Research in Nursing and Health, 9,* 249–255.

Spielberger, C. D., Gorsuch, R. L., Lushene, R., Vagg, P. R., & Jacobs, G. A. (1983). *Manual for the state-trait anxiety inventory.* Palo Alto, CA: Consulting Psychologists Press.

Stern, P. N., Tilden, V. P., & Maxwell, E. K. (1980). Culturally-induced stress during childbearing: The Philippino-American experience. *Issues in Health Care of Women, 2*(3–4), 67–81.

Sund, K., & Ostwald, S. K. (1985). Dual-earner families' stress levels and personal and life-style-related variables. *Nursing Research, 34,* 357–361.

Tentoni, S. C., & High, K. A. (1980). Culturally induced postpartum depression. *Journal of Obstetric, Gynecologic, and Neonatal Nursing, 9,* 246–249.

Thomas, S. P., & Groer, M. W. (1986). Relationship of demographic, life-style, and stress variables to blood pressure in adolescents. *Nursing Research, 35,* 169–172.

Tilden, V. P. (1983). The relation of life stress and social support to emotional disequilibrium during pregnancy. *Research in Nursing and Health, 6,* 167–174.

Tilden, V. P. (1984). The relation of selected psychosocial variables to single status of adult women during pregnancy. *Nursing Research, 33,* 102–107.

Walker, L. O. (1989a). A longitudinal analysis of stress process among mothers of infants. *Nursing Research, 38,* 339–343.

Walker, L. O. (1989b). Stress process among mothers of infants: Preliminary model testing. *Nursing Research, 38,* 10–16.

White, M., & Dawson, C. (1981). The impact of the at-risk infant on family solidarity. In R. Lederman & B. Raff (Eds.), *Perinatal parental behavior.* New York: Liss. March of Dimes Birth Defects Foundation. *Birth Defects, Original Article Series, 17*(6), 253–284.

White, M., & Ritchie, J. (1984). Psychological stressors in antepartum hospitalization: Reports from pregnant women. *Maternal-Child Nursing Journal, 13,* 47–56.

Wilford, B., & Andrews, C. (1986). Sibling preparation classes for preschool children. *Maternal-Child Nursing Journal, 15,* 171–185.

Woods, N. F. (1985). Relationship of socialization and stress to premenstrual symptoms, disability, and menstrual attitudes. *Nursing Research, 34,* 145–149.

Yarcheski, A., & Mahon, N. E. (1986). Perceived stress and symptom patterns in early adolescents: The role of mediating variables. *Research in Nursing and Health, 9,* 289–297.

Zahr, L. K., Khoury, M., & Nugent, K. (1988). Neonatal behavior on prenatally stressed Lebanese infants. *Image, 20,* 200–202.

Zigrossi, S. T., & Riga-Ziegler, M. (1986). The stress of medical management on pregnant diabetics. *MCN, The American Journal of Maternal/Child Nursing 11,* 320-323.

CHAPTER 4

Parent-Infant Nursing Research on Coping

DEFINITIONS AND DESCRIPTIONS OF COPING

DEFINING COPING

Common to most definitions of coping is the focus on efforts of the individual to deal with a stressful situation (Table 4–1). Those efforts may be directed at the situation itself or at the distress engendered within the individual by the situation (Panzarine, 1985). Most theorists define coping as the response to an event or situation that exceeds or taxes an individual's usual behavior patterns. For example, Lazarus and Folkman (1984) define coping as "constantly changing cognitive and behavioral efforts to manage specific external and/or internal demands that are appraised as taxing or exceeding the resources of the person" (p. 141). Thus, coping is usually seen as conceptually distinct from habits that have been adopted to resolve recurrent problems of daily living. To what extent is coping as defined here an aspect of pregnancy and parenting? Despite assertions that pregnancy can be stressful (Table 3–1), little parent-infant nursing research has focused on coping itself.

This chapter also includes the concept of control. Control has many potential meanings, but it is used in pregnancy and childbirth literature primarily to denote either ways in which women perceive their situations (Gara & Tilden, 1984) or women's views about their ability to influence decisions made about their reproductive experience (Humenick, 1981). These two dimensions of control closely parallel the phenomena of cognitive appraisal/reappraisal and instrumental coping.

Table 4–1
DEFINITIONS AND DESCRIPTIONS OF COPING

"Coping responses were defined as efforts to prevent, avoid, or control emotional distress." (Collins & Post, 1986, p. 309.)

"Coping is help actors provide to themselves, that is, behavior by which people facilitate their progress toward a goal or behavior by which they redefine their goals and reconcile themselves to a likely state of affairs." (Brickman et al. [in press] as cited in Cronenwett & Brickman, 1983, p. 84.)

"Cognitive and emotional processes are equally important to the coping process, and each is a result of the cognitive appraisal of the environment." (Gasper, 1987, p. 230.)

THEORETICAL MODELS OF COPING

Within a research context, investigators may either conceptualize coping as a stable (traitlike) or dynamic (processlike) phenomenon. If viewed as stable, investigators emphasize intrapersonal resources or patterns that are typically used in dealing with stressful situations. In contrast, if copying is viewed as a dynamic process, then investigators emphasize the specific strategies directly used in managing a stressful encounter. (See Chapter 2 for a discussion of coping resources versus coping processes.)

Coping may also precede a stressful event. For example, intervention studies may emphasize the learning of coping skills prior to a stressful encounter. Panzarine (1985) has called this "anticipatory coping" (p. 50). Studies of preparation for childbirth are noteworthy in this regard. Humenick (1981) further explicated the role of coping within a mastery model of childbirth: Coping skills are one potential support that offsets stressors during childbirth so that women achieve a sense of mastery of their experiences.

Within a practice context, the concept of coping takes on still other meanings. For example, in a theoretical paper on helping and coping in childbirth, Cronenwett and Brickman (1983) have outlined four models of coping within the context of helping relationships. In the moral model, responsibility for actions is placed on individuals; that is, self-help is fundamental to coping. The compensatory model also stresses the role of the individual in solving problems but permits the use of resources to overcome obstacles not created by the individual. In the medical model, coping is shaped by dependency on experts to solve problems. Finally, the enlightened model also stresses that solutions come from expert helpers who provide new, "enlightened" solutions to problems. Each model construes differently client coping and the helping relationship vis-à-vis coping. Each model of coping and helping stems from judgments that are largely philosophical in nature, but the empirical assessment of the utility of each model within existing care delivery systems would add substance to the comparative evaluation of the model.

Table 4–2
MEASURES/TOOLS FOR THE CONCEPT OF COPING

Tool	Source Described in	Studies Using Tool
Chronicity Impact & Coping Instrument: Parent Questionnaire: One hundred sixty-seven item scale	Hymovich (1981, 1983, 1984)	—
Parental Coping Scale: Eighty-one-item scale for coping with a handicapped child	Damrosch, Lenz, & Perry (1985)	Damrosch & Perry (1989)
Coping Responses Inventory: Fifty-nine-item scale for employed women with children	Collins & Post (1986)	—
Coping Responses Scale: Thirty-three-item inventory	Moos, Cronkite, Billings, & Finney (1984)	Roberts et al. (1987)*
McNett Coping Effectiveness Questionnaire: Eighteen-item scale of attributes of effective coping	McNett (1987)	McNett (1987)*
Ways of Coping Checklist: Sixty-eight-item scale for coping in a specific situation	Folkman & Lazarus (1980)	Gass (1987)* McNett (1987)*
Jalowiec Coping Scale: Forty-item scale of coping strategies	Jalowiec & Powers (1981) Jalowiec, Murphy, & Powers (1984)	Yarcheski & Mahon (1986)* Powers & Jalowiec (1987)*
Family Coping Inventory: Twenty-eight-item or ninety-item scale	McCubbin, Boss, Wilson, & Lester (1978)	Ventura (1982) Ventura & Boss (1983) Ventura (1986)
Means-Ends Problem-Solving Procedure: Story completion (middle segment) test of alternative generation	Platt & Spivack (1975)	Gennaro (1986)

Multidimensional Health Locus of Control Scale: Eighteen-item scale of locus of control related to health	K. A. Wallston, B. S. Wallston, & DeVellis (1978)	Littlefield & Adams (1987) Lewallen (1989) Fullerton (1982)
Pregnancy Attitude Index: Twenty-four-item scale of expectancy control related to pregnancy and childbirth	O'Connell (1983)	—
Attitude Toward Issues of Choice in Childbirth Scale: Eighteen-item scale of attitudes toward control in childbirth	Fullerton (1982)	Fullerton (1982)
Prenatal Attitude Towards Childbirth Participation Scale: Ten-item scale of perceptions about control in childbirth and life	Humenick & Bugen (1981b)	Humenick & Bugen (1981b)
Neuromuscular Dissociation Relaxation Rating Scale: Six-item scale for rating relaxation	Humenick & Marchbanks (1981)	Humenick & Marchbanks (1981)
Schroeder Labor Locus of Control Scale: Twenty-item scale with pre- and post-labor versions	Schroeder (1985)	Schroeder (1985)
Labour Agentry Scale (forms A–D): Scale for personal control in labor	Hodnett & Simmons-Tropea (1987)	Hodnett & Osborn (1989) Hodnett (1982) Hodnett & Abel (1986)
Labor Agency Scale: Nine-item scale of perceived control during labor	Humenick & Bugen (1981b)	Humenick & Bugen (1981b) Humenick & Bugen (1981a)
Delivery Agency Scale: Ten-item scale of perceived control during delivery	Humenick & Bugen (1981b)	Humenick & Bugen (1981b) Humenick & Bugen (1981a)

*Not a parent-infant population.

MEASUREMENT

GENERAL STRATEGIES

Because coping is largely an intrapersonal phenomenon, its measurement relies heavily on self-report methods of measurement. Particularly when individuals use various internal thought processes, such as internal monologues, to manage a stressful situation, only the individual may be aware of the use. However, methods of measuring coping may vary with the way the stressful situation is delimited. That is, tools may address characteristic coping patterns across any number of situations or they may focus specifically on coping with a particular stressor. These two approaches to measuring coping approximate trait versus process orientations to the concept of coping (Lazarus & Folkman, 1984; Panzarine, 1985). If the former, survey questionnaires which cover a broad range of coping strategies and which have reliability and validity with a wide range of populations are needed. If the latter, measurement of coping may involve questionnaires which are situation-specific, as well as other methods such as diaries, checklists, and repeated interviews. For a general review of coping instruments and related issues, see Cohen (1987).

SPECIFIC TOOLS

Table 4–2 presents examples of tools relevant to assessing coping and related concepts such as control and problem solving. A number of tools are specifically designed for use with expectant mothers; they include the Neuromuscular Dissociation Relaxation Rating Scale (Humenick & Marchbanks, 1981), the Labour Agentry Scale (Hodnett & Simmons-Tropea, 1987), the Schroeder Labor Locus of Control Scale (Schroeder, 1985), and the Pregnancy Attitude Index (O'Connell, 1983). Table 4–2 cites studies in which coping tools were used with parents or other populations. The preponderance of tools are self-report questionnaires of one form or another.

SUMMARY OF RESEARCH

SCOPE OF COPING RESEARCH

Overall, compared to the number of studies of stress (Chapter 3), fewer studies have investigated coping during pregnancy, childbirth, and early parenting. Also unlike stress research, research on coping has been rather evenly divided between studies focused on intervention and studies focused on description or prediction (Table 4–3). Because there are only a limited number of studies of coping during pregnancy and early parenting, those studies are mainly isolated research efforts. A notable exception is the interrelated set of studies on interventions with analogued labor pain. (For other studies on psychological processes in pregnancy and childbirth, see Chapters 11 and 12.)

Table 4–3
COPING RESEARCH IN PREGNANCY, LABOR, AND EARLY PARENTING

DESCRIPTIVE
Coping Strategies Identified
Griffith (1983), women 25 to 65 y of age
Killien & Brown (1987), adult women in four role patterns
Coping Patterns
Gara & Tilden (1984), pregnancy as positive
Gasper (1987), persistent anemia during pregnancy
Sandelowski & Bustamante (1986), cesarean birth
Stewart & Glazer (1986), women with in vitro fertilization
Differences in Coping Patterns
Damrosch & Perry (1989), mothers vs. fathers of handicapped children
Fullerton (1982), mothers with in- vs. out-of-hospital births
Killien & Brown (1987), women in four role patterns
Ventura (1982), mothers vs. fathers
Ventura (1986), mothers vs. fathers
Ventura & Boss (1983), mothers vs. fathers
RELATIONSHIPS AMONG VARIABLES/PREDICTIVE MODELS
Humenick & Bugen (1981b), mastery variables in childbirth
Ventura (1982), coping and parent and infant factors
Ventura (1986), coping and parent and infant factors
Willmuth et al. (1978), control and childbirth satisfaction
*INTERVENTION TO ENHANCE COPING**
Bernardini et al. (1983), components of Lamaze
Durham & Collins (1986), music during classes and labor
Geden et al. (1986), pain management strategies
Geden et al. (1985), components of Lamaze
Geden et al. (1984), pain-coping strategies
Hodnett (1982), type of fetal monitor
Manderino & Bzdek (1984), pain-reducing strategies
Spaulding (1969), tape recordings
Timm (1979), prenatal classes
Worthington et al. (1982), components of childbirth classes

*Interventions aimed at teaching parenting skills are presented in the chapter on role attainment unless coping terminology is specifically used by authors.

DESCRIPTIVE RESEARCH

Coping Strategies Identified

Data about coping among women in the childbearing years has been provided by a study of stress and coping among women between 25 and 65 years of age. Griffith (1983) used a self-report questionnaire to gather data from 579 women on coping patterns. Women rated how often they used 13 coping methods to handle problems. The three most prevalent coping methods in the 25- to 34-year-old group were talking with friends/associates, consumption of food, and working. Significant differences in coping methods were found across age groups. For women over 45 years of age, working and religion were the most prevalent coping methods.

In a related study of coping strategies, Killien and Brown (1987) investigated coping strategies used for daily hassles experienced by 92 adult women in four role configurations (e.g., married working mothers and homemakers). For 48 percent of the hassles, women made no response to the hassles. For the remaining hassles, the two most prevalent coping strategies were problem solving (19.2 percent) and emotional responses (10.5 percent). Although differences occurred in the rank ordering of coping strategies for the four role configurations, doing nothing and problem solving were the two most prevalently used coping strategies for all four groups.

Coping Patterns

Stewart and Glazer (1986) described the results of a pilot study (n = 3) focused on expectations and coping with in vitro fertilization. Open-ended interviews revealed that support from the in vitro fertilization team and the spouse facilitated coping. In a descriptive case study of responses of a primipara to persistent anemia (Gasper, 1987), six types of coping responses were identified; they included conditional compliance, expressing affective states, monitoring, using support, replenishing, and using knowledge.

In a study using grounded theory methods, Gara and Tilden (1984) sought to explain why some women view their pregnancies in a positive manner. From interviews of 32 pregnant women, the investigators generated the core category of "adjusted control." During data collection, perception of control was identified as influencing attitude toward pregnancy: "The greater a woman's perception of having control in her life, the more positive seemed her perception of her pregnancy" (p. 430). The idea of control was further refined as adjusted control, wherein women achieved a sense of control by construing their pregnancies as reasonable to themselves. Four subdimensions of adjusted control include: physical/biological, emotional, social, and financial.

In another qualitative study, Sandelowsi and Bustamante (1986) investigated the experience of cesarean birth among 50 low-income women outside "the natural childbirth culture." Based on analysis of interviews, four coping patterns were identified: (1) prenatal avoidance of the idea of a cesarean birth, (2) postpartal avoidance of blame for the cesarean birth, (3) evaluating the cesarean birth in terms of the outcomes, and (4) comparing and contrasting physical aspects of vaginal and cesarean childbirth. Overall, women in the sample demonstrated neutrality in their feelings toward their child-birth experiences: "The women were neither depressed nor happy, but simply 'OK,'" (p. 87).

Differences in Coping

In addition to the research of Killien and Brown (1987) on differences in coping for different role configurations reported above, Ventura (1982, 1986; Ventura & Boss, 1983) has investigated differences in coping between mothers and fathers of infants. In a sample of 100 mothers and 100 fathers, Ventura (1982; Ventura & Boss, 1983) compared coping behaviors used by parents when infants were 2 to 3 months old. Coping behaviors were gathered by adapting the 28-item version of the Family Coping Inventory for use with new parents. Of 28 behaviors, mothers found 17 more helpful than fathers; examples were seeking understanding from friends, shopping with friends, keeping in shape, and talking to someone (Ventura & Boss, 1983, p. 872). Fathers found only one behavior more helpful than mothers: engaging in social activities. With factor analysis of coping behaviors, three broad coping patterns were identified. Mothers perceived two of those coping patterns more helpful than fathers did: (1) social support and self-development and (2) being religious, thankful, and content (Ventura, 1982). In a subsequent replication study (N = 47 couples), mothers' and fathers' coping were again compared. In this second sample, mothers found one coping pattern more helpful than fathers did: social support and self-development (Ventura, 1986).

Fullerton (1982) sought to determine whether women (n = 33) who sought out-of-hospital births differed on control variables in comparison to those who sought in-hospital births (n = 33). The two groups were matched retrospectively on age, parity, and marital status. Both health- and childbirth-specific measures of control were used. Significant differences on four of five subscales indicated that women who sought out-of-hospital births had a more internal locus of control related to health and childbirth than those who sought in-hospital births.

Damrosch & Perry (1989) compared mothers' and fathers' patterns of response to parenting a child with Down's syndrome. The children with Down's syndrome ranged from infants to adults. Fathers reported a recovery pattern of steady, gradual improvement while mothers more frequently reported a peaks-and-valleys pattern. Mothers reported more frequent chronic sorrow than fathers. Finally, compared to fathers, mothers more frequently used the following coping patterns: expression of negative emotion, self-blaming, communication of feelings, and special feelings such as embarrassment in public.

RELATIONAL/PREDICTIVE RESEARCH

Control and Childbirth

To test the relationship between sense of personal control and satisfaction with childbirth, Willmuth, Weaver, and Borenstein (1978) conducted a survey of new mothers. As predicted, women who both attended prepared childbirth classes and were very satisfied with childbirth had a more internal locus of control than those who were less satisfied. That mothers had attended prepared childbirth classes did not, considered as a single variable, predict satisfaction with childbirth.

In a study of mastery during childbirth, Humenick and Bugen (1981b) assessed mothers' (N = 33) attitudes toward active participation in labor, instrumentality, expressiveness, control perceptions, and evaluation of labor and delivery. Prenatal attitude toward participation was significantly related to childbirth satisfaction but not control perceptions. Postnatal, but not prenatal, instrumentality and expressiveness were significantly related to perceptions of control in labor and delivery.

Parental Coping

Ventura (1982) also correlated parental coping patterns with infant temperament and parental functioning variables. Coping patterns were related, in part, to parental functioning (particularly depression) and also were modestly related to infant temperamental characteristics. In a replication study, Ventura (1986) found that in mothers coping was unrelated to parental functioning but in fathers one coping pattern (social support and self-development) was inversely related to depression and anxiety. Relationships between parental coping and selected infant temperamental characteristics were also found.

INTERVENTION RESEARCH

Panzarine (1985, pp. 54–55) indicated that clinical intervention studies of coping have employed two types of intervention: (1) those focused on preparatory information, and (2) those focused on instruction and rehearsal in specific coping strategies. Intervention studies of coping during pregnancy and early parenting have included both forms of intervention. The majority of coping studies in parent-infant nursing have focused on the labor and delivery experience.

Preparation for Childbirth

Timm (1979) tested the effect of prenatal education on two outcomes, medication use in labor and infant birth weight. Low-income pregnant women (N = 118) were randomly assigned to one of three groups (6 weeks of prenatal education classes, 6 weeks of knitting classes, or no classes). The prenatal education classes covered information on changes in pregnancy and postpartum, coping techniques during labor, and medications, and included a hospital tour. Knitting classes covered information on basic knitting techniques and how to knit a baby shirt. No differences in infant birth weights were found among the three groups. Women in the prenatal education group used significantly less medication in labor than women in the other two groups.

Bernardini, Maloni, and Stegman (1983) studied the impact of three variables (method of instruction, regular practice, and goal-directed statements) on neuromuscular control during labor. Women (N = 92) were selected for the study on the basis of their intent to use the Lamaze method during labor. Observed during labor for a minimum of two 10-minute periods, women's neuromuscular control was rated on a five-point, six-item scale. Women who attended Lamaze classes had better neuromuscular control than self-taught women. Also, the amount of practice and having a goal for labor were associated with neuromuscular control. The quasi-experimental nature of this study (no random assignment and no manipulation of independent variables by the investigators) weakens the strength of conclusions that may be drawn about the effects of the variables studied.

Durham and Collins (1986) tested the effect of self-selected music on the use of pain medication in labor. Both the treatment group (n = 15) and the control group (n = 15) participated in prepared childbirth classes. In addition, the treatment group, to which subjects were assigned randomly, listened to music during classes and labor. The two groups did not differ statistically in their use of pain medication in labor.

Coping with Analoged Labor Pain

A number of studies have tested the effects of various techniques to enhance coping during labor by using an analog to labor pain as the stressor. Worthington, Martin, and Shumate (1982) conducted two such experiments with nulliparous female volunteers. Immersing the forearm in ice water (0 to 1°C) was used as the pain stimulator. In experiment 1, a factorial design (12 groups plus 1 no-treatment control group) was used to test the individual and combined effects of structured breathing, effleurage, and rehearsal on pain tolerance. Pain tolerance was measured by total number of seconds that subjects' hands were immersed in ice water. Among the 12 experimental groups, significant main effects were found for structured breathing, no effleurage, and rehearsal. When experimental groups were compared with the no-treatment control group, three of four groups using rehearsal had significantly better pain tolerance than the control group.

In experiment 2 (N = 52), the individual and combined effects of coaching and coping-skill training were tested by using pain tolerance as the outcome variable. Both main effects for coaching and coping-skill training were significant. The group receiving both coping-skill training and coaching fared significantly better than the control group, the coaching-only group, or the coping-skills-only group.

In another labor-pain analog study (N = 60), Manderino and Bzkek (1984) compared the effects of four pain-reducing treatments on self-reported pain and physiological variables. The four treatment groups were videotaped modeling, videotaped information and modeling, videotaped information, and a control videotape. Using a pain stimulator as the labor analog, group comparisons revealed that the group receiving both information and modeling reported significantly less pain. No significant differences in physiological variables were found.

Geden, Beck, Brouder, Glaister, and Pohlman (1985) conducted a labor-pain analog study (N = 80) of individual and combined effects of three Lamaze components (relaxation, informational lectures, and breathing exercises). Using a pain stimulator as the labor analog, effects of treatments were measured by self-reported pain and physiological variables. Study outcomes indicated that, overall, relaxation was the most therapeutically active component as evidenced by pain reports, EMG, and heart rate outcomes.

In a related study (N = 100), Geden, Beck, Hauge, and Pohlman (1984) tested the effects of 10 treatment conditions on reported pain and physiological variables. Treatment conditions included (1) pleasant imagery, (2) pleasant imagery plus relaxation, (3) sensory transformation, (4) sensory transformation plus relaxation, (5) neutral imagery, (6) neutral imagery plus relaxation, (7) combined cognitive strategies, (8) combined cognitive strategies plus relaxation, (9) relaxation only, and (10) no treatment. Subjects in the sensory transformation group reported significantly less pain than those in the neutral imagery or no-treatment groups. Other group differences were not statistically significant for reported pain. No significant treatment effects for the physiological variables were found.

In still another labor-pain analog study (N = 120), Geden, Beck, Anderson, Kennish, and Mueller-Heinze (1986) tested the effects of five cognitive and one pharmacologic approaches to pain reduction. Cognitive approaches included systematic desensitization, sensory description, sensory transformation, modeling, and relaxation. Twelve groups were formed to test individual and combined effects of approaches plus control conditions. Outcomes were measured by using self-reported pain and physiological variables. At the end of 20 pain trials, 2 groups had significantly less pain than the no-treatment control group: (1) sensory transformation and (2) combined cognitive strategies plus pharmacologic strategy. No significant treatment effects were found for physiological variables.

Other

Hodnett (1982) compared the effects of two types of fetal monitoring on perceived control in labor in a sample of 30 primigravidas. Women were randomly assigned to either the control group receiving electronic fetal monitoring or the experimental group receiving radiotelemetric fetal monitoring. The experimental group experienced greater control in labor than the control group. In addition, the experimental group spent more time out of bed, had more positive labor experiences, and used less anesthesia than the control group.

In a postpartum study, Spaulding (1969) tested the effects of tape recordings on coping with mothering tasks. While on the postpartum ward, primiparas (N = 99) were assigned to one of three groups (nurses' teaching tape, mothers' teaching tape, or control). Mothers in the two experimental groups listened to tape recordings of either nurses' or mothers' comments about caring for babies. A week later mothers were interviewed at home about their mothering practices and were rated on three developmental tasks. Overall, the tape recordings had little or no impact on mothering practices or ratings of developmental tasks.

FUTURE DIRECTIONS

Coping is an important construct in parent-infant nursing. Studies of coping, however, are less abundant than might be expected. Fortunately, there is an increasing battery of tools for measuring coping, particularly in relation to control during pregnancy and childbirth. Most descriptive and correlational studies of coping have used cross-sectional designs or longitudinal designs with very small sample sizes. Thus, a well-confirmed knowledge base about coping during pregnancy and early parenting is not yet available. Consequently, descriptive and correlational studies which incorporate larger samples and a longitudinal perspective are needed to provide a clearer picture of coping responses to stress during pregnancy and early parenting. Unanswered at this time are questions about what are the optimal patterns of coping during pregnancy and early parenting. Also unanswered are questions about the dynamics and consequences associated with different coping patterns such as women's tendency to smoke more than men in response to distress (Biener, 1987).

At present, parent-infant intervention studies of coping have focused almost exclusively on coping with the labor and delivery experience. Continued systematic research that draws on existing knowledge is needed to maintain the momentum on this topic. (See Coussens and Coussens [1984] for a critical review of research on the effectiveness of childbirth education.) Still needed are new interventions to facilitate coping with other stressors occurring during pregnancy and early parenting. Also, both short- and long-term effects of the use of various coping strategies should be studied to determine what, if any, are the adaptive costs of various forms of coping. For example, Johnson, Christman, and Stitt (1985) reported that coping techniques showed a different pattern of effects after discharge than during hospitalization among surgical patients.

REFERENCES

Bernardini, J. Y., Maloni, J. A., & Stegman, C. E. (1983). Neuromuscular control of childbirth-prepared women during the first stage of labor. *Journal of Obstetric, Gynecologic, and Neonatal Nursing, 12,* 105–111.

Biener, L. (1987). Gender differences in the use of substances for coping. In R. C. Barnett, L. Biener, & G. K. Baruch (Eds.), *Gender and stress* (pp. 330–349). New York: Free Press.

Cohen, F. (1987). Measurement of coping. In S. V. Kasl & C. L. Cooper (Eds.), *Stress and health: Issues in research methodology* (pp. 283–305). New York: Wiley.

Collins, C., & Post, L. (1986). An instrument to measure coping responses in employed mothers: Preliminary results. *Research in Nursing and Health, 9,* 309–316.

Coussens, W. R., & Coussens, P. D. (1984). Maximizing preparation for childbirth. *Health Care for Women International, 5,* 335–353.

Cronenwett, L., & Brickman, P. (1983). Models of helping and coping in childbirth. *Nursing Research, 32,* 84–88.

Damrosch, S. P., Lenz, E. R., & Perry, L. A. (1985). Use of parental advisors in the development of a parental coping scale. *Maternal-Child Nursing Journal, 14,* 103–109.

Damrosch, S. P., & Perry, L. A. (1989). Self-reported adjustment, chronic sorrow, and coping of parents of children with Down's syndrome. *Nursing Research, 38,* 25–30.

Durham, L., & Collins, M. (1986). The effect of music as a conditioning aid in prepared childbirth education. *Journal of Obstetric, Gynecologic, and Neonatal Nursing, 15,* 268–270.

Folkman, S., & Lazarus, R. S. (1980). An analysis of coping in a middle-aged community sample. *Journal of Health and Social Behavior, 21,* 219–239.

Fullerton, J. D. T. (1982). The choice of in-hospital or alternative birth environment as related to the concept of control. *Journal of Nurse-Midwifery, 27,* 17–22.

Gara, E. O., & Tilden, V. P. (1984). Adjusted control: An explanation for women's positive perceptions of their pregnancies. *Health Care for Women International, 5,* 427–436.

Gasper, M. L. (1987). The response of one primigravida to the situation of persistent anemia during pregnancy. *Maternal-Child Nursing Journal, 16,* 227–249.

Gass, K. A. (1987). The health of conjugally bereaved older widows: The role of appraisal, coping and resources. *Research in Nursing and Health, 10,* 39–47.

Geden, E., Beck, N. C., Anderson, J. S., Kennish, M. E., & Mueller-Heinze, M. (1986). Effects of cognitive and pharmacologic strategies on analogued labor pain. *Nursing Research, 35,* 301–306.

Geden, E., Beck, N. C., Brouder, G., Glaister, J., & Pohlman, S. (1985). Self-report and psychophysiological effects of Lamaze preparation: An analogue of labor pain. *Research in Nursing and Health, 8,* 155–165.

Geden, E., Beck, N., Hauge, G., & Pohlman, S. (1984). Self-report and psychophysiological effects of five pain-coping strategies. *Nursing Research, 33,* 260–265.

Gennaro, S. (1986). Anxiety and problem-solving ability in mothers of premature infants. *Journal of Obstetric, Gynecologic, and Neonatal Nursing, 15,* 160–164.

Griffith, J. W. (1983). Women's stress responses and coping patterns according to age groups: 2. *Issues in Health Care of Women, 6,* 327–340.

Hodnett, E. (1982). Patient control during labor: Effects of two types of fetal monitors. *Journal of Obstetric, Gynecologic, and Neonatal Nursing, 11,* 94–99.

Hodnett, E. D., & Abel, S. M. (1986). Person-environment interaction as a determinant of labor length variables. *Health Care for Women International, 7,* 341–356.

Hodnett, E. D., & Osborn, R. W. (1989). Effects of continuous intrapartum professional support on childbirth outcomes. *Research in Nursing and Health, 12,* 289–297.

Hodnett, E. D. & Simmons-Tropea, D. A. (1987). The labour agentry scale: Psychometric properties of an instrument measuring control during childbirth. *Research in Nursing and Health, 10,* 301–310.

Humenick, S. S. (1981). Mastery: The key to childbirth satisfaction? A review. *Birth and the Family Journal, 8*(2), 79–83.

Humenick, S. S., & Bugen, L. A. (1981a). Correlates of parent-infant interaction: An exploratory study. In R. P. Lederman, B. S. Raff, & P. Carroll (Eds.), *Perinatal parental behavior: Nursing research and implications for newborn health.* New York: Alan R. Liss for the March of Dimes Birth Defects Foundation. *Birth Defects, Original Article Series*, 17(6), 181–199.

Humenick, S. S., & Bugen, L. A. (1981b). Mastery: The key to childbirth satisfaction? A study. *Birth and the Family Journal, 8*(2), 84–90.

Humenick, S. S., & Marchbanks, P. (1981). Validation of a scale to measure relaxation in childbirth education classes. *Birth and the Family Journal, 8*(3), 145–150.

Hymovich, D. P. (1981). Assessing the impact of chronic childhood illness on the family and parent coping. *Image, 13(3),* 71–74.

Hymovich, D. P. (1983). The chronicity impact and coping instrument: Parent questionnaire. *Nursing Research, 32,* 275–281.

Hymovich, D. P. (1984). Development of the chronicity impact and coping instrument: Parent questionnaire (CICI:PQ). *Nursing Research, 33,* 218–222.

Jalowiec, A., Murphy, S. P., & Powers, M.J. (1984). Psychometric assessment of the Jalowiec coping scale. *Nursing Research, 33,* 157–161.

Jalowiec, A., & Powers, M. J. (1981). Stress and coping in hypertensive and emergency room patients. *Nursing Research, 30,* 10–14.

Johnson, J. E., Christman, N. J., & Stitt, C. (1985). Personal control interventions: Short- and long-term effects on surgical patients. *Research in Nursing and Health, 8,* 131–145.

Killien, M., & Brown, M. A. (1987). Work and family roles of women: Sources of stress and coping strategies. *Health Care for Women International, 8*(2–3), 169–184.

Lazarus, R. S., & Folkman, S. (1984). *Stress, appraisal, and coping.* New York: Springer.

Lewallen, L. P. (1989). Health beliefs and health practices of pregnant women. *Journal of Obstetric, Gynecologic, and Neonatal Nursing, 18,* 245–246.

Littlefield, V. M., & Adams, B. N. (1987). Patient participation in alternative perinatal care: Impact on satisfaction and health locus of control. *Research in Nursing & Health, 10,* 139–148.

Manderino, M. A., & Bzdek, V. M. (1984). Effects of modeling and information on reactions to pain: A childbirth-preparation analogue. *Nursing Research, 33,* 9–14.

McCubbin, H., Boss, P., Wilson, L., & Lester, G. (1978). *Family coping inventory.* (Available from H. McCubbin, Family Social Sciences, University of Minnesota, 290 McNeal Hall, St. Paul, MN 55108.)

McNett, S. C. (1987). Social support, threat, and coping responses and effectiveness in the functionally disabled. *Nursing Research, 36,* 98–103.

Moos, R. H., Cronkite, R. C., Billings, A. G., & Finney, J. W. (1984). *Health and daily living form manual.* Palo Alto, CA: Social Ecology Laboratory, Dept. of Psychiatry, Stanford University Veterans Administration Hospital.

O'Connell, M. L. (1983). Locus of control specific to pregnancy. *Journal of Obstetric, Gynecologic, and Neonatal Nursing, 12,* 161–164.

Panzarine, S. (1985). Coping: Conceptual and methodological issues. *Advances in Nursing Science, 7*(4), 49–57.

Platt, J., & Spivack, G. (1975). *Manual for the means-ends problem-solving procedure (MEPS).* Philadelphia: Department of Mental Health Sciences, Hahnemann Medical College and Hospital.

Powers, M. J., & Jalowiec, A. (1987). Profile of the well-controlled, well-adjusted hypertensive patient. *Nursing Research, 36,* 106–110.

Roberts, J. G., Browne, G., Steiner, D., Byrne, C., Brown, B., & Love, B. (1987). Analysis of coping responses and adjustment. Stability of conclusions. *Nursing Research, 36,* 94–97.

Sandelowski, M., & Bustamante, R. (1986). Cesarean birth outside the natural childbirth culture. *Research in Nursing and Health, 9,* 81–88.

Schroeder, M. A. (1985). Developing and testing a scale to measure locus of control prior to and following childbirth. *Maternal-Child Nursing Journal, 14,* 111–121.

Spaulding, M. R. (1969). The effectiveness of tape recordings with primiparas of the lower socio-economic group in coping with mothering tasks. *Communicating Nursing Research, 2,* 107–128.

Stewart, S., & Glazer, G. (1986). Expectations and coping of women undergoing in vitro fertilization. *Maternal-Child Nursing Journal, 15,* 103–113.

Timm, M. M. (1979). Prenatal education evaluation. *Nursing Research, 28,* 338–342.

Ventura, J. N. (1982). Parent coping behaviors, parent functioning, and infant temperament characteristics. *Nursing Research, 31,* 269–273.

Ventura, J. N. (1986). Parent coping, a replication. *Nursing Research, 35,* 77–80.

Ventura, J. N., & Boss, P. G. (1983). The family coping inventory applied to parents with new babies. *Journal of Marriage and the Family, 45,* 867–875.

Wallston, K. A., Wallston, B. S., & DeVellis, R. (1978). Development of the multidimensional health locus of control (MHLC) scales. *Health Education Monographs, 6*(2), 160–170.

Willmuth, R., Weaver, L., & Borenstein, J. (1978). Satisfaction with prepared childbirth and locus of control. *Journal of Obstetric, Gynecologic, and Neonatal Nursing, 7*(3), 33–37.

Worthington, E. L., Martin, G. A., & Shumate, M. (1982). Which prepared-childbirth coping strategies are effective? *Journal of Obstetric, Gynecologic, and Neonatal Nursing, 11,* 45–51.

Yarcheski, A., & Mahon, N. E. (1986). Perceived stress and symptom patterns in early adolescents: The role of mediating variables. *Research in Nursing and Health, 9,* 289–297.

CHAPTER 5

Parent-Infant Nursing Research on Social Support

DEFINITIONS AND DESCRIPTIONS OF SOCIAL SUPPORT

DEFINING SOCIAL SUPPORT

Social support is a concept that has been of great theoretical interest in nursing (Roberts, 1988; Norbeck, 1981; Gardner, 1979; Dimond & Jones, 1983). Despite that, MacElveen-Hoehn and Eyres (1984) have concluded that lack of clarity about the definition and manner of operation of social support poses major problems for the study of families and children. Thus, analysis of the meaning of social support is needed, as is knowledge of how social support works to protect health and parenting.

Despite the widespread use of social support in parent-infant nursing science, most definitions of it are adopted from other fields. One commonly used definition is that of House (1981), who describes social support as interpersonal transactions that include one or more of the following: emotional support, appraisal support, informational support, or instrumental support (see Brown, 1986b; MacElveen-Hoehn & Eyres, 1984; Cronenwett & Kunst-Wilson, 1981). Mercer and Ferketich (1988) further partitioned social support into three constructs: social embeddedness, perceived support, and enacted support (see Table 5–1 for definitions).

Table 5–1
DEFINITIONS AND DESCRIPTIONS OF SOCIAL SUPPORT IN PREGNANCY AND EARLY PARENTING

Definitions of Social Support Constructs

"Social embeddedness, or network support, refers to connections that individuals have with others in their environment." (Mercer & Ferketich, 1988, p. 27.)

"Perceived support refers to a person's belief that help or empathy is readily available if needed." (Mercer & Ferketich, 1988, p. 27.)

"Enacted or received support assesses what persons do when they provide support (provide or receive tangible, emotional, informational, or appraisal help), and such support is likely to be provided when individuals face a crisis." (Mercer & Ferketich, 1988, p. 27.)

Definitions of Family

"The family was defined as a dynamic system that functions as a whole, made up of subsystems of individuals and dyads. Individuals included the expectant mother, expectant father, unborn infant, and dyads included the mother-father, mother-unborn infant and father-unborn infant." (Mercer et al., 1988a, p. 268.)

The family is "a psychosocial unit composed of two or more people who have a commitment to each other and who live together." (Lasky et al., 1985, p. 42.)

The concept of social support is usually used in reference to the support available to or perceived by parents, but a broader view would encompass support for the young infant. Supportive parenting in infancy and early childhood is often seen as fundamental to healthy psychosocial development later in life. Thus, Richardson (1982) summarized the psychoanalytic position about early family relationships as follows: "Successes and failures in mothering often reflect a long chain of similar mother-child interactions from one generation to the next" (p. 9). Presumably, the same conclusions would be drawn about cross-generational similarities in fathering. Thus, social support is a concept relevant to both parents and infants.

Indeed, social support is an important aspect of family relationships in general. (See Table 5–1 for definitions of the family.) Because one may experience social support from other than family members, however, the concepts of family and social support are identical. Nevertheless, supportive family relationships are of paramount importance in pregnancy and early parenting (Richardson, 1982). During pregnancy, the mother-to-be redefines her relationships with and responsibilities to significant others as part of her preparation for motherhood: "She comes to view them differently and to depend on them in different ways because of her pregnancy and anticipated motherhood" (Richardson, 1982, p. 17). In turn, reactions of significant others to her take on new meaning: "Responses of significant others to her pregnancy provide much information concerning the ease or difficulty with which she will make the important life transition" (p. 17). Thus, social support is tied closely to psychological adaptations made by women during pregnancy and following childbirth.

Table 5–2
TENETS OF SUPPORT IN FAMILY-CENTERED MATERNITY CARE

"The essence of nursing . . . is support: of families in crisis, in need of health guidance, or in whatever they declare as their health need." (Kuhn, 1984, p. 95.)

"The quality of support can only be evaluated by the reciprocant." (Kuhn, 1984, p. 95.)

"The nurse must be willing to invest in effort directed away from self." (Kuhn, 1984, p. 96.)

The antecedents of support are goodness of fit, an identifiable need or goal, and availability. (Kuhn, 1984, pp. 96–97.)

Criteria for the evaluation of support provided by nurses include perceived presence, accommodation, cue identification, and reliability. (Kuhn, 1984, pp. 98–99.)

Finally, definitions of social support have focused primarily on support in the existing natural social system of parents. Social support as a dimension of parent-nurse relationships has less often been considered. Indeed, some have noted that social support may not be desirable in formal health care systems because it may impair the client's movement toward self-care and autonomy (MacElveen-Hoehn & Eyres, 1984, p. 28). Others would disagree, however. Kuhn (1984), for one, has stated that support is fundamental to nursing. (See Table 5–2 for a summary of key tenets in Kuhn's analysis of support in family-centered maternity care.) Some of the apparent discrepancies between the two positions may stem from failure to distinguish between supportive acts of care providers and the care providers becoming continuing members of clients' social networks. However, questions about what types of social support are appropriately and effectively provided by nurses still remain.

THEORETICAL MODELS OF SOCIAL SUPPORT

Several theoretical models of social support have been proposed for parent-infant nursing. Crawford (1985) proposed a theoretical model focused on conflict within the social network of new mothers. Besides age and socioeconomic status, Crawford included the concepts of partiality, multiplexity, and reciprocity as influences upon social network conflict.

Focusing on fathers, Cronenwett and Kunst-Wilson (1981) developed a model of the transition to fatherhood which included social support as a conditioning factor. Using House's categories of emotional, instrumental, informational, and appraisal support, each support category was operationally defined in terms of the transition to fatherhood.

An additional theoretical model of social support is inherent in a number of parent-infant studies which have focused on social support as an intervening variable in the stress-illness relationship. Although the exact manner by which social support operates is unclear, two broad hypotheses, the direct-effect hypothesis and the buffering hypothesis, prevail

(Chapter 2). In the direct-effect hypothesis, social support is related directly to health or other outcomes regardless of the level of stress present. In the buffering hypothesis, however, social support "explains significant differences in health outcomes only under conditions of high stress" (MacElveen-Hoehn & Eyres, 1984, p. 26).

MEASUREMENT

GENERAL STRATEGIES

For some time, nurses have been interested in capturing the phenomena of support and family relations. Rich (1978), for example, proposed use of sociograms to measure support systems in pregnancy. More recently, nurse researchers have turned to quantitative instruments designed in interview or questionnaire format. As of this date, observational methods for measuring social support are rare.

Measurement of social support plays a big part in interpreting research findings. There is no one accepted definition of social support to guide measurement. As a result, a large number of tools measuring different facets of support have been developed (Heitzmann & Kaplan, 1988). Unfortunately, the developers and users of those tools have given uneven attention to reliability and validity issues (D. L. Rock, Green, Wise, & R. D. Rock, 1984; Heitzmann & Kaplan, 1988). Because the concept of social support at present is composed of multiple complex components (Chapter 2), investigators should clearly delineate which component is most salient to their work before selecting a measure of social support (Barrera, 1986). Researchers and clinicians may be attracted to measures of perceived social support if they are interested in subjective perceptions of parents. If actual resources available to parents are of concern, then measures of social network and reports of support actually received may be more relevant. For thoughtful analyses of conceptual and measurement issues related to social support in the context of nursing, see Tilden (1985) and Stewart (1989).

SPECIFIC TOOLS

A number of tools for measuring social support exist. Table 5–3 presents social support measures used in parent-infant nursing research. Of these, the Norbeck Social Support Questionnaire (Norbeck, Lindsey, & Carrieri, 1981), the Social Network Inventory (Cronenwett, 1984), and the Personal Resources Questionnaire (Brandt & Weinert, 1981) are widely used tools that were developed by nurses. Readers interested in a critical analysis of these and other social support measures should see the reviews by Heitzmann and Kaplan (1988), House and Khan (1985), Barrera (1986), and Payne and Jones (1987).

Table 5–3
MEASURES/TOOLS FOR THE CONCEPT OF SOCIAL SUPPORT

Tool	Source Described in	Studies Using Tool
	SOCIAL SUPPORT TOOLS	
Norbeck Social Support Questionnaire: Includes functional and network subscales	Norbeck, Lindsey, & Carrieri (1981) Norbeck, Lindsey, & Carrieri (1983) Norbeck (1984)	Capuzzi (1989) Koniak-Griffin (1988) Curry (1987) Norbeck & Anderson (1989a) Coleman et al. (1989) Dormire et al. (1989) Norbeck & Anderson (1989b)
Influence of Specific Referents: Seven items for rating each referent	Kaufman & Hall (1989)	Kaufman & Hall (1989)
Instrumental support interview: Structured interview	Thoits (1982)	Lenz, Parks, Jenkins, & Jarrett (1986)
Personal Resources Questionnaire: Two-part tool of multidimensional aspects of social support	Brandt & Weinert (1981) Weinert (1984)	Brandt (1984a) Brandt (1984b) Aaronson (1989) Barnard, Magyary, et al. (1988) Booth et al. (1987) Booth et al. (1989) Barnard et al. (1987) Albrecht & Rankin (1989)
Inventory of Socially Supportive Behaviors: Forty-item scale	Barrera (1981)	Mercer & Ferketich (1988) Mercer et al. (1988a) Ferketich & Mercer (1989) Mercer, Ferketich, May, DeJoseph, & Sollid (1988b)

Table 5–3
MEASURES/TOOLS FOR THE CONCEPT OF SOCIAL SUPPORT *(Continued)*

Tool	Source Described in	Studies Using Tool
	SOCIAL SUPPORT TOOLS (Continued)	
Support Behaviors Inventory: Six-point scale of partner and other support	Brown (1986b)	Brown (1986a) Brown (1986c) Brown (1987a) Kemp & Hatmaker (1989)
Support Importance Scale: Forty-five-item scale	Brown (1987b)	Brown (1987b)
Social Network Inventory: Tool for social network	Cronenwett (1984) Cronenwett (1985a)	Cronenwett (1984) Cronenwett (1985a) Cronenwett (1985b) Jordan (1987)
Social network checklist: Twenty-six-item list to assess size and membership of social network	Mercer et al. (1988b)	Mercer et al. (1988b)
Social Support Questionnaire: Scale for subfacets of social support	Schaefer, Coyne, & Lazarus (1981)	Tilden (1983b) Norbeck & Tilden (1983) Tilden (1984)
Nursing Support in Labor Questionnaire: Twenty-item scale	Kintz (1987)	Kintz (1987)
	SOCIAL COMPETENCE TOOLS*	
Community Life Skills Scale: Thirty-two-item scale of skills needed for community living	Booth et al. (1989)	Booth et al. (1987) Booth et al. (1989) Barnard, Magyary, et al. (1988)

Social Skills Scale (also called Adult Conversational Skills Scale): Sixty-three-item scale for observing verbal and nonverbal skills	Booth, et al. (1989)	Booth et al. (1987) Booth et al. (1989) Barnard, Magyary, et al. (1988)
	RELATIONSHIP AND FAMILY TOOLS	
Relationship Change Scale: Twenty-six-item questionnaire	Guerney (1977)	Rankin et al. (1985) Rankin & Campbell (1983) Lenz, Soeken, Rankin, & Fischman (1985)
Dyadic Adjustment Scale: Thirty-two-item dyadic adjustment scale	Spanier (1976)	Lamm (1983) Cranley (1984) Porter & Demeuth (1979) Rankin et al. (1985) Tomlinson (1987) Lenz et al. (1985)
Intimate Relationship Scale: Twelve-item scale for changes in intimate aspects of marital relationship	Lenz et al. (1985)	Lenz et al. (1985)
Marriage Role Expectation Inventory: Seventy-one-item scale of role expectations	Dunn (1963)	Meleis & Swendsen (1978)
Marital Adjustment Test: Scale for marital adjustment	Locke & Wallace (1959)	Ferketich & Mercer (1989) Dooher (1980) Hangsleben (1983) Mercer et al. (1988b)

Table 5–3
MEASURES/TOOLS FOR THE CONCEPT OF SOCIAL SUPPORT *(Continued)*

Tool	Source Described in	Studies Using Tool
	RELATIONSHIP AND FAMILY TOOLS (Continued)	
Marital Satisfaction Scale: Forty-eight-item scale	Roach, Frazier, & Bowden (1981)	Jordan (1987) Majewski (1986)
Kansas Marital Satisfaction Scale: Three-item satisfaction scale	Schumm, Scanlon, Crow, Green, & Buckler (1983)	Saunders & Robins (1987)
Marital Relationship Scale: Scale for feelings, attitudes, and behaviors during pregnancy	Wapner (1976)	Cranley (1981) Weaver & Cranley (1983)
Braiker & Kelly Scale: Scale to assess conflict, ambivalence, love, and communication	Braiker & Kelley (1979)	Saunders & Robins (1987)
Family Solidarity Scale: Nineteen-item scale of family solidarity	White & Dawson (1981)	White & Dawson (1981)
Feetham Family Functioning Survey: Twenty-one-item scale of family relationships	Roberts & Feetham (1982)	Mercer et al. (1988a) Barnard et al. (1987) Ferketich & Mercer (1989) Mercer et al (1988b)
Family Dynamics Measure: Six-subscale tool for holistic family assessment	Lasky et al. (1985)	Brackbill, White, Wilson & Kitch (1990)
Focused Interview and Observational Field Schedules: Tool focused on grandmother functions	Flaherty et al. (1987)	Flaherty et al. (1987)

*Because social support and social competence are closely linked, several tools used in parent-infant nursing research to measure competence are included.

Further, because family relationships can be a major source of social support or conflict to parents, Table 5-3 also includes several tools that have been used to study marital and family relationships in nursing studies. Finally, if studies using these tools with other clinical populations were found, they also are included for comparative purposes.

SUMMARY OF RESEARCH

SCOPE OF SOCIAL SUPPORT RESEARCH

Studies of social support during pregnancy and parenting were important in the early development of the field of social support research (e.g., Nuckolls, Cassel, and Kaplan, 1972; Gottlieb, 1978). Parent-infant nursing research has added to the vast literature on social support by describing (1) types and sources of support used by parents, (2) dimensionality of social support during pregnancy, (3) differences in social support associated with subpopulations, and (4) relationships between social support variables and many health-related and parenting variables (Table 5-4).

Nurses have also examined family relationships—a key source of support—during pregnancy and early parenting. Finally, nurses have conducted interventions in which support served as a key variable. In those interventions support has been treated either as an independent variable or as an outcome of intervention. (*Note:* Research on family relationships during pregnancy that emphasizes a role attainment paradigm is located in Chapter 11, on the antepartal period.)

DESCRIPTIVE RESEARCH

Types and Sources of Support

Brown (1987b) conducted a survey of 313 expectant couples to determine how important specific types of supportive behaviors were during pregnancy. Both mothers and fathers rated emotionally supportive behaviors highest in importance. Lowest in importance were behaviors related to information and advice. One area in which men differed significantly from women was in the importance that men ascribed to having acceptance of their work schedules; women ascribed greater importance to reassurance about being attractive.

In a study of social support among mothers of handicapped young children, Brandt (1984a) identified sources of support. Mothers reported that the major sources of support for a variety of problems were their partners.

Kintz (1987) conducted a survey of 78 postpartum women to assess the helpfulness of various types of nursing support behaviors during labor.

Table 5–4
SOCIAL SUPPORT RESEARCH IN PREGNANCY AND EARLY PARENTING

DESCRIPTIVE

Sources and Types of Support
Brandt (1984a), mothers of handicapped young children
Brown (1987b), expectant couples
Cronenwett (1985b), new parents
Kintz (1987), women during labor
Majewski (1987), first-time new mothers
Mercer et al. (1984), teen mothers
Nikolaisen & Williams (1980), parents experiencing SIDS
Pridham (1984), new mothers

Dimensionality of Social Support
Brown (1986b), expectant parents

Social Support Patterns
Flaherty (1988), mothers of adolescent mothers
Flaherty et al. (1987), mothers of adolescent mothers
Mackey & Lock (1989), women's expectations of nurses during labor

Partner Status and Pregnancy
Tilden (1983a)

Differences in Social Support
Brown (1986a), fathers vs. mothers
Brown (1987a), employed vs. homemaking mothers
Capuzzi (1989), mothers of handicapped vs. nonhandicapped infants
Cronenwett (1985b), antepartum vs. postpartum parents
Jordan (1987), employed vs. nonemployed mothers
Kemp & Hatmaker (1989), low- vs. high-risk mothers
Mercer & Ferketich (1988), high- vs. low-risk mothers and fathers
Tilden (1984), single vs. partnered pregnant women

RELATIONSHIPS AMONG VARIABLES/PREDICTIVE MODELS

Negative Life Events as Predictors of Support
Brandt (1984a)

Social Network and Perceived Support
Cronenwett (1984)

Support, Attachment, and Other Parenting Variables
Capuzzi (1989)
Cranley (1984)
Cronenwett (1985a)
Dormire et al. (1989)
Koniak-Griffin (1988)
Mercer et al. (1984)

Table 5–4
(Continued)

RELATIONSHIPS AMONG VARIABLES/PREDICTIVE MODELS (Cont.)
Family and Marital Relationships Ellis & Hewat (1985) Porter & Demeuth (1979) Rankin et al. (1985) White & Dawson (1981)
Social Support and Health Practices Aaronson (1989) Albrecht & Rankin (1989) Coleman et al. (1989) Kaufman & Hall (1989) Stephens (1985)
Support in Relation to Stress Effects on Health Brown (1986c) Ferketich & Mercer (1989) Lenz et al. (1986) Mercer & Ferketich (1988) Norbeck & Anderson (1989a) Norbeck & Anderson (1989b) Norbeck & Tilden (1983) Nuckolls et al. (1972) Tilden (1983b)
Support in Relation to Stress Effects on Parenting/Children Bee, Hammond, Eyres, Barnard, & Snyder (1986) Brandt (1984b) Curry (1987) Mercer et al. (1988a)
INTERVENTION RELATED TO SOCIAL SUPPORT AND RELATIONSHIPS
Barnard, Snyder, & Spietz (1984), postnatal interventions Barnard et al. (1985), postnatal interventions; antenatal interventions Barnard, Booth, et al. (1988), postnatal interventions Barnard, Magyary, et al. (1988), antenatal interventions Booth et al. (1987), antenatal interventions Booth et al. (1989), antenatal interventions Cronenwett (1980), postpartum support groups Hodnett & Osborn (1989), continuous professional support in labor Krutsky (1985), siblings at birth Mitchell et al. (1988), antenatal interventions Moore (1983), Lamaze classes

Nursing support behaviors were categorized into the broad areas of affective, affirmative, and aid support. All behaviors in all three categories were rated as helpful during labor. Most helpful were the following: coaching, praising effort, friendly/personal care, accepting behavior, being respectful, and making the patient feel cared about.

Majewski (1987) interviewed first-time mothers to assess sources and types of support received. The majority of mothers reported their mates to be the most supportive persons in their transitions. Further, mothers reported that mates most frequently rendered support by providing physical assistance. Mothers who attended a parent support group were rated as having more difficult transitions than nonattenders.

Pridham (1984) investigated types of help that new mothers used to solve infant problems. The type of help varied with the nature of the problem encountered. Two of the most frequently reported sources of help were partners and books. Books were used particularly for problems related to growth and development.

Cronenwett (1985b) assessed parents for their perceptions of changes in types of support needed 5 months after the births of their children. The majority of mothers expressed an increased need for all four types of support assessed: emotional, instrumental, informational, and appraisal. Overall, fewer fathers than mothers expressed an increased need for the various types of support, but only the differences between mothers and fathers about an increased need for emotional and appraisal support were statistically significant.

Mercer, Hackley, and Bostrom (1984) examined sources of support for teenaged mothers from the immediate postpartal period to 1 year after childbirth. Mothers of teenagers were the persons most frequently identified as most helpful during the immediate postpartal period; at 1 year, the persons identified as most helpful shifted to the mates of teenaged mothers.

Finally, Nikolaisen and Williams (1980) conducted a retrospective survey of support among parents who had experienced sudden infant death syndrome. Sources of support rated as most helpful were, in descending order, mates, relatives, others, friends and nurses (tied), hospital, literature, and clergy. Rated as least helpful were relatives and others.

Dimensionality of Support in Pregnancy

To test whether social support is a unidimensional or multidimensional phenomenon during pregnancy, Brown (1986b) developed and tested the Support Behaviors Inventory (SBI). The SBI was constructed using House's (1981) conceptualization of social support. Discriminant validity of subscales and factor analysis of items were used to assess the number of dimensions inherent in the SBI. Both methods supported a unidimensional structure of social support among expectant parents.

Support Patterns

In a qualitative study of infant care functions of black grandmothers, the investigators (Flaherty, Facteau, & Garver, 1987; Flaherty, 1988) conducted focused interviews with black women whose daughters were adolescent mothers. Through analysis of interviews, seven types of grandmothers' caring functions were identified: managing, caretaking, coaching, assessing, nurturing, assigning, and patrolling.

Using interviews to gather information about women's expectations of nursing support during childbirth, Mackey and Lock (1989) identified different patterns of desired support. Women were about evenly divided into three levels of desired support: (1) limited nurse involvement, (2) moderate nurse involvement, and (3) extensive nurse involvement. The three levels of nurse involvement were described, respectively, as technical, observational, and participant. Nurse involvement was further described in terms of seven areas of nursing activity: presence, decision making, assistance, physical assessment, information, comfort, and support.

Partner Status and Pregnancy

To explore the psychological and social experience of pregnancy among single adult women, Tilden (1983a) interviewed 15 partnered and 15 single pregnant women. Both partnered and single women experienced concerns about psychosocial developmental tasks of pregnancy such as safe passage for self and baby. Areas of concern specific to single mothers included decision making, particularly related to continuing the pregnancy and becoming a single mother, disclosure of the pregnancy, seeking social support, and managing such future legal issues as the baby's last name.

Differences in Support

In a comparison of satisfaction with partner support among pregnant couples having their first child, expectant mothers and fathers did not differ significantly in their overall satisfaction with support (Brown, 1986a). Social support differences between expectant parents also were studied by Cronenwett (1984). Mothers and fathers did not differ in the social network variables of size of network, density, and mean frequency of contact. However, there were more men in fathers' networks and more women in mothers' networks.

In assessing changes in social network structure from antepartum to 8 months postpartum, Cronenwett (1985b) found that fathers' social networks shrank in size and increased in overlap with their wives' networks. In mothers' social networks, contacts shifted from coworkers to friends with preschool children.

In comparing employed and homemaking expectant mothers, Brown

(1987a) found that homemakers were less satisfied with nonspouse support and, further, valued support more than employed women did. Employed women specifically valued instrumental support—help with household tasks—to a greater extent than homemakers. In a comparison of homemaking and employed women who were giving birth to their second children, Jordan (1987) found employed mothers had more coworkers in their networks whereas homemakers had more kin. The two groups did not differ, however, in amount of perceived social support or marital satisfaction.

Comparing social support among high-risk expectant mothers and fathers, Mercer and Ferketich (1988) found no significant gender differences for size of social network, although expectant mothers did report greater received and perceived social support than fathers. Among low-risk expectant mothers and fathers, Mercer and Ferketich (1988) found no gender differences in perceived social support, but mothers reported greater social support networks and received more social support than fathers. Overall, expectant mothers reported their mothers, mates, female friends, and nurses as being in their networks more often than did fathers. In turn, expectant fathers reported fathers-in-law and male friends in their networks more frequently than did mothers (Mercer & Ferketich, 1988). In comparing social support levels of women with low- and high-risk pregnancies, those with high-risk pregnancies received greater support; among the mates, however, partners of high-risk mothers received less support than their low-risk counterparts (Mercer & Ferketich, 1988). In another study, Kemp and Hatmaker (1989) failed to find differences in social support between low- and high-risk expectant mothers.

Tilden (1984) examined partnered (n = 116) and single women (n = 25) in a study of psychosocial variables during pregnancy. Single pregnant women had lower tangible support than partnered women, but both groups had comparable levels of informational and emotional support. In addition, single women reported more negative life event stress and more state anxiety.

In a comparison of social support given mothers of handicapped (n = 15) and nonhandicapped infants (n = 21), Capuzzi (1989) found that mothers differed in prenatal social support. Postnatally, there were no differences in social support when infants were 1 and 6 months corrected age. At 12 months, however, mothers of handicapped infants reported less social support in the form of aid than did mothers of nonhandicapped infants.

RELATIONAL/PREDICTIVE RESEARCH

Negative Life Events as Predictors of Support

In a study of 91 mothers of developmentally delayed children 6 months to 3 years old, Brandt (1984a) examined the relation of negative life events to social support. Of three measures of social support, two—perceived support and average satisfaction with support obtained—were related to negative life events. The third, number of resources, was not related to negative life events.

Social Network and Perceived Support

To explore the relation between social network and perceived social support, Cronenwett (1984) studied 54 expectant couples. After measuring network and perceived support variables, eight regression analyses were carried out by using network variables to predict perceived social support. Of network variables, size most consistently served as a predictor of support in five of eight regressions.

Support, Attachment, and Other Parenting Variables

Several investigations examined the relation of social support to attachment, role attainment, and other parenting variables. (For other studies of attachment and role attainment, see Chapters 13 and 14.) Cranley (1984) conducted two studies about the relationship between social support and parents' prenatal attachment to their fetuses. In the first study (N = 30), social support was positively related to expectant mothers' fetal attachment. The second study, which included 326 expectant couples, examined the relationship between marital adjustment and parental-fetal attachment. As predicted, marital adjustment was significantly related to fetal attachment among both mothers and fathers.

In assessing the relations between antepartal social networks and postnatal responses to parenthood, Cronenwett (1985a) followed 50 expectant couples from pregnancy to 6 weeks after childbirth. Network or support variables predicted two of seven responses to parenthood for both mothers and fathers: confidence in ability to cope with parenting and infant care and satisfaction with parenting and infant care. For both mothers and fathers, emotional support best predicted satisfaction with parenting and infant care.

Mercer et al. (1984) studied the relation of social support to maternal role attainment in 66 teenaged mothers at the immediate postpartal period and at 1, 4, 8, and 12 months after childbirth. In the immediate postpartal period, there was only one significant correlation between social support and role attainment measures. At 1 month, physical, emotional, and informational support were significantly correlated with one or more role attainment measures. At 4 months, only physical support correlated significantly with role attainment, and at 8 months there were no significant correlations between support and role attainment. Finally, at 1 year, only emotional support correlated significantly with role attainment measures.

In another study of adolescents, Koniak-Griffin (1988) examined social support and other variables as they were related to prenatal fetal attachment. Neither total social support nor its components were significantly related to adolescents' attachment to their fetuses. Taken together in multiple regression analysis, however, four variables were significant predictors of fetal attachment: total functional support, total network, whether pregnancy was planned, and whether mothers planned to keep their babies.

Dormire, Strauss, and Clarke (1989) examined the relation of social support to parent-infant synchrony and parenting stress in 18 adolescent mothers of term, healthy infants. Based on observations at 1 month postpartum, social support was significantly related to parent-infant synchrony. Overall parenting stress was not related to either overall parent-infant synchrony or overall social support. Several relations at the level of subscales were found.

Family and Marital Relationships

Rankin, Campbell, and Soeken (1985) examined instrumental social support (e.g., child care) and the marital relationship among first-time parents. Mothers' prenatal estimates of postnatal assistance with child care and household tasks exceeded that actually received. For mothers, but not for fathers, support with child care and household tasks was related to satisfaction with changes in the marital relationship.

Ellis and Hewat (1985) conducted a survey of postpartal women to assess mothers' perceptions of spousal relationships following birth. The majority reported that changes in their relationships were either positive or neutral. However, sexual interest declined more for women than for their partners. Tiredness was identified by women as a factor that contributed to changes in sexual interest. Of mothers who were breast-feeding, most reported no effect of breast feeding on sexual relations.

To assess the relation between marital adjustment and the psychological acceptance of pregnancy, Porter and Demeuth (1979) surveyed 25 expectant couples. As expected, for both mothers and fathers, greater marital adjustment was associated with greater pregnancy acceptance.

White and Dawson (1981) studied the impact of at-risk infants on family solidarity. Infants were of low, moderate, and high risk. Measurements of family solidarity and other variables were taken when infants were 3 and 6 months old. A family solidarity scale was developed and covered the areas of togetherness, communication, team performance, and ritual. Because the majority of parents reported high family closeness and satisfaction, most analyses of family solidarity were focused on discrete items. For example, as risk status increased, parents went out less and ate together at home more. Also, parents of high-risk infants reported more sexual dissatisfaction than other parents. Of note, parental depression was associated with communication items on the family solidarity scale.

Social Support and Health Practices

Several studies examined relations between social support and health behaviors. (For other studies of health behaviors, see Chapter 8.) Albrecht and Rankin (1989) examined the relations between anxiety, health behaviors (smoking, alcohol intake, nutrition, and breast self-examination), and support systems in 47 low-risk pregnant women. Data were collected via questionnaire after 6 to 30 weeks of gestation. Both state and trait anxiety were negatively related to social support. In examining relations to specific health behaviors, higher alcohol intake was related to lower social support. In addition, smoking was related to higher alcohol intake, but smoking was not related to trait or state anxiety.

Stephens (1985) examined the relations of general expressive support, pregnancy-specific expressive support, and instrumental support to alcohol consumption during pregnancy. There were 311 pregnant women in the final sample. Two support measures, general expressive and pregnancy-specific, predicted prepregnancy alcohol consumption. By contrast, none of the three support measures predicted alcohol consumption during actual pregnancy.

In an additional study of changes in alcohol consumption and social support during pregnancy, Coleman, Ryan, and Williamson (1989) surveyed 153 women in the third trimester. Three measures of support were used: general, instrumental, and pregnancy-specific. General and instrumental support had low but significant correlations with decreased alcohol consumption. Oddly, pregnancy-specific support was correlated with consumption but not in the expected direction; that is, the greater the support, the greater the increase in use.

In a related study, Aaronson (1989) examined the relations between various aspects of social support and abstaining from alcohol, cigarettes, and caffeine during pregnancy. In Aaronson's survey of 529 women, social support was assessed by a general measure of perceived support, three measures of perceived support specific to the three abstentions, and three measures of received support specific to the three abstentions. Each health practice was predicted at statistically significant levels by its respective specific perceived and received social support measures. General social support did not predict any of the three health practices during pregnancy.

Kaufman and Hall (1989) examined the relations of social network to (1) the decision to breast-feed and (2) the duration of breast feeding among mothers of preterm infants. The 125 participating mothers completed scales measuring wishes of seven social referents related to breast feeding and also responded to a measure of social network support. Mothers who chose to breast-feed were more influenced by referents' views about breast feeding than those bottle feeding. Of referents, the baby's father was most influential. Of 88 breast-feeding mothers, 62 abandoned breast feeding or hand expression of milk over a period of months. As the number of persons providing support for breast feeding increased, so did the mothers' duration of breast feeding.

Direct and Stress-Buffering Effects of Social Support

The capacity of social support to buffer (i.e., protect) people from the harmful effects of stress has been of great interest to investigators in nursing and other fields. (See Chapter 2 for a discussion of social support as a stress buffer.) In nursing studies of stress, investigators have tested the direct and buffering effects of social support on mental health, physical health, family functioning, parenting, and child development. Because of their complexity and scope, these studies are summarized in Table 5–5. In several of the 13 studies presented in Table 5–5, difficulties were encountered in accounting for a substantial amount of variance in outcome measures when testing the originally proposed theoretical models (e.g., Curry, 1987; Mercer & Ferketich, 1988; and Mercer, Ferketich, DeJoseph, May, and Sollid, 1988a). In another study, model testing was hampered by problems of multicollinearity (Brandt, 1984b). In addition, in about one-half of the studies the stress-buffering hypothesis (interaction of stress and social support) was not examined within the entire sample (e.g., Bee et al., 1986; Curry, 1987). With these limitations in mind, 11 of 13 studies found at least some evidence of a relationship between social support, either as a direct effect or as a buffering effect, and health status or other outcomes. In particular, social support demonstrated direct effects on emotional health among low-risk women (Tilden, 1983b; Norbeck & Tilden, 1983; Norbeck & Anderson, 1989a; Mercer & Ferketich, 1988).

INTERVENTION RESEARCH

Interventions Related to Childbirth

Three interventions related to childbirth are reported here. In two, the impact of interventions on family outcome variables was examined, and in one support was used as an intervention variable.

Krutsky (1985) examined the impact of sibling presence at birth on 16 couples. Parents primarily chose to have siblings present to benefit the siblings' development and to enhance family sharing. No comparison group was included. The main effect of sibling presence as reported by both mothers and fathers was that it added to family unity. All 32 parents reported they would choose to have siblings present for any future births.

Table 5–5
PARENT-INFANT NURSING STUDIES OF STRESS/LIFE EVENTS, SOCIAL SUPPORT, AND PARENT/INFANT OUTCOMES

		SOCIAL SUPPORT		
Study	**Sample**	**Direct Effect Found?**	**Buffer/Interaction Effect Found?**	**Parent/Infant Outcomes**
Bee et al. (1986)	From a longitudinal sample of 193 mother-infant pairs, 177 were in 1-y and 169 in 4-y follow-up	Not reported for overall sample	Not reported for overall sample	Home environment at 1 y
		Not reported for overall sample	Not reported for overall sample; for low-support mothers, two of three outcomes were related to life change events	Child development: IQ, receptive language, behavior problems
Brandt (1984b)	Ninety-one mothers of children with developmental delays, aged 7–39 mo	No, for overall sample regression analysis	Trend in overall sample regression analysis	Maternal discipline
		Yes, for mothers with high-acute stress		Maternal discipline
		Yes, for mothers with high-chronic stress		Maternal discipline
		No, for mothers with low-acute stress		Maternal discipline
		No for mothers with low-chronic stress		Maternal discipline

Table 5–5
PARENT-INFANT NURSING STUDIES OF STRESS/LIFE EVENTS, SOCIAL SUPPORT, AND PARENT/INFANT OUTCOMES *(Continued)*

		SOCIAL SUPPORT		
Study	**Sample**	**Direct Effect Found?**	**Buffer/Interaction Effect Found?**	**Parent/Infant Outcomes**
Brown (1986c)	Three hundred thirteen expectant couples	Yes, for expectant fathers	Not tested	Index of good and ill health
		Yes for expectant mothers	Not tested	Index of good and ill health
Curry (1987)	Seventy-five women hospitalized for high-risk pregnancies	No, for four of four maternal outcomes	Not tested	Maternal outcomes: relationship with mother; acceptance of pregnancy; identification with motherhood; maternal-fetal attachment
Ferketich & Mercer (1989)	One hundred forty-seven fathers (pregnancy to 8 mo postpartum)	No, but some evidence of indirect effects in causal modeling	Not tested	Perceived health status
Lenz et al. (1986)	One hundred fifty-five mothers of 6 mo old infants	Yes, for three of five support variables	No	Number of illnesses
Mercer & Ferketich (1988)	One hundred fifty-three high-risk pregnant women and 75 mates; 218 low-risk pregnant women and 147 mates	No, for three of three measures for high-risk women	Not tested	Anxiety

		Yes, for one of three measures for low-risk women	Not tested	Anxiety
		Yes, for one of three measures for mates of high-risk women	Not tested	Anxiety
		Yes, for one of three measures for mates of low-risk women	Not tested	Anxiety
		No, for three of three measures for high-risk women	Not tested	Depression
		Yes, for one of three measures for low-risk women	Not tested	Depression
		Yes, for one of three measures for mates of high-risk women	Not tested	Depression
		No, for three of three measures for mates of low-risk women	Not tested	Depression
Mercer et al. (1988a)	Same as above sample	No, for high-risk women	Not tested	Family functioning
		Yes, for mates of high-risk women	Not tested	Family functioning
		Yes, for low-risk women	Not tested	Family functioning

Table 5–5
PARENT-INFANT NURSING STUDIES OF STRESS/LIFE EVENTS, SOCIAL SUPPORT, AND PARENT/INFANT OUTCOMES *(Continued)*

		SOCIAL SUPPORT		
Study	**Sample**	**Direct Effect Found?**	**Buffer/Interaction Effect Found?**	**Parent/Infant Outcomes**
		Yes, for mates of low-risk women	Not tested	Family functioning
Norbeck & Anderson (1989a)	Two hundred sixty-one low-risk pregnant women during 2nd trimester; 190 again at 3rd trimester	Yes, in two of three regressions	Yes, in two of three regressions	State anxiety
Norbeck & Anderson (1989b)	Triethnic sample of 208 low-income, low-risk pregnant women (59 black, 73 white, 76 Hispanic)	No, for black women	No, for black women	Birth weight
		No, for white women	No, for white women	Birth weight
		No, for Hispanic women	No, for Hispanic women	Birth weight
		Yes, partner support for black women	No, for black women	Gestational age
		No, for white women	No, for white women	Gestational age
		No, for Hispanic women	No, for Hispanic women	Gestational age
		Yes, partner and mother support for black women	No, for black women	Total gestational complications

		Yes, mother and friend support for black women (friend support related opposite of predicted direction)	No, for black women	Total labor complications
		No, for black women	No, for black women	Total infant complications
		Yes, for mother support for black women	No, for black women	Long labor
		Yes, for mother support for black women	No, for black women	Caesarean section
		No, for white women	No, for white women	Total gestational complications
		No, for white women	No, for white women	Total labor complications
		Yes, for mother support for white women (mother support related in opposite of predicted direction)	Yes, for white women (opposite of predicted direction)	Long labor
		No, for white women	Yes, for white women (opposite predicted direction)	Caesarean section
Norbeck & Tilden (1983)	One hundred seventeen low-risk pregnant women	Yes, for one of two social support measures	No	Emotional disequilibrium

Table 5–5
PARENT-INFANT NURSING STUDIES OF STRESS/LIFE EVENTS, SOCIAL SUPPORT, AND PARENT/INFANT OUTCOMES ***(Continued)***

		SOCIAL SUPPORT		
Study	**Sample**	**Direct Effect Found?**	**Buffer/Interaction Effect Found?**	**Parent/Infant Outcomes**
		No, in seven of seven analyses	Yes, in three of seven analyses	Pregnancy complications
Nuckolls et al (1972)	One hundred seventy primigravidas married to enlisted men	No	Yes	Pregnancy/neonatal complications
Tilden (1983b)	One hundred forty-one low-risk pregnant women	Yes	No	Emotional disequilibrium

Moore (1983) compared the impact of two methods of childbirth education (Lamaze and hospital-taught classes) on the marital relationship. Couples (N = 105) selecting either form of childbirth preparation completed a marital conflict scale at two prenatal testings and one postpartal testing. Only one significant group difference was found for marital conflict: Fathers in the Lamaze group had lower conflict at the second prenatal testing. In addition, Lamaze mothers had longer labors, used less medication, and more often chose rooming-in than did hospital-taught mothers. Overall, parents, regardless of group, experienced progressively less interpersonal conflict from the first prenatal to the postpartal testing.

Hodnett and Osborn (1989) conducted a stratefied (general prenatal vs. Lamaze classes), randomized (control vs. experimental) trial of continuous professional support during labor. Subjects were 103 low-risk women with vaginal births who were accompanied by husbands/partners during labor. The experimental intervention consisted of professional support (emotional, informational, tangible, and advocacy) provided by lay midwives and midwives in training. They met with parents prenatally to initiate relationships and were present with them from the onset of labor at home to 1 hour after delivery in the hospital. Comparable prenatal contact occurred for the control group. Follow-up interviews were conducted by a person blind to group assignment. Women selecting general versus Lamaze classes differed prenatally on expected control during childbirth and commitment to an unmedicated birth. There were no prenatal significant differences between groups based on control versus experimental assignment.

Compared to women in the control group, women in the experimental group used analgesia or anesthesia for labor and birth less frequently, had more intact perineums, and had more oxytocics. No significant differences in any indicators of length of labor were found. Type of classes or treatment did not have a significant main effect on postpartal perceptions of control in labor. In regression analysis, prenatal expectations for control in labor and a classification variable (experimental group and had no medication) accounted for 30 percent of the variance in experienced control in labor.

Intervention during the Postpartal Period

Cronenwett (1980) conducted a descriptive analysis of postpartum support groups offered to families taking Lamaze childbirth classes. No comparisons with those not attending were conducted. Current and former group participants were surveyed with a 73 percent response rate. All were married and white. Sixty percent began participation in the support groups when their infants were 2 to 3 months old. Groups were evenly divided as to whether babies were present during meetings. None of the groups chose to include husbands. The initial reason most often given for joining the group was a wish to talk with others experiencing the same kind of situation. In rating the importance of topics covered in groups, negative feelings about parenting was most important while babies were under 6 months old. After 6 months, issues related to working outside the home were most important. Length of time in the groups was associated with employment; the employed mothers often continued in support groups for a year or more (cf. L. Wandersman, A. Wandersman, & Kahn, 1980).

Programmatic Research on Supportive Interventions

Because the research of Barnard and associates on supportive nursing interventions represents a program of research (Barnard et al., 1985), individual research articles and chapters are presented together to give a coherent review of the program. First, the Newborn Nursing Models Project, a postnatal set of interventions, will be presented (Barnard, Snyder, & Spietz, 1984; Barnard et al., 1985; Barnard, Booth, Mitchell, & Telzrow, 1988). Second, the Clinical Nursing Models Project, a set of two interventions begun during pregnancy will be presented (Barnard et al., 1985; Barnard et al., 1988; Booth, Barnard, Mitchell, & Spieker, 1987; Booth, Mitchell, Barnard & Spieker, 1989; Mitchell, Magyary, Barnard, Sumner, & Booth, 1988).

The Newborn Nursing Models project was an experimental field test of three alternative approaches to intervention, assigned at random, to families during the postnatal period (Barnard, Booth, et al., 1988). Selection criteria for participation in the project included nonoptimal infant (prematurity, low birth weight, perinatal complications) and parent characteristics (lower social class, lower educational level). Infant characteristics emphasized biological risk while those of parents emphasized social risk (Barnard et al., 1984). Interventions were conducted with infants and parents from birth to 3 months in the home setting (Barnard et al., 1984).

Three interventions were tested in the Newborn Nursing Models Project: Nursing Parent and Child Environment (NPACE), Nursing Support Infant Bio-Behavioral (NSIBB), and Nursing Standard Approach to Care (NSTAC). NPACE provided individualized, supportive care based on systematic assessment of parents and infants. Approximately 15 different assessment tools covering parent, infant, and environment were incorporated into the intervention. They included questionnaires, interviews, infant behavioral records kept by mothers, and observations of mothers and infants. Based on assessments, individualized care was provided. Establishing a caring relationship was a significant component of the NPACE intervention. NSIBB was a more standardized intervention in which nurses taught parenting skills and knowledge of infant development. Mothers learned about infant cues, sleep-wake patterns, massage, infant exercise, and related issues. More narrowly focused than NPACE, NSIBB emphasized infant behaviors and interaction between parent and infant. The third intervention, NSTAC, consisted of general support services offered by the local health department. NSTAC emphasized assessment of health status, client-identified problems, and environmental resources (Barnard et al., 1984; Barnard et al., 1985; Barnard, Booth, et al., 1988). On average, the three interventions comprised 8, 5, and 1 hours per case, respectively (Barnard, Booth, et al., 1988). (For detailed descriptions of the goals of each intervention, see Barnard et al., 1985, pp. 261–266.)

The sample was 185 mothers and their infants from the caseload of the Seattle–King County Health Department. Fifty percent were first-time mothers, 38 percent were without partners/husbands, and 42 percent had less than 12 years of formal education. Gestational age of infants ranged from 34 to 41.5 weeks (Barnard, Booth, et al., 1988).

At 3, 10, and 24 months, infants were tested on the Bayley Infant Scales, and observations were made of parent-infant interaction and home stimulation (Barnard, Booth, et al., 1988). No significant differences among intervention groups were found for infant development, parent-infant interaction, or home stimulation. To determine if the three interventions improved interaction or development over what would be expected, study outcomes were compared with normative data and findings from nonintervention studies. First, two-way ANOVA showed a significant time effect indicating a significant decline in mental development from 3 to 24 months. Next, mental development for Newborn Models infants was compared to extant data from a nonintervention sample of infants with low-education mothers. The Newborn Models infants had significantly lower mental development at 10 and 24 months than the comparison group (Barnard, Booth, et al., 1988).

For parent-infant interaction, the three Newborn Models groups showed a significant time effect, with significant increases occurring from 3 to 24 months. Compared again to extant data for a nonintervention group, Newborn Models mothers were equivalent with the comparison group on interaction at 3 months, dropped below them at 10 months, and surpassed them at 24 months. By contrast, Newborn Models infants were lower in interaction than the comparison group at 3 months and 10 months but were equivalent to them by 24 months. Finally, for home stimulation, Newborn Models families were significantly lower at 3 months than the comparison group, equivalent to them at 10 months, and surpassed them by 24 months. In conclusion, the three interventions as a whole appeared to have positive effects on the parent-child relationship over time but did not improve infants' mental development (Barnard, Booth, et al., 1988). The investigators explained these discrepant findings by proposing "that the interventions were not powerful enough to produce the amount of improvement in the mothers necessary to foster concomitant improvement in the child" (Barnard, Booth, et al., 1988, p. 76).

Based on the findings of the Newborn Nursing Models Project, Barnard et al. (1985) concluded that the "newborn period was a difficult time in which to establish a relationship with the mother and therefore a poor choice of time to begin intervention with a socially at-risk parent"

(p. 255). Thus, in the Clinical Nursing Models Project, the period of intervention was moved to the prenatal period and extended through the infant's first birthday. The earlier experience with the deficit or problematic social relationships of at-risk mothers also led to a greater emphasis on a therapeutic relationship component in the Clinical Nursing Models Project (Barnard et al., 1985).

The Clinical Nursing Models Project was a field experiment in which two alternative models for providing nursing services in the home were tested. Mothers were randomly assigned to one of the two intervention conditions. Initiated at midpregnancy, the intervention lasted through the end of the infant's first year; data collection on mothers and infants continued until children were 3 years old (Mitchell et al., 1988). An extensive battery of maternal, infant, environmental, and related qualities was assessed during midpregnancy through the child's third year. Data collectors were blind to group assignments of families.

The two interventions, the Mental Health Model (MH) and the Information and Resource Model (IR), were designed for high-risk families during the prenatal and infancy periods. Both programs were delivered along with companion prenatal and infant health care services, including nutritional counseling. Home visiting was the setting for providing the interventions. A consistent intervenor was assigned to each family during the course of the intervention. Each intervention was guided by written protocols and specific objectives for the different phases of the intervention (from prenatal to infancy) (Mitchell et al., 1988).

The IR group served as the comparison group receiving traditional public health nursing care. This approach emphasized providing information, particularly about promoting and maintaining physical health of mother and infant, and making referrals to community agencies and resources for needed services (Mitchell et al., 1988).

By contrast, the MH group emphasized a therapeutic relationship between client and nurse. This model thus emphasized process, focusing on family problems and developmental issues. Although physical health was covered in the MH model, its aim was to focus more intently on psychosocial aspects of health and maternal competence. Brammer's (1973) view of the helping relationship partially guided the development of the nurse-client relationship. Because many clients had deficits in social interaction, they received attention in order to build the therapeutic relationship. In addition, nurse-intervenors in the MH condition had biweekly consultation with a clinical psychologist to discuss client situations (Mitchell et al., 1988). For more detailed descriptions of the MH and IR intervention protocols, see Mitchell et al. (1988) and Barnard, Magyary, et al. (1988).

Mothers were recruited into the study through the local health department. They had one or more social risk factors, such as history of child abuse or neglect with their children, addiction, psychiatric problems, low income, or education. Mothers' mean age was 21 years; 92 percent were white and 27 percent were married and living with spouses. Most infants were born at term (Booth et al., 1987).

In all, 68 mothers participated in the MH intervention and 79 in the IR intervention. Of these, 95 (65 percent) remained in the study at the completion of the intervention phase. In comparing those remaining at 1 year with dropouts, there were no differences on demographic factors; dropouts were, however, less socially competent based on intake assessments. The remaining members of the two intervention groups did not differ on demographic or initial social competence measures (Barnard, Magyary, et al., 1988).

At 1 year, the MH and IR mothers did not differ on social skills or mother-infant interaction (Booth et al., 1989). MH mothers had less depression at 1 and 2 years than IR mothers. MH mothers also perceived they had more support, had more positive teaching interactions, and provided more positive home stimulation to infants than IR mothers. In contrast, children of MH and IR mothers had few differences. For example, no differences were found on 13-month security of attachment or 2-year Bayley motor or mental scores. Overall, only 45 percent of children were securely attached, which was considerably lower than expected (Barnard, Magyary, et al., 1988).

To further examine intervention effects, MH and IR families were partitioned according to various characteristics at entry into the project. Statistical analyses showed that families with lower-IQ mothers benefited more from the MH intervention than those with lower-IQ mothers in the IR intervention: Children of lower-IQ-MH mothers were more often securely attached; mother-child interaction was more positive at 2 years; home stimulation was more positive; Bayley motor scores were higher; and stability of attachment was greater. In turn, families with higher-IQ mothers benefited more from the IR intervention: Infants of higher-IQ IR mothers were more often securely attached and had greater stability of attachment from 13 to 20 months than infants with higher-IQ mothers in the MH intervention (Barnard, Magyary, et al., 1988). For further analyses of the process aspects of the interventions and their relationship to maternal and infant variables, see Booth et al. (1987, 1989).

FUTURE RESEARCH DIRECTIONS

In the span of less than 10 years, social support has become a key construct considered in parent-infant nursing research. Nurses' interest in support was no doubt influenced by Nuckolls's et al. (1972) finding of the stress-buffering effects of social support among pregnant women. The intensity of research on social support in the last decade stimulated extensive tool development and critical reviews of the concept. Those reviews occurred in both nursing and other fields (Barrera, 1986; Dimond & Jones,

1983; Heitzmann & Kaplan, 1988; House & Kahn, 1985; Payne & Jones, 1987; Roberts, 1988; Rock et al., 1984; Stewart, 1989; Tilden, 1985).

Still, issues of conceptualization and measurement remain important. To give coherence to findings from future research, investigators should give special attention to several matters in selecting measures of social support. Tools used in research should match the theoretical definitions of support. Although social support may take many forms, not all will be equally relevant to specific stressors or phenomena under study. Future investigators need to do careful theoretic work to define the elements of social support particularly pertinent in specific investigations before selecting research instruments (Barrera, 1986). Thus, to continue to advance knowledge, investigators of social support can no longer arbitrarily select a social support tool. Instead, they should carefully consider (1) why the component of support they select to measure is particularly suited to their study and (2) how it operates in influencing parent-infant phenomena. Indeed, several recent studies have demonstrated this clarity of approach in instrument selection (e.g., Aaronson, 1989).

Reliability and validity should be given equal emphasis in tool selection. Low reliability leads to attenuated correlations among measures. In that regard, Heitzmann and Kaplan (1988) have simulated the effect of measurement error on the correlation of four social support tools with five health indicators. As expected, correlations diminished as reliability decreased. Furthermore, demonstrated construct validity is essential to make inferences from social support data to hypotheses about support. Evidence for construct validity should include both convergent evidence and discriminant evidence (Heitzmann & Kaplan, 1988).

Although there are a number of tools to measure parents' social network and perceived support, Tilden (1985) has noted the dearth of social support tools to measure reciprocity of social support (giving *and* receiving) and the cost of support (negative vs. positive support). Further instrument development is therefore needed to capture the full gamut of the social support phenomenon.

In a related vein, compared to knowledge about the benefits of social support, less is known about circumstances in which social support is harmful. For example, in their review of the social support literature, House and Kahn (1985, p. 93) suggest that women may serve as support providers more often than men. Because women are more responsive to events in the lives of others than men, women may disproportionately experience the negative costs of support giving compared to men (Belle, 1982). Research is needed to determine to what extent this may be true of pregnant women, new mothers, and their partners.

Some past parent-infant nursing studies have contained serious methodological problems. Future investigators doing correlational studies should be vigilant about problems of (1) method variance, including multicollinearity of similar measures and (2) design limitations. Instruments measuring different concepts may share methods and have similar items. For example, if social support is used to predict mental health, care should be taken to select measures of social support that are unconfounded by symptoms (B. S. Dohrenwend, B. P. Dohrenwend, Dodson, and Shrout, 1984; Lazarus, DeLongis, Folkman, & Gruen, 1985). Hobfoll (1986) has also cautioned investigators about the pitfalls of confounding life events and social support. Further, the issue of direction of influence is inherent in all one-panel correlational studies of social support (Dooley, 1985). Longitudinal studies are preferred. Even they pose problems of inference, however, when subject attrition occurs.

To balance the quality of design with the cost of future research, new approaches to social support research may be needed. Multiple sources of funding may be needed to ensure that conclusions are based on high-quality data. Coordination of social support research with other research programs in institutions may also prove useful.

Because the largest number of studies of social support have been descriptive or predictive in nature, support-based nursing interventions are less abundant. The program of research initiated by Barnard and associates at the University of Washington is a model for future investigators interested in supportive interventions for parents and infants. Particularly noteworthy in that research is the cumulative building of knowledge that spans specific projects. Additional programmatic research in supportive nursing interventions are needed.

REFERENCES

Aaronson, L. S. (1989). Perceived and received support: Effects on health behavior during pregnancy. *Nursing Research, 38,* 4–9.

Albrecht, S. A., & Rankin, M. (1989). Anxiety levels, health behaviors, and support systems of pregnant women. *Maternal-Child Nursing Journal, 18,* 49–60.

Barnard, K. E., Booth, C. L., Mitchell, S. K., & Telzrow, R. W. (1988). Newborn nursing models: A test of early intervention to high-risk infants and families. In E. D. Hibbs (Ed.), *Children and families: Studies in prevention and intervention* (pp. 63–81). Madison, CT: International Universities Press.

Barnard, K. E., Hammond, M., Mitchell, S. K., Booth, C. L., Spietz, A., Snyder, C., & Elsas, T. (1985). Caring for high-risk infants and their families. In M. Green (Ed.), *The psychosocial aspects of the family* (pp. 245–266). Lexington, MA: Heath.

Barnard, K. E., Hammond, M. A., Sumner, G. A., Kang, R., Johnson-Crowley, N., Snyder, C., Spietz, A., Blackburn, S., Brandt, P., & Magyary, D. (1987). Helping parents with preterm infants: Field test of a protocol. *Early Child Development and Care, 27,* 255–290.

Barnard, K. E., Magyary, D., Sumner, G., Booth, C. L., Mitchell, S. K., & Spieker, S. (1988). Prevention of parenting alterations for women with low social support. *Psychiatry, 51*(3), 248–253.

Barnard, K. E., Snyder, C., & Spietz, A. (1984). Supportive measures for high-risk infants and families. In K. E. Barnard, P. A. Brandt, B. S. Raff, & P. Carroll (Eds.), *Social support and families of vulnerable in-*

fants. White Plains, NY: March of Dimes Birth Defects Foundation. *Birth Defects, Original Article Series, 20*(5), 291–315.

Barrera, M. (1981). Social support in the adjustment of pregnant adolescents. In B. H. Gottlieb (Ed.), *Social networks and social support* (pp. 69–96). Beverly Hills, CA: Sage.

Barrera, M. (1986). Distinctions between social support concepts, measures, and models. *American Journal of Community Psychology, 14,* 413–445.

Bee, H. L., Hammond, M. A., Eyres, S. J., Barnard, K. E., & Snyder, C. (1986). The impact of parental life change on the early development of children. *Research in Nursing & Health, 9,* 65–74.

Belle, D. (1982). The stress of caring: Women as providers of social support. In L. Goldberger & S. Breznitz (Eds.), *Handbook of stress* (pp. 496–505). New York: Free Press.

Booth, C. L., Barnard, K. E., Mitchell, S. K., & Spieker, S. J. (1987). Successful intervention with multi-problem mothers: Effects on the mother-infant relationship. *Infant Mental Health Journal, 8,* 288–306.

Booth, C. L., Mitchell, S. K., Barnard, K. E., & Spieker, S. J. (1989). Development of maternal social skills in multiproblem families: Effects on the mother-child relationship. *Developmental Psychology, 25,* 403–412.

Brackbill, Y., White, M., Wilson, M., & Kitch, D. (1990). Family dynamics as predictors of infant disposition. *Infant Mental Health Journal, 11,* 113–126.

Braiker, H. B., & Kelley, H. H. (1979). Conflict in the development of close relationships. In R. L. Burgess & T. L. Huston (Eds.), *Social exchange in developing relationships* (pp. 135–168). New York: Academic Press.

Brammer, L. M. (1973). *The helping relationship: Process and skills.* Englewood Cliffs, NJ: Prentice-Hall.

Brandt, P. A. (1984a). Social support and negative life events of mothers with developmentally delayed children. In K. E. Barnard, P. A. Brandt, B. S. Raff, & P. Carroll (Eds.), *Social support and families of vulnerable infants.* White Plains, NY: March of Dimes Birth Defects Foundation. *Birth Defects, Original Article Series, 20*(5), 205–223.

Brandt, P. A. (1984b). Stress-buffering effects of social support on maternal discipline. *Nursing Research, 33,* 229–234.

Brandt, P. A., & Weinert, C. (1981). The PRQ—A social support system. *Nursing Research, 30,* 277–280.

Brown, M. A. (1986a). Marital support during pregnancy. *Journal of Obstetric, Gynecologic, and Neonatal Nursing, 15,* 475–483.

Brown, M. A. (1986b). Social support during pregnancy: A unidimensional or multidimensional construct? *Nursing Research, 35,* 4–9.

Brown, M. A. (1986c). Social support, stress, and health: A comparison of expectant mothers and fathers. *Nursing Research, 35,* 72–76.

Brown, M. A. (1987a). Employment during pregnancy: Influences on women's health and social support. *Health Care for Women International, 8*(2-3), 151–167.

Brown, M. A. (1987b). How fathers and mothers perceive prenatal support. *MCN, The American Journal of Maternal/Child Nursing, 12,* 414–418.

Capuzzi, C. (1989). Maternal attachment to handicapped infants and the relationship to social support. *Research in Nursing and Health, 12,* 161–167.

Coleman, M., Ryan, R., & Williamson, J. (1989). Social support and the alcohol consumption patterns of pregnant women. *Applied Nursing Research,* 2, 154–160.

Cranley, M. S. (1981). Roots of attachment: The relationship of parents with their unborn. In R. P. Lederman, B. S. Raff, & P. Carroll (Eds.), *Perinatal parental behavior: Nursing research and implications for newborn health.* New York: Alan R. Liss for the March of Dimes Birth Defects Foundation. *Birth Defects, Original Article Series, 17*(6), 59–83.

Cranley, M. S. (1984). Social support as a factor in the development of parents' attachment to their unborn. In K. E. Barnard, P. A. Brandt, B. S. Raff, & P. Carroll (Eds.), *Social support and families of vulnerable infants.* White Plains, NY: March of Dimes Birth Defects Foundation. *Birth Defects, Original Article Series, 20*(5), 100–109.

Crawford, G. (1985). A theoretical model of support network conflict experienced by new mothers. *Nursing Research, 34,* 100-102.

Cronenwett, L. R. (1980). Elements and outcomes of a postpartum support group program. *Research in Nursing and Health, 3,* 33-41.

Cronenwett, L. R. (1984). Social networks and social support of primigravida mothers and fathers. In K. E. Barnard, P. A. Brandt, B. S. Raff, & P. Carroll (Eds.), *Social support and families of vulnerable infants.* White Plains, NY: March of Dimes Birth Defects Foundation. *Birth Defects, Original Article Series, 20*(5), 168-186.

Cronenwett, L. R. (1985a). Network structure, social support, and psychological outcomes of pregnancy. *Nursing Research, 34,* 93-99.

Cronenwett, L. R. (1985b). Parental network structure and perceived support after birth of first child. *Nursing Research, 34,* 347-352.

Cronenwett, L. R., & Kunst-Wilson, W. (1981). Stress, social support, and the transition to fatherhood. *Nursing Research, 30,* 196-201.

Curry, M. A. (1987). Maternal behavior of hospitalized pregnant women. *Journal of Psychosomatic Obstetrics and Gynaecology, 7,* 165-182.

Dimond, M., & Jones, S. L. (1983). Social support: A review and theoretical integration. In P. L. Chinn (Ed.), *Advances in nursing theory development* (pp. 235-249). Rockville, MD: Aspen.

Dohrenwend, B. S., Dohrenwend, B. P., Dodson, M., & Shrout, P. E. (1984). Symptoms, hassles, social supports, and life events: Problems of confounded measures. *Journal of Abnormal Psychology, 93,* 222-230.

Dooher, M. E. (1980). Lamaze method of childbirth. *Nursing Research, 29,* 220-224.

Dooley, D. (1985). Causal inference in the study of social support. In S. Cohen & S. L. Syme (Eds.), *Social support and health* (pp. 109-125). New York: Academic Press.

Dormire, S. L., Strauss, S. S., & Clarke, B. A. (1989). Social support and adaptation to the parent role in first-time adolescent mothers. *Journal of Obstetric, Gynecologic, and Neonatal Nursing, 18,* 327-337.

Dunn, M. S. (1963). *A marriage role expectation inventory.* New York: Family Life Publications.

Ellis, D. J., & Hewat, R. J. (1985). Mother's postpartum perceptions of spousal relationships. *Journal of Obstetric, Gynecologic, and Neonatal Nursing, 14,* 140-146.

Ferketich, S. L., & Mercer, R. T. (1989). Men's health status during pregnancy and early fatherhood. *Research in Nursing & Health, 12,* 137-148.

Flaherty, M. J. (1988). Seven caring functions of black grandmothers in adolescent mothering. *Maternal-Child Nursing Journal, 17,* 191-207.

Flaherty, M. J., Sr., Facteau, L., & Garver, P. (1987). Grandmother functions in multigenerational families: An exploratory study of black adolescent mothers and their infants. *Maternal-Child Nursing Journal, 16,* 61-73.

Gardner, K. G. (1979). Supportive nursing: A critical review of the literature. *Journal of Psychiatric Nursing and Mental Health Services, 17*(10), 10-16.

Gottlieb, B. H. (1978). The development and application of a classification scheme of informal helping behaviours. *Canadian Journal of Behavioural Science, 10,* 105-115.

Guerney, B. (1977). *Relationship enhancement skill training program for therapy, prevention and enrichment.* San Francisco: Jossey-Bass.

Hangsleben, K. L. (1983). Transition to fatherhood: An exploratory study. *Journal of Obstetric, Gynecologic, and Neonatal Nursing, 12,* 265-270.

Heitzmann, C. A., & Kaplan, R. M. (1988). Assessment of methods for measuring social support. *Health Psychology, 7,* 75-109.

Hobfoll, S. (1986). Social support: Research, theory, and applications from research on women. In S. E. Hobfoll (Ed.)., *Stress, social support, and women* (pp 239-256). New York: Harper & Row.

Hodnett, E. D., & Osborn, R. W. (1989). Effects of continuous intrapartum professional support on childbirth outcomes. *Research in Nursing and Health, 12,* 289-297.

House, J. S. (1981). *Work stress and social support.* Reading, MA: Addison-Wesley.

House, J. S., & Kahn, R. L. (1985). Measures and concepts of social support. In S. Cohen & S. L. Syme. (Eds.), *Social support and health* (pp. 83–108). New York: Academic Press.

Jordan, P. L. (1987). Differences in network structure, social support, and parental adaptation associated with maternal employment status. *Health Care for Women International, 8*(2-3), 133–150.

Kaufman, K. J., & Hall, L. A. (1989). Influences of the social network on choice and duration on breast-feeding in mothers of preterm infants. *Research in Nursing and Health, 12,* 149–159.

Kemp, V. H., & Hatmaker, D. D. (1989). Stress and social support in high-risk pregnancy. *Research in Nursing and Health, 12,* 331–336.

Kintz, D. L. (1987). Nursing in labor. *Journal of Obstetric, Gynecologic, and Neonatal Nursing, 16,* 126–130.

Koniak-Griffin, D. (1988). The relationship between social support, self-esteem, and maternal-fetal attachment in adolescents. *Research in Nursing and Health, 11,* 269–278.

Krutsky, C. D. (1985). Siblings at birth: Impact on parents. *Journal of Nurse-Midwifery, 30,* 269–276.

Kuhn, J. (1984). Updating family-centered maternity care: Application of a conceptual analysis of support. *Health Care for Women International, 5*(1-3), 93–101.

Lamm, N. H. (1983). The second high-risk birth: Impact on maternal dyadic adjustment. *Issues in Health Care of Women, 4,* 251–259.

Lasky, P., Buckwalter, K. C., Whall, A., Lederman, R., Speer, J., McLane, A., King, J. M., & White, M. A. (1985). Developing an instrument for the assessment of family dynamics. *Western Journal of Nursing Research, 7,* 40–57.

Lazarus, R. S., DeLongis, A., Folkman, S., & Gruen, R. (1985). Stress and adaptational outcomes. *American Psychologist, 40,* 770–779.

Lenz, E. R., Parks, P. L., Jenkins, L. S., & Jarrett, G. E. (1986). Life change and instrumental support as predictors of illness in mothers of 6-month-olds. *Research in Nursing & Health, 9,* 17–24.

Lenz, E. R., Soeken, K. L., Rankin, E. A., & Fischman, S. H. (1985). Sex-role attributes, gender, and postpartal perceptions of the marital relationship. *Advances in Nursing Science. 7*(3), 49–62.

Locke, H. J., & Wallace, K. M. (1959). Short marital-adjustment and prediction tests: Their reliability and validity. *Marriage and Family Living. 21,* 251–255.

MacElveen-Hoehn, P., & Eyres, S. J. (1984). Social support and vulnerability: State of the art in relation to families and children. In K. E. Barnard, P. A. Brandt, B. S. Raff, & P. Carroll (Eds.), *Social support and families of vulnerable infants.* White Plains, NY: March of Dimes Birth Defects Foundation. *Birth Defects, Original Article Series, 20(5),* 11–29.

Mackey, M. C., & Lock, S. E. (1989). Women's expectations of the labor and delivery nurse. *Journal of Obstetric, Gynecologic, and Neonatal Nursing, 18,* 505–512.

Majewski, J. L. (1987). Social support and the transition to the maternal role. *Health Care for Women International, 8,* 397–407.

Majewski, J. L. (1986). Conflicts, satisfactions, and attitudes during transition to the maternal role. *Nursing Research, 35,* 10–14.

Meleis, A. I., & Swendsen, L. A. (1978). Role supplementation: An empirical test of a nursing intervention. *Nursing Research, 27,* 11–18.

Mercer, R. T. & Ferketich, S. L. (1988). Stress and social support as predictors of anxiety and depression during pregnancy. *Advances in Nursing Science, 10*(2), 26–39.

Mercer, R. T., Ferketich, S. L. DeJoseph, J., May, K. A., & Sollid, D. (1988a). Effect of stress on family functioning during pregnancy. *Nursing Research, 37,* 268–275.

Mercer, R. T., Ferketich, S., May, K., DeJoseph, J., & Sollid, D. (1988b). Further exploration of maternal and paternal fetal attachment. *Research in Nursing & Health, 11,* 83–95.

Mercer, R. T., Hackley, K. C., & Bostrom, A. (1984). Social support of teenage mothers. In K. E. Barnard, P. A. Brandt, B. S. Raff, & P. Carroll (Eds.), *Social support and families of vulnerable infants.* White Plains, NY: March of Dimes Birth Defects Foundation. *Birth Defects, Original Article Series, 20*(5), 245–272.

Mitchell, S. K., Magyary, D., Barnard, K. E., Sumner, G. A., & Booth, C. L. (1988). A comparison of home-based prevention programs for families of newborns. In L. A. Bond (Ed.), *Families in transition: Primary prevention programs that work* (pp. 73–98). Newbury Park, CA: Sage.

Moore, D. (1983). Prepared childbirth and marital satisfaction during the antepartum and postpartum periods. *Nursing Research, 32,* 73–79.

Nikolaisen, S. M., & Williams, R. A. (1980). Parent's view of support following the loss of their infant to sudden infant death syndrome. *Western Journal of Nursing Research, 2,* 593–601.

Norbeck, J. S. (1981). Social support: A model for clinical research and application. *Advances in Nursing Science, 3*(4), 43–59.

Norbeck, J. S. (1984). The Norbeck social support questionnaire. In K. E. Barnard, P. A. Brandt, B. S. Raff, & P. Carroll, (Eds.), *Social support and families of vulnerable infants.* White Plains, NY: March of Dimes Birth Defects Foundation. *Birth Defects, Original Article Series, 20*(5), 45–57.

Norbeck, J. S., & Anderson, N. J. (1989a). Life stress, social support, and anxiety in mid- and late-pregnancy among low income women. *Research in Nursing and Health, 12,* 281– 287.

Norbeck, J. S., & Anderson, N. J. (1989b). Psychosocial predictors of pregnancy outcomes in low-income black, hispanic, and white women. *Nursing Research, 38,* 204–209.

Norbeck, J. S., Lindsey, A. M., & Carrieri, V. L. (1981). The development of an instrument to measure social support. *Nursing Research, 30,* 264–269.

Norbeck, J. S., Lindsey, A. M., & Carrieri, V. L. (1983). Further development of the Norbeck Social Support Questionnaire. *Nursing Research, 32,* 4–9.

Norbeck, J. S., & Tilden, V. P. (1983, March). Life stress, social support, and emotional disequilibrium in complications of pregnancy: A prospective, multivariate study. *Journal of Health and Social Behavior, 24,* 30–46.

Nuckolls, K. B., Cassel, J., & Kaplan, B. H. (1972). Psychological assets, life crisis and the prognosis of pregnancy. *American Journal of Epidemiology, 95,* 431-441.

Payne, R. L., & Jones, J. G. (1987). Measurement and methodological issues in social support. In S. V. Kasl & C. L. Cooper (Eds.), *Stress and health: Issues in research methodology* (pp. 167–205). New York: Wiley.

Porter, L. S. & Demeuth, B. R. (1979). The impact of marital adjustment on pregnancy acceptance. *Maternal-Child Nursing Journal, 8,* 103–113.

Pridham, K. F. (1984). Information needs and problem solving of parents of infants. In K. E. Barnard, P. A. Brandt, B. S. Raff, & P. Carroll (Eds.), *Social support and families of vulnerable infants.* White Plains, NY: March of Dimes Birth Defects Foundation. *Birth Defects, Original Article Series, 20*(5), 125–149.

Rankin, E. A. D., & Campbell, N. D. (1983). Perception of relationship changes during the third trimester of pregnancy. *Issues in Health Care of Women, 6,* 351–359.

Rankin, E. A. D., Campbell, N. D., & Soeken, K. L. (1985). Adaptations to parenthood: Differing expectations of social supports for mothers versus fathers. *Journal of Primary Prevention, 5*(3), 145–153.

Rich, O. J. (1978). The sociogram: A tool for depicting support in pregnancy. *Maternal-Child Nursing Journal, 7,* 1–9.

Richardson, P. (1982). Significant relationships and their impact on childbearing: A review. *Maternal-Child Nursing Journal, 11,* 17–40.

Roach, A. J., Frazier, L. P., & Bowden, S. R. (1981). The marital satisfaction scale: Development of a measure for intervention research. *Journal of Marriage and the Family, 43,* 537–546.

Roberts, C. S., & Feetham, S. L. (1982). Assessing family functioning across three areas of relationships. *Nursing Research, 31,* 231–235.

Roberts, S. J. (1988). Social support and help seeking: Review of the literature. *Advances in Nursing Science, 10*(2), 1–11.

Rock, D. L., Green, K. E., Wise, B. K., & Rock, R. D. (1984). Social support and social network scales: A psychometric review. *Research in Nursing and Health, 7,* 325–332.

Saunders, R. B., & Robins, E. (1987). Changes in the marital relationship during the first pregnancy. *Health Care for Women International, 8,* 361–377.

Schaefer, C., Coyne, J. C., & Lazarus, R. (1981). The health related functions of social support. *Journal of Behavioral Medicine, 4,* 381-406.

Schumm, W. R., Scanlon, E. D., Crow, C. L., Green, D. M., & Buckler, D. L. (1983). Characteristics of the Kansas marital satisfaction scale in a sample of 79 married couples. *Psychological Reports, 53,* 583–588.

Spanier, G. (1976). Measuring dyadic adjustment: New scales for assessing the quality of marriage and similar dyads. *Journal of Marriage and the Family, 38,* 15–28.

Stephens, C. J. (1985). Identifying social support components in prenatal populations: A multivariate analysis on alcohol consumption. *Health Care for Women International, 6,* 285–294.

Stewart, M. J. (1989). Social support instruments created by nurse investigators. *Nursing Research, 38,* 268–275.

Thoits, P. A. (1982). Conceptual, methodological, and theoretical problems in studying social support as a buffer against life stress. *Journal of Health and Social Behavior, 23,* 145–159.

Tilden, V. P. (1983a). Perceptions of single vs. partnered adult gravidas in the midtrimester. *Journal of Obstetric, Gynecologic, and Neonatal Nursing, 12,* 40–48.

Tilden, V. P. (1983b). The relation of life stress and social support to emotional disequilibrium during pregnancy. *Research in Nursing and Health, 6,* 167–174.

Tilden, V. P. (1984). The relation of selected psychosocial variables to single status of adult women during pregnancy. *Nursing Research, 33,* 102–107.

Tilden, V. P. (1985). Issues of conceptualization and measurement of social support in the construction of nursing theory. *Research in Nursing and Health, 8,* 199–206.

Tomlinson, P. S. (1987). Spousal differences in marital satisfaction during transition to parenthood. *Nursing Research, 36,* 239–243.

Wandersman, L., Wandersman, A. & Kahn, S. (1980). Social support in the transition to parenthood. *Journal of Community Psychology, 8,* 332–342.

Wapner, J. (1976). The attitudes, feelings and behaviors of expectant fathers attending Lamaze classes. *Birth and the Family Journal, 3,* 5–13.

Weaver, R. H., & Cranley, M. S. (1983). An exploration of paternal-fetal attachment behavior. *Nursing Research, 32,* 68–72.

Weinert, C. (1984). Evaluation of the personal resource questionnaire: A social support measure. In K. E. Barnard, P. A. Brandt, B. S. Raff, & P. Carroll (Eds.), *Social support and families of vulnerable infants* White Plains, NY: March of Dimes Birth Defects Foundation. *Birth Defects, Original Article Series, 20*(5), 59–78.

White, M., & Dawson, C. (1981). The impact of the at-risk infant on family solidarity. In R. P. Lederman & B. S. Raff (Eds.), *Perinatal parental behavior: Nursing research and implications for newborn health* New York: Liss. March of Dimes Birth Defects Foundation. *Birth Defects, Original Article Series, 17*(6), 253–284.

PART THREE

Health

CHAPTER 6

The Paradigm of Health

OVERVIEW

The focus of this chapter is the paradigm of health in nursing. The origins of its association with nursing have been traced to Nightingale (Tripp-Reimer, 1984). In contemporary nursing theory, health is one of the four concepts in the nursing metaparadigm (Fawcett, 1989). Of all the paradigms covered in this book, however, none is more nebulous and more subject to debate than the meaning of "health."

Both as a discipline and a profession, nursing has struggled with defining "health" and its relationship to illness. Indeed, some would argue that conceptualizations of health and disease represent fundamentally different and incompatible paradigms (e.g., Hall & Allan, 1986). Others such as Rogers (1970) stress the common origins of health and disease: "Health and sickness [i.e. pathological processes], however defined, are expressions of the process of life. What meaning they may have is derived out of an understanding of the life process in its totality" (p. 85). Achieving clear understanding of what is health is complicated by the abstract nature of many of its definitions, particularly if it is defined in a more substantive manner than the absence of disease. (See Table 6–1 for examples of definitions of health and related concepts in nursing.)

Parent-infant nursing in particular has a strong tradition of emphasizing health and wellness care during pregnancy and infancy. Care of women and infants with at-risk status or with complications of pregnancy and birth also are central concerns to nurses. Thus, the practice of parent-infant nursing requires views of health which capture the full range of health states from wellness to illness and disability. However, the preventable nature of many illnesses or disabilities related to pregnancy, childbirth, and infancy continues to energize prevention efforts with mothers and infants. Still further, the promotion of maternal and infant health and healthy lifestyles is seen as setting the stage for long-term positive development and

Table 6–1
DEFINITIONS OF HEALTH AND RELATED CONCEPTS FROM NURSING LITERATURE

Health Definitions

"A dynamic state of being in which the developmental and behavioral potential of an individual is realized to the fullest extent possible." (American Nurses' Association, 1980, p. 5.)

"A state of existence reflecting the totality of the system in interaction with the environment." (Bilitski, 1981, p. 19.)

"The expansion of consciousness." (Newman, 1986, p. 3.)

"The actualization of inherent and acquired human potential through goal directed behavior, competent self-care, and satisfying relationships with others while adjustments are made as needed to maintain structural integrity and harmony with the environment." (Pender, 1987b, p. 27.)

Related Definitions

Health promotion: "Health care directed toward high-level wellness through processes that encourage alteration of personal habits or the environment in which people live." (Brubaker, 1983, p. 12.)

Disease: "A morbid physical condition identified by its syndrome of signs and symptoms." (Smith, 1983, p. 33.)

Disease: "Malfunctioning or maladaptation of biological and psychological processes in the individual." (Tripp-Reimer, 1984, p. 103.)

Illness: "A subjective phenomenon in which individuals who perceive themselves as not feeling well modify their normal behavior. In contrast to disease (a concept of biology), illness is a personal phenomenon concerning an individual's altered perception of self." (Tripp-Reimer, 1984, p. 104.)

Risk: "The presence of potentially stressful factors in a person's environment." (Rose & Killien, 1983, p. 62.)

Risk factors: "Characteristics that increase the probability of a disease condition being detected, but they do not lead to prediction with any certainty." (Dixon & Dixon, 1984, p. 2.)

Vulnerability: "A dynamic continuum . . . that . . . is affected by both constitutional and acquired factors." (Rose & Killien, 1983, p. 64.)

well-being. In addition, health patterns of other family members, particularly fathers, are increasingly of concern. Thus, as a field, parent-infant nursing captures many facets of health: wellness, risk, and disability/disease, prevention of disease and promotion of health, and health-related behavior patterns of mothers and other family members.

In this chapter the paradigm of health is considered from two standpoints: health status and health behaviors. Health status includes concepts of health as well as illness, disease, risk, and symptoms patterns. Health behaviors include conceptualizations of health promotion, behavioral aspects of disease prevention, and health-related life-style. Partitioning the health paradigm in this way is done to organize topical material. Clearly, there is evidence of a relationship between health behaviors and health status (US Department of Health, Education, and Welfare, 1979). Models of health status and health behaviors represent alternative ways of understanding the link between the two broad concepts. (*Note:* It is beyond the scope of this chapter to examine concepts of health as defined in various conceptual models of nursing. Readers are referred to Fawcett [1989] and Fitzpatrick and Whall [1983].)

KEY CONCEPTS AND RELATIONSHIPS

HEALTH STATUS

Conceptualizations of Health

The study of health status requires a view of what health is. The nature of health has been a topic of debate and theorizing since the early Greek times (Smith, 1983). Even today there are many views that define and describe the nature of health, but there is no consensus on exactly what health is. Fortunately, the complex and diverse definitions of health have been carefully studied by two nurses. The first, Keller (1981), gathered 42 definitions of health published by health professionals and non-healthcare professionals. She then completed a conceptual analysis of the definitions of health by identifying the subconcepts embedded in them. The frequency of occurrence of 21 subconcepts within definitions of health was tabulated and rank-ordered.

Table 6–2 presents the rank and frequency of mention of the 21 subconcepts in the 42 definitions of health. Most noteworthy is the high rate at which "physical/biological" and "emotional/psychological" subconcepts of health were mentioned. Also ranked high are "environment," "social," and "opposite of disease, pain." What Keller's analysis does not do is provide a clear idea about the relations of health and disease beyond indicating that the concepts are often seen as opposite.

In the second analysis, carried out by Smith (1981, 1983), health was identified as one end of a health-illness continuum. Health was explicated as both a comparative concept (more or less present) and a relative term (as the standard of health changes, so also may appraisals of its presence). Smith proposed that the standards or models of health used for health appraisal are of four types: eudaemonistic, adaptive, role performance, and clinical. For each model of health, the health-illness continuum is anchored by distinctive standards of health and illness (Fig. 6–1).

In the eudaemonistic model, health is viewed as general well-being and self-realization. Health in essence is actualizing one's full intrinsic potential. In turn, illness in the eudaemonistic model is a condition that blocks or impairs realizing one's potential.

Table 6–2
Ranking of 21 Subconcepts Included in 42 Definitions/Descriptions

Rank	Subconcepts	Mentions
1	Physical/biological	22
2	Emotional/psychological	20
4	Environment	13
4	Social	13
4	Opposite of (or freedom from) disease, pain	13
6	Integrated functioning	11
7	Optimum capability	10
8	Adaptation	9
9.5	Daily living/activities	5
9.5	Spiritual	5
13	Cultural	4
13	Wellness	4
13	Relationships	4
13	Purposeful direction	4
13	Meaning in life, one's values	4
17	Well-being	3
17	Harmony	3
17	Heredity	3
19.5	Balance	2
19.5	Self-knowledge, self-realization	2
21	(W)Holistic	1

Reprinted from Advances in Nursing Science, Vol. 4, No. 1, p. 49, with permission of Aspen Publishers, Inc., © 1981.

In the adaptive model, health is represented by interactions between persons and the environment, social and physical, that are effective. Because flexible patterns of response increase the likelihood of fit with the environment, they are the key to an adaptive view of health. Illness, by contrast, is marked by alienation of persons from their environment and ineffective patterns of response.

The role-performance model construes health as the capacity to fulfill social roles; illness is present when people are incapable of fulfilling their roles. Although work roles are central to the role-performance model, other roles such as parent also are relevant to this model.

The focus of the clinical model is on removing morbid physical and mental problems and the pain associated with them. Health is equated with the absence of disease and its symptoms. Presence of the signs and symptoms of disease indicates illness.

The four models of health are alternative, but not mutually exclusive, ways of viewing health and illness. The clinical model provides the narrowest view of health, and the eudaemonistic model provides that most expan-

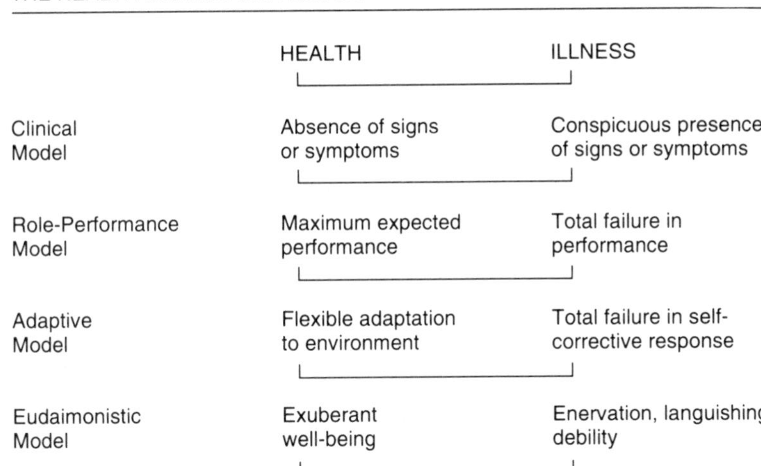

Figure 6–1
The health-illness continuum. (Reprinted by permission of the publisher from Smith, Judith A., THE IDEA OF HEALTH: IMPLICATIONS FOR THE NURSING PROFESSIONAL. [New York: Teachers College Press, © 1983 by Teachers College, Columbia University. All rights reserved.] p. 32.)

sive. The emphasis of each model is distinct. That does not, however, prevent the models from being used in conjunction with one another.

Smith's analysis of health provides alternative, but not mutually exclusive, ways to view health status within the context of parent-infant nursing. Her analysis of health covers the diverse range of health states found in the practice of parent-infant nursing. When Smith's analysis is used, symptom patterns during pregnancy and childbirth most clearly fall under a clinical model of health. Mastery of the skills associated with the parenting role and flexibly adjusting to demands of parenthood and a new baby reflect the role-performance and adaptive models, respectively. Exhibiting a sense of well-being and zest for life during pregnancy and early parenting would, in turn, reflect the eudaemonistic model of health. In infant care, both the clinical and the adaptive models have high relevance to risk screening and parent-infant interaction, respectively.

Most theoretical work on health has focused on defining health, but the writings of Newman (1979, 1986, 1987) contain a more substantive view of health and its relation to human life process. Newman's view of health is a "synthesis of disease and non-disease" (1979, p. 56). Key assumptions of Newman's theoretical position are presented in Table 6–3. Her framework for understanding health is phrased in terms of the fundamental concepts of movement, time, space, and consciousness. She describes the relationship of nursing and health as follows:

> *This framework provides a view of health as the totality of life process and therefore one which encompasses disease as a meaningful aspect. In this context, the goal of nursing is not to make people well, or to prevent their getting sick, but to assist people to utilize the power that is within them as they evolve toward higher levels of consciousness. (1979, p. 67)*

Newman elaborates her ideas about patterns of health as expanding consciousness in her more recent writings (Newman, 1986, 1987). Her work has potential relevance to several phenomena in parent-infant nursing: symptom patterns during pregnancy and postpartum, the experience of subjective time during labor and postpartum. The utility of her theoretical work for parent-infant nursing has yet to be developed and tested in research, however.

Disease and Illness

Understanding health status requires an understanding of the concepts of disease and illness and their interrelations. Tripp-Reimer (1984) provides one of the most lucid analyses of these correlative concepts. According to Tripp-Reimer, disease represents a biomedical (etic) perspective in which there is malfunctioning of biological and psychological processes of persons. Illness, by contrast, is the subjective (emic) experience of alternations in personal well-being and social functioning.

Table 6–3
ASSUMPTIONS OF NEWMAN'S THEORETICAL FRAMEWORK

1. "Health encompasses conditions heretofore described as illness, or in medical terms, pathology." (p. 56.)
2. "These 'pathological' conditions can be considered a manifestation of the total pattern of the individual." (p. 57.)
3. "The pattern of the individual that eventually manifests itself as pathology is primary and exists prior to structural or functional changes." (p. 57.)
4. "Removal of the pathology in itself will not change the pattern of the individual." (p. 57.)
5. "If becoming 'ill' is the only way an individual's pattern can manifest itself, then that is health for that person." (p. 58.)
6. "Health is the expansion of consciousness." (p. 58.)

Source: Theory Development in Nursing (pp. 56–58) by M. A. Newman, 1979, Philadelphia: FA Davis. Copyright 1979 by FA Davis Company. Adapted by permission.

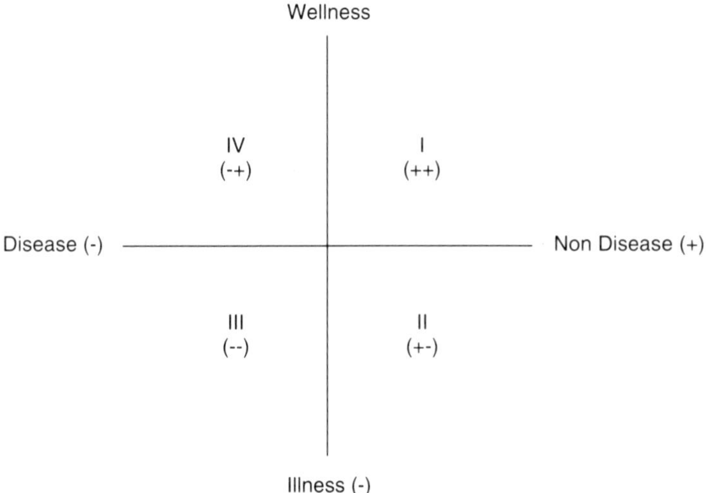

Figure 6–2
Emic-etic health grid. (From "Reconceptualizing the construct of health: Integrating emic and etic perspectives" by T. Tripp-Reimer, 1984, *Research in Nursing and Health, 7,* p. 104. Copyright © 1984 by John Wiley & Sons, Inc. Reprinted by permission of John Wiley & Sons, Inc.)

Biomedical diagnoses rendered by physicians constitute an etic perspective; the opposite of disease is nondisease. In turn, laypersons' subjective views of their state of being and functioning reflect an emic one; the opposite of illness is wellness.

Tripp-Reimer constructed an emic-etic health grid to bring together the concepts of disease and illness (Fig. 6–2). The grid contains four quadrants, two of which are concordant views between the client and health practitioner about the client's health state and two of which are discordant views. The conceptual distinctions made by Tripp-Reimer are particularly relevant when nurses engage in reseach with populations whose views of disease and illness may differ from those of health care providers.

Risk

The concept of risk is related to health, particularly if health is defined in terms of a disease orientation. In parent-infant nursing, the concepts of risk and risk assessment are prevalent in prenatal and perinatal care. The meaning of risk is intertwined with the interaction of persons and their environments (Rose & Killien, 1983). As Rose and Killien note, risk is described in nursing literature as "both environmental and personal factors that contribute to health problems" (1983, p. 61). Arguing for a distinction between the terminology for environmental and personal risk factors, they recommend that *risk* be used to refer to environmental hazards and *vulnerability* be used to refer to personal characteristics (see definitions in Table 6–1).

Although risk and vulnerability represent *probabilistic* relations between a person's current and future health, both concepts have theoretical and practical importance. At the theoretical level, the concepts of risk and vulnerability serve as predictors of health outcomes. At a practical level, developing and refining nursing measures of risk and vulnerability may facilitate research on health status and provide ways to improve client assessment.

Risk and vulnerability are especially congruent with the clinical and adaptive models of health. Because risk and vulnerability typically are related to health problems rather than well-being, they fit with clinical definitions of health. Risk and vulnerability also are related to each other in a dynamic way, so that personal characteristics may offset or intensify environmental hazards. Thus, there are similarities to the adaptive model of health.

HEALTH BEHAVIORS

In her 1984 review of health promotion and illness prevention, Pender identified health behaviors as both (1) health-promoting actions and (2) health-protecting (preventive) actions. While health-promoting actions target enhancing and maintaining well-being and self-actualization, health-protecting actions focus on guarding against a specific disease or injury (Pender, 1984, 1987b).

A number of midrange models of health behaviors have been proposed, and they reflect different definitions of health and include alternative predictors of behavioral outcomes. Several models of health behaviors have been used in or proposed for nursing research. Among them are the health belief model (e.g., Becker, 1974), the health promotion model (Pender, 1987b) and the interactional model of client behavior (Cox, 1980).

Reflecting a strong emphasis on subjective perceptions, the health belief model predicts likelihood of action (preventive health behaviors) based on individual perceptions and modifying factors. The individual perceptions center on perceived susceptibility to a given disease and perceived seriousness of that disease. Other factors that play a role in predicting the likelihood of taking action are demographic, sociopsychologic, and structural variables, perceived threat of the disease, cues to action, and perceived benefits and barriers (Becker et al., 1977). Clearly, the health belief model assumes a clinical model of health and primarily relates to health-protecting (preventive) behaviors. The health belief model has also been used to study adherence in chronic illness (Redeker, 1988). For a critical review of the health belief model, see Mikhail (1981).

As a complement to models of health protection, Pender proposed the health promotion model (1987b). Pender's view of health promotion encompasses "a multidimensional pattern of self-initiated actions and perceptions that serve to maintain or enhance the level of wellness, self-actualization, and fulfillment of the individual" (Walker, Sechrist, & Pender, 1987, p. 77). Instead of predicting the likelihood of disease-avoiding behavior, Pender's model predicts the likelihood of taking health-promotive actions. Likelihood of action is predicted by cues to action and sets of both modifying factors and cognitive-perceptual factors. Among the modifying factors are demographic characteristics and situational factors. The cognitive-perceptual factors include such variables as perceived health status, definition of health, and perceived barriers and benefits of health-promoting behaviors. (See Fig. 6–3 for a diagram of the health promotion model.)

Existing models of health behaviors have usually omitted the care provider as a variable. To incorporate the client-profession relationship explicitly into a predictive model of client health behavior, Cox (1980) proposed the interaction model of client health behavior. This model

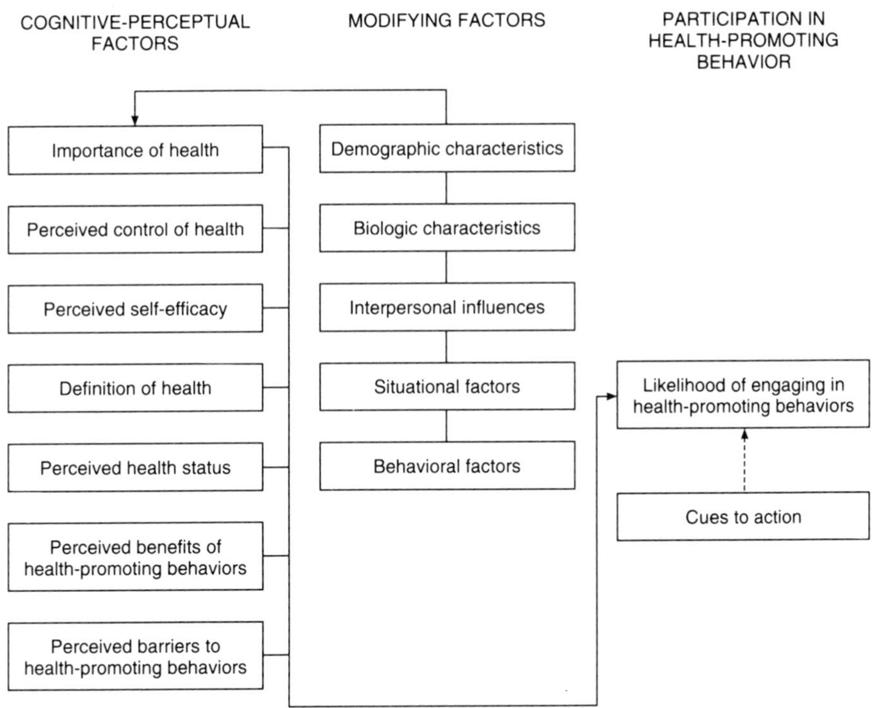

Figure 6–3
Health promotion model. (From *Health Promotion in Nursing Practice* [p. 58] by N. J. Pender, 1987, Norwalk, CT: Appleton & Lange. Copyright 1987 by Appleton & Lange. Reprinted by permission.)

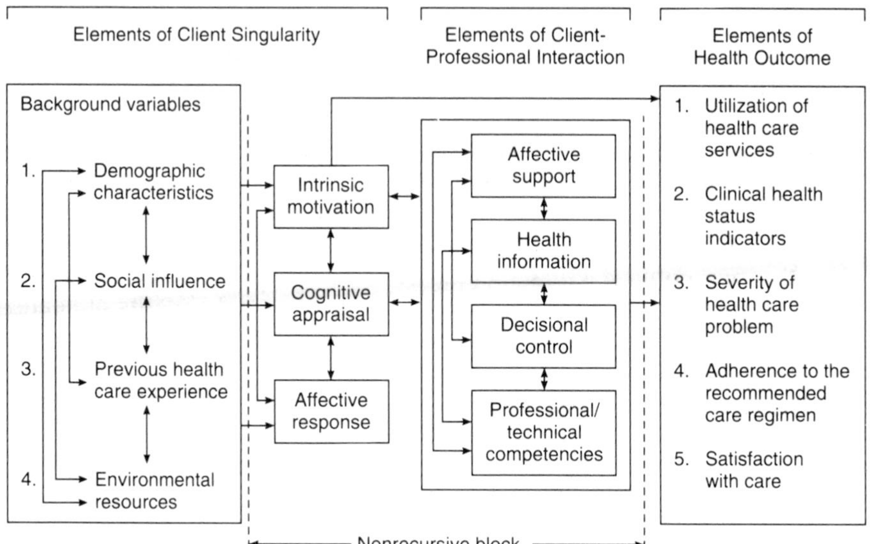

Figure 6–4
Interaction of client health behavior. (Reprinted from Advances in Nursing Science, Vol. 5, No., 1, p. 47, with permission of Aspen Publishers, Inc., © 1982).

assumes that the client initiates contact with the health care provider. Cox's model has three types of components: elements of client singularity, client-professional interaction, and health outcomes. Included in client singularity are background variables, motivation, appraisal of health care concern, and affective response to the concern. The elements of client-professional interaction include affective support, health information, decisional control, and professional/technical competencies. Five types of elements, including health status indicators, comprise the outcomes of the model (Figure 6–4).

In contrast to health status where there are many abstract definitions of health but few guidelines for midrange theories, the area of health behaviors offers multiple midrange theories for consideration. The models reviewed briefly here, and others in the literature (Cox, 1980; Pender, 1987a), provide a rich variety of choices for factors to be emphasized in predicting behavior and the type of behavior to be predicted.

METHODOLOGY

Although there are numerous definitions of health and a wide variety of tools for measuring health in the literature, the coordination among definitions and measurement is often lacking (Beckstrand, 1978). Validly measuring health is one of the major issues facing nursing research. A major gap exists between theoretical concepts of health and the manner in which these are operationalized in research (Reynolds, 1988). In an analysis of research reports on health in major nursing journals, Reynolds found most nurse researchers measured health through indices of illness, disability, or symptoms. She noted that although nurses often subscribe to definitions of health which incorporate more than the absence of disease, their actual research reflects a clinical (disease) model of health. In a further breakdown of most commonly used approaches of measuring health, Reynolds reported the following as predominating: physical aspects, single measures, and self-report.

To improve the congruence between theoretical and operational aspects of investigations of health, a clear definition of the view of health guiding the research is needed. This should be followed by critical review of possible indicators. (For a review of rating scales and questionnaire for measuring various aspects disability and health, see McDowell and Newell [1987].) Selecting appropriate tools for measuring health is not solely a function of theoretic concerns, however. Engel (1984) has pointed out that life stage may also be an important consideration. Thus, tools developed for use with older adults may not be suitable for use with younger adults.

If suitable indicators are not available for measuring theoretic aspects of health, instrument development may be warranted. That is particularly true of emerging concepts of health. According to Pender (1984), "Defining health operationally and developing indices for measuring health as a positive state in all its complexity must be a high priority for nurse researchers" (p. 99).

The distinction between etic and emic perspectives provided by Tripp-Reimer (1984) also is relevant to measuring health status. Particularly when etic and emic views are likely to be discordant, multiple measures of health status may be needed to capture both biomedical and client categories. To facilitate capturing the emic perspective, Tripp-Reimer has provided a general interview guide for client assessment (p. 107) suitable for a number of situations.

Measurement of risk and vulnerability related to health status also requires careful consideration. In designing or selecting instruments to assess risk and vulnerability, key concerns are adequate specificity and sensitivity. For a lucid discussion of methodological issues in risk measurement, see Frankenburg (1985).

In addition to improving measurement of health, more information is needed about how to promote healthy life-styles among parents and young children. Testing of health promotion models with pregnant women and new parents is needed to determine the empirical validity of models for these populations. Still further, models for intervening to improve health behaviors—and ultimately health status—are needed. Clearly, long-term programs of research, and not isolated projects, are required if advances

Table 6–4
GUIDING QUESTIONS FOR PROGRAMMATIC RESEARCH ON HEALTH BEHAVIORS

Phase	Guiding Question
Hypothesis	Given that a significant problem or goal involving health behavior has been identified, what exactly is the problem or goal? What biological, psychological and environmental factors contribute to development, maintenance, and change of the behavior?
Method	Can nursing and behavioral theory, methods, and data be used to construct cost-effective methods for developing healthy behaviors or changing unhealthy behaviors? If so, which methods may be practical for widespread dissemination?
Controlled Trials	Can these methods be efficacious when studied under controlled research conditions?
Defined Populations	Will these methods be effective if disseminated, and what variables influence their effectiveness in the "real world"?
Dissemination	Are these methods in fact effective when implemented as ongoing services in the community?

Source: Adapted from "Health behavior and health promotion" by J. A. Best, R. Cameron, and M. Grant, 1986, *American Journal of Health Promotion;* 1 (2): pp. 51–52. Copyright 1986 by American Journal of Health Promotion. Adapted by permission.

are to be made in this extremely complex area of investigation. Table 6–4 contains a series of questions, adapted from Best, Cameron, and Grant (1986), to guide the phases of programmatic nursing research in health behaviors.

REFERENCES

American Nurses' Association. (1980). *Nursing: A social policy statement.* Kansas City, Mo: American Nurses' Association.

Becker, M. H. (Ed.). (1974). *The health belief model and personal health behavior.* Thorofare, NJ: Slack.

Becker, M. H., Haefner, D. P., Kasl, S. V., Kirscht, J. P., Maiman, L. A., & Rosenstock, I. M. (1977). Selected psychosocial models and correlates of individual health-related behaviors. *Medical Care, 15,* 27–46.

Beckstrand, J. K. (1978). *A conceptual and logical analysis of selected health indicators.* Unpublished doctoral dissertation. Austin, TX: The University of Texas at Austin.

Best, J. A., Cameron, R., & Grant, M. (1986). Health behavior and health promotion. *American Journal of Health Promotion, 1,* 48–57.

Bilitski, J. S. (1981). Nursing science and the laws of health: The test of substance as a step in the process of theory development. *Advances in Nursing Science, 4*(1), 15–29.

Brubaker, B. H. (1983). Health promotion: A linguistic analysis. *Advances in Nursing Science, 5*(3), 1–14.

Cox, C. L. (1980). An interaction model of client health behavior: Theoretical prescription for nursing. *Advances in Nursing Science, 5*(1), 41-56.

Dixon, J. K., & Dixon, J. P. (1984). An evolutionary-based model of health and viability. *Advances in Nursing Science, 6*(3), 1-18.

Engel, N. S. (1984). On the vicissitudes of health appraisal. *Advances in Nursing Science, 7*(1), 12-23.

Fawcett, J. (1989). *Analysis and evaluation of conceptual models of nursing* (2nd ed.). Philadelphia: Davis.

Fitzpatrick, J. J., & Whall, A. L. (1983). *Conceptual models of nursing: Analysis and application.* Bowie, MD: Brady.

Frankenburg, W. K. (1985). The concept of screening revisited. In W. K. Frankenburg, R. N. Emde, & J. W. Sullivan (Eds.), *Early identification of children at risk: An international perspective* (pp. 3-17). New York: Plenum.

Hall, B. A., & Allan, J. D. (1986). Sharpening nursing's focus by focusing on health. *Nursing and Health Care, 7,* 315-320.

Keller, M. J. (1981). Toward a definition of health. *Advances in Nursing Science,4*(1), 43-64.

McDowell, I., & Newell, C. (1987). *Measuring health: A guide to rating scales and questionnaires.* New York: Oxford.

Mikhail, B. (1981). The health belief model: A review and critical evaluation of the model, research, and practice. *Advances in Nursing Science, 4*(1), 65-82.

Newman, M. A. (1979). *Theory development in nursing.* Philadelphia: Davis.

Newman, M. A. (1986). *Health as expanding consciousness.* St. Louis, MO: Mosby.

Newman, M. A. (1987). Patterning. In M. E. Duffy & N. J. Pender (Eds.), *Conceptual issues in health promotion: Report of proceedings of a wingspread conference* (pp. 36-50). Indianapolis: Sigma Theta Tau.

Pender, N. J. (1984). Health promotion and illness prevention. *Annual Review of Nursing Research, 2,* 83-105.

Pender, N. J. (1987a). Health and health promotion: The conceptual dilemmas. In M. E. Duffy & N. J. Pender (Eds.), *Conceptual issues in health promotion: Report of proceedings of a wingspread conference* (pp. 7-23). Indianapolis: Sigma Theta Tau.

Pender, N. J. (1987b). *Health promotion in nursing practice* (2nd ed.). Norwalk: CN: Appleton & Lange.

Redeker, N. S. (1988). Health beliefs and adherence in chronic illness. *Image,* 20, 31-35.

Reynolds, C. L. (1988). The measurement of health in nursing research. *Advances in Nursing Science, 10*(4), 23-31.

Rogers, M. E. (1970). *An introduction to the theoretical basis of Nursing.* Philadelphia: FA Davis.

Rose, M. H., & Killien, M. (1983). Risk and vulnerability: A case for differentiation. *Advances in Nursing Science, 5*(3), 60-73.

Smith, J. A. (1981). The idea of health: A philosophical inquiry. *Advances in Nursing Science, 3*(3), 43-50.

Smith, J. A. (1983). *The idea of health.* New York: Teachers College Press.

Tripp-Reimer, T. (1984). Reconceptualizing the construct of health: Integrating emic and etic perspectives. *Research in Nursing and Health, 7,* 101-109.

U. S. Department of Health, Education, and Welfare. (1979). *Health people: The surgeon general's report on health promotion and disease prevention* (DHEW Publication No. 79-55071). Washington, D.C.: GPO.

Walker, S. N., Sechrist, K. R., & Pender, N. J. (1987). The health-promoting lifestyle profile: Development and psychometric characteristics. *Nursing Research, 36,* 76-81.

CHAPTER 7

Parent-Infant Nursing Research on Health Status

DEFINITIONS AND DESCRIPTIONS OF HEALTH STATUS

DEFINING HEALTH STATUS

Theoretical definitions of health and health status during pregnancy, early parenting, and infancy are virtually absent in parent-infant nursing research. One notable exception is Brown (1988), who proposed the following definition: "Health is a broad multidimensional construct that can include a wide range of dimensions, from lack of illness symptoms to indices of quality of life" (p. 531). Most commonly, however, health status is defined only operationally by virtue of health-related variables or instruments incorporated into studies. For the most part, symptoms—rather than health in a positive sense—have been the object of parent-infant nursing studies. For an excellent historical perspective on the study of symptomatology in expectant mothers and fathers, see Brown (1988).

To capture the wide scope to research on health status, the following working definition guided development of this chapter: Health status was defined as a complex phenomenon with both general and specific dimensions of well-being and health problems manifested in overall level of physical and/or psychological well-being; risk levels for pregnancy-specific health problems; emotional and physical symptom expression and symptom syndromes; specific biological parameters of gestation, physical condition, size and functioning; and biological and psychosocial functional status of parents and infants.

THEORETICAL MODELS OF HEALTH STATUS

The model most widely used by parent-infant nurses for studying health status is one which views health as the end stage or outcome of stress-related events. In this type of model, health status is operationally defined in terms of manifestations of disease or other pathology-related indicators such as physical or emotional symptoms. Stress models often incorporate social support and other moderating factors in the prediction of health outcomes. Because stress models assume that in some way stress has weakened normal defenses or set in motion processes that lead to poor health, measuring amounts of symptoms, complications, and negative emotional states such as anxiety and depression follows logically. Indeed, childbearing, particularly pregnancy, is often identified by nurses as a stressful event (Table 3–1). Viewing health status during childbearing in terms of negative (or disease indicators) may in part be explained by Nuckolls, Cassel, and Kaplan's (1972) research linking high stress and low psychosocial assets to pregnancy complications. See Chapter 2 for an overview of stress models and Chapters 3 and 5 for research that examines the relation of stress and social support to health outcomes.

MEASUREMENT

GENERAL STRATEGIES

Ware, Brook, Davies, and Lohr (1981) state there are at least five reasons for studying health status. Adapted for parent-infant nursing, these reasons translate into five purposes for studying health status: (1) measuring the effectiveness of nursing interventions, (2) assessing quality of nursing care, (3) estimating health needs of populations served by parent-infant nurses, (4) improving clinical decision making with specific nursing clients, and (5) understanding the causes and consequences of differences in health status among parent-infant populations. Each of these purposes may somewhat alter the requirements of health status indicators used in specific investigations. For example, general health ratings are sensitive measures of individual differences in health status, but they fail to provide a detailed analysis of specific effects of experimental intervention protocols (Ware, 1984).

Theoretic reasons also guide requirements for health status indicators used in specific studies. As Smith's (1981, 1983) analysis of health presented in Chapter 6 suggests, measurement of health is not limited to documenting the absence of disease. For example, low scores on scales measuring psychological distress or physical symptoms do not capture health as a distinct, positive attribute. If health as well-being or other positive state is the phenomenon of interest, then the qualities measured should be congruent with the conceptual orientation of the study. Thus, indicators of self-esteem and well-being may instead become the focal point of health measurement. A shift in the model of health requires a corresponding shift in the attributes measured.

Parent-infant nurses have relied heavily on questionnaires and checklists for self-report measures of health status. These are efficient methods for gathering data from large samples in cross-sectional studies. Other self-report methods may be more suitable if the interplay of health-related events in sequential order is under intensive study. See Woods (1981) for advantages and problems of an alternate measurement method: health diaries.

SPECIFIC TOOLS

As the material in Chapter 6 revealed, health is a multifaceted construct. It includes both traditional clinical symptoms and diagnoses as well as "positive" components. Table 7-1 presents measures of health status from parent-infant nursing research. The health status measures in Table 7-1 reflect the diverse range of operational meanings of health. Such traditional clinical indicators as symptoms, anxiety, and depression, as well as more positive components of health such as self-esteem are included. Also, some measures of health status included here—complication, emotional distress, and biological and anthropometric measures—could also be construed as indicators of stress responses. That is in keeping with the models of stress that define stress in terms of resultant effect on mental or physical health status. Indicators of stress that flow from a stimulus or interactional model of stress are presented in Chapter 3. (For a thorough review of 50 health-related tools, including functional status, well-being, social health, quality of life, pain, and general health, see McDowell and Newell [1987]. For suggested guidelines in selecting measures of health status, see Ware et al. [1981].)

In addition, several tools used with other populations are included in Table 7-1 because of their potential relevance to parent-infant nursing. Citations to nursing research in which these tools have been used with other clinical populations also are provided.

One health status indicator, depression, raises some special methodological issues. Recent methodological studies suggest that investigators should be cautious and not equate self-report survey findings about depressive symptoms with diagnosable clinical depression (Davis & Jensen, 1988; Gotlib, Whiffen, Mount, Milne, & Cordy, 1989). Using the Beck Depression Inventory, Gotlib et al. (1989) reported a 24.8 percent prevalence of postpartum depressive symptoms. Based on a companion diagnostic

Table 7–1
MEASURES/TOOLS FOR THE CONCEPT OF HEALTH STATUS

Tool	Source Described in	Studies Using Tool
	ANXIETY, AFFECT, AND MOOD MEASURES	
State-Trait Anxiety Inventory: Forty-item self-report scale (some studies only use part of scale)	Spielberger, Gorsuch, & Lushene (1970) Spielberger, Gorsuch, Lushene, Vagg, & Jacobs (1983)	Consolvo (1986) R. P. Lederman, E. Lederman, Work, and McCann (1979) Norbeck & Tilden (1983) Tilden (1983) Tilden (1984) Mercer & Ferketich (1988) Norbeck & Anderson (1989a) Cranley (1981) Hodnett & Osborn (1989) Norbeck & Anderson (1989b) Gennaro (1986) Gennaro (1988) Ferketich & Mercer (1989) Gibby (1988) Brouse (1988) Hodnett & Abel (1986) Mercer, Ferketich, May, DeJoseph, & Sollid (1988a) Mercer et al. (1988b) Gaffney (1986) Blank (1986) Humenick & Bugen (1981)
Taylor Manifest Anxiety Scale: Fifty-item trait anxiety scale	Taylor (1953)	Schroeder-Zwelling & Hock (1986) Meleis & Swendsen (1978) Glazer (1980) Avant (1981)

Table 7–1
MEASURES/TOOLS FOR THE CONCEPT OF HEALTH STATUS *(Continued)*

Tool	Source Described in	Studies Using Tool
ANXIETY, AFFECT, AND MOOD MEASURES (Continued)		
Center for Epidemiologic Studies Depression Scale: Twenty-item scale for depressive symptoms	Radloff (1977)	Mercer & Ferketich (1988) Ferketich & Mercer (1989) Mercer et al. (1988a) Mercer et al. (1988b)
Lubin Depression Adjective Checklist: Thirty-two-item scale of affective state	Lubin (1967)	Tilden (1983) Tilden (1984) Norbeck & Tilden (1983) Gennaro (1988)
Beck Depression Inventory: Twenty-one-item depression scale	Beck, Ward, Mendelson, Mock, & Erbaugh (1961)	White & Dawson (1981) Booth, Barnard, Mitchell, & Spieker (1987) Booth et al. (1989) Barnard et al. (1988) Fawcett & York (1986) Hangsleben (1983)
Multiple Affect Adjective Checklist: One hundred thirty-two-item scale of mood states	Zuckerman & Lubin (1965)	Muhlenkamp & Joyner (1986)* Strickland (1987) Brooten et al. (1988)
Affects Balance Scale: Forty-item scale of positive and negative affect	Derogatis (1975a)	Northouse & Swain (1987)*
Affect Balance Scale: Ten-item scale of positive and negative affect	Bradburn (1969)	Engel (1984)*
Profile of Mood States: Sixty-five-item adjective checklist of mood states	McNair, Lorr, & Droppleman (1971)	Fehring (1983)* Dorinsky (1984)*

SYMPTOM, RISK, AND COMPLICATION MEASURES		
Questionnaire on nausea and vomiting: Sixteen-item tool	Alley (1984)	Alley (1984)
Questionnaire on nausea and vomiting: Fifteen-item tool	Dilorio (1985)	Dilorio (1985)
Expectant Father's Monthly Health Diary: Two-hundred eighty-item tool for couvade symptoms and related data	Clinton (1986)	Clinton (1986) Schodt (1989)
Brief Symptom Inventory: Fifty-three-item scale	Derogatis (1975b)	Ventura (1986)
Somatic Symptoms Checklist: Twenty-four-item scale	Longobucco & Freston (1989)	Longobucco & Freston (1989)
Health and Physical History Scale: Scale of men's symptoms during their wives' pregnancy and related health questions	Weaver & Cranley (1983)	Weaver & Cranley (1983)
Symptom Checklist: Thirty-two-item scale	Strickland (1987)	Strickland (1987)
Symptoms Checklist: Scale of 23 symptoms	Fawcett & York (1986)	Fawcett & York (1986)
Pregnancy Discomfort Checklist: Twenty-nine-item symptom scale	Wallace et al. (1986)	Wallace et al. (1986)
Hopkins Symptom Checklist (SCL-90) or (SCL-90-R): Measure of psychological distress	Derogatis (1977)	Bonachick (1984)* Bernstein et al. (1988)
Expectant Father's Preliminary Health Interview: One hundred ninety-four item tool of potential risk factors for couvade	Clinton (1986)	Clinton (1986)

Table 7–1
MEASURES/TOOLS FOR THE CONCEPT OF HEALTH STATUS *(Continued)*

Tool	Source Described in	Studies Using Tool
SYMPTOM, RISK, AND COMPLICATION MEASURES (Continued)		
Pregnancy risk assessment: Biomedical risk-factor screening tool	Hobel et al. (1973)	Mercer & Ferketich (1988) Mercer et al. (1988a) Mercer et al. (1988b) Riesch (1984)
Obstetric and infant complications	Norbeck & Anderson (1989b)	Norbeck & Anderson (1989b)
Obstetric complications: Scoring manual	Littman & Parmelee (1974a)	Slager-Earnest et al. (1987) Brown (1979) White-Traut & Nelson (1988) Anderson (1981)
Glazer & Abraham Obstetrical Complications Checklist: Thirty-one-item scale of complications related to anxiety	Glazer & Abraham (1987)	
High-risk pregnancy index: Index based on risk factors	Trotter, Chang, & Thompson (1982)	Trotter et al. (1982)
Postnatal complications: Scoring manual	Littman & Parmelee (1974b)	Slager-Earnest et al. (1987) Brown (1979) White-Traut & Nelson (1988) Barnard et al. (1987) Anderson (1981)
Child Behavior Checklist (2–3 y): Parent report of child adjustment	Thomas Achenbach, Ph.D. University of Vermont Dept. of Psychiatry 1 South Prospect Street Burlington, VT 05401	Barnard et al. (1988)

HEALTH CARE EPISODES		
Number of rehospitalizations		Brooten et al. (1986) Brown et al. (1989)
Acute care visits		Brooten et al. (1986)
Length of hospitalization		Kearney & Cronenwett (1989)
Length of time in neonatal intensive care		Schraeder (1986) Schraeder, Rappaport, & Courtwright (1987)
Number of days on mechanical ventilation		Schraeder (1986) Schraeder et al. (1987)
BIOLOGICAL AND ANTHROPOMETRIC MEASURES		
Monoclonal antibody test for chlamydia		Abel & Unwerth (1988)
Maternal weight gain		Sweeney et al. (1985) Aaronson & Macnee (1989) Taffel (1986)
Pulse		Sibley, Ruhling, Cameron-Foster, Christensen, & Bolen (1981)
Blood pressure		Sibley et al. (1981)
Respiratory gas analysis during treadmill test		Sibley et al. (1981)
Apgar Score	Apgar (1966)	Kirgis, Woolsey, & Sullivan (1977) Lederman et al. (1981) Hutti & Johnson (1988) Stein (1983)
		Holz, Cooney, & Marchese (1989) Kearney & Cronenwett (1989) Mitchell, Bee, Hammond, & Barnard (1985) Bee et al. (1982)

Table 7–1
MEASURES/TOOLS FOR THE CONCEPT OF HEALTH STATUS *(Continued)*

Tool	Source Described in	Studies Using Tool
	BIOLOGICAL AND ANTHROPOMETRIC MEASURES (Continued)	
Gestational age		Stein (1983) Trotter et al. (1982)
Dubowitz gestational age estimate	L. Dubowitz, V. Dubowitz, & Goldberg (1970)	Mitchell et al. (1985) Bee et al. (1982)
Gestational length		Brown et al. (1989) Aaronson & Macnee (1989)
Birth weight		Holz et al. (1989) Sweeney et al. (1985) Brown et al. (1989) Aaronson & Macnee (1989) Taffel (1986) Trotter et al. (1982) Schraeder (1986) Schraeder, Rappaport, & Courtwright (1987)
Ponderal index		Sweeney et al. (1985)
Body mass		Aaronson & Macnee (1989)
Edema		Aaronson & Macnee (1989)
Fetal heart rate		Lederman et al. (1981) Lederman et al. (1985) Sibley et al. (1981)
Presence of intraventricular hemorrhage		Schraeder (1986) Schraeder et al. (1987)

Length of labor		Lederman et al. (1979) Lederman et al. (1985) Lederman et al. (1978) Holz et al. (1989) Hodnett & Abel (1986)
Labor curve	Friedman (1978)	Halfar (1985)
Montevideo units: Index of amplitude/ frequency of labor contractions	Caldeyro-Barcia & Poseiro (1959)	Lederman et al. (1979) Lederman et al. (1985) Lederman et al. (1978)
MULTIDIMENSIONAL FUNCTIONAL STATUS & ADAPTATION MEASURES		
Inventory of Functional Status after Childbirth, (formerly Childbirth Impact Profile): Scale of 36 items about resuming activities after childbirth	Fawcett, Tulman, & Myers (1988)	Tulman & Fawcett (1988)
Postpartum Adaptation Scale: Ninety-six-item scale covering physical, social, and other areas of status	Nichols (1989)	—
HEALTH-ORIENTED & WELL-BEING MEASURES		
Health Responses Scale: Fifty-item scale for illness and wellness during pregnancy	Brown (1986)	Brown (1986) Brown (1987) Brown (1988)
Health Perceptions Questionnaire (32 items) or General Health Index (22 items): Self-report measures of general health	Davies & Ware (1981) Ware (1976)	Engel (1984)* Ferketich & Mercer (1989) Mercer et al. (1988a) Mercer et al. (1988b)
Index of Well-Being: Nine-item scale of life satisfaction	Campbell, Converse, & Rodgers (1976)	Reed (1986)*

Table 7–1
MEASURES/TOOLS FOR THE CONCEPT OF HEALTH STATUS *(Continued)*

Tool	Source Described in	Studies Using Tool
SELF-ESTEEM AND SELF-CONCEPT MEASURES		
Self-esteem Scale: Ten-item self-report scale	Rosenberg (1965, 1979)	Cranley (1981) Mercer & Ferketich (1988) Tilden (1983) Tilden (1984) Norbeck & Tilden (1983) Ferketich & Mercer (1989) Wallace et al. (1986) Roberts (1983) Cox & Smith (1982) Mercer et al. (1988a) Mercer et al. (1988b) Kemp & Page (1987)
Tennessee Self Concept Scale: One-hundred-item, multifactorial scale of self concept	Fitts (1965)	Mercer (1986a) Mercer (1986b) Lee (1982) Mercer et al. (1983) Curry (1983) Brouse (1985) Gaffney (1986) Curry (1982)
Coopersmith Self-Esteem Inventory: Fifty-eight-item scale	Coopersmith (1967)	Koniak-Griffin (1988)

*Data are not from a parent-infant population.

interview, however, they estimate the true prevalence of diagnosable depression to be approximately 13 percent. Thus, depressive symptoms measured by survey tools should not be directly equated with clinical depression according to diagnostic criteria.

METHODOLOGICAL STUDIES OF HEALTH STATUS MEASUREMENT

Hepworth et al. (1987) examined the utility of gynecologic age as a predictor or explanatory variable in research with adolescents. Particularly when chronologic age has little or no variance in a sample, gynecologic age (chronologic age minus age at menarche) may be more useful. Secondary analyses of two data sets gathered on adolescent mothers were used to illustrate the utility of gynecologic age. In both data sets, after partialling out chronologic age, adolescents' maternal behaviors were correlated with gynecologic age at higher-than-chance proportions. Findings supported the proposal that gynecologic age may add variability to age-related analyses when the range of chronologic age is restricted.

Kavanaugh, Meier, and Engstrom (1989) compared intrarater and interrater reliability of infant-weighing procedures on electronic and mechanical scales. Interrater reliability was assessed by having each rater weigh an infant on each scale once before a feeding. Intrarater reliability was assessed by having one rater weigh an infant twice on each scale following a feeding. Intrarater and interrater reliabilities were higher on the electronic scale than on the mechanical scale. Intrarater discrepancies exceeding 5 g were 4 and 34 percent on electronic and mechanical scales, respectively. Interrater discrepancies exceeding 5 g were 0 and 66 percent on electronic and mechanical scales, respectively.

To construct more accurate models of estimating infant birth weight prior to birth, Engstrom and Chen (1984) tested the predictive utility of a set of maternal variables and extrauterine measurements during labor. The predictor set included maternal height, pregravid weight, weight gain during pregnancy, fundal height, McDonald's measurement, uterine width, uterine height, abdominal girth, and station of the fetal head. Data from 44 nulliparous women in labor were used in the predictive equation. Of the actual infant birth weight, 69.6 percent was predicted by a set of five variables: maternal height, weight gain during pregnancy, fundal height, abdominal girth, and station. Accuracy of estimates based on the predictive equation exceeded that of estimates based on palpation of the maternal abdomen.

Marshall (1989) tested the predictive accuracy of two obstetric risk tools in estimating complications in labor. One tool was developed by Hobel, Hyvarinen, Okada, and Oh (1973), and the other was developed by the Maternity Center Association (MCA) in New York. Data from 699 clinic patients assessed for risk at 37 to 42 weeks of gestation were used in the comparison. Sensitivity (true positives) and specificity (true negatives) were 33 and 65 percent, respectively, for the Hobel risk assessment; for the MCA risk assessment, sensitivity and specificity were 88 and 10 percent, respectively. Thus, neither tool was an effective predictor of intrapartal complications among women at term.

Watters and Kristiansen (1989) developed a battery of instruments to evaluate postnatal nursing care. The battery did not directly measure clinical health status; instead, it measured areas, such as patient satisfaction and self-rated maternal competence, likely to influence health outcomes. Tested on 200 women during hospitalization for childbirth, psychometric findings provided support of the reliability and validity of the battery.

SUMMARY OF RESEARCH

SCOPE OF HEALTH STATUS RESEARCH

For the most part, studies dealing with the relation between health status and stress, coping, social support, and health behaviors are located in Chapters 3, 4, 5, and 8, respectively. Health status instrumentation from those studies is included in Table 7–1 to demonstrate the full range of health indicators being used in parent-infant nursing research.

Table 7–2 presents parent-infant studies of health status excluding those already reviewed in Chapters 3 and 5. Descriptive accounts of health status have almost exclusively focused on studying symptom occurrence in childbearing samples. Qualitative studies are rare except for one on childbearing in prison. A number of studies have examined differences in symptoms or health status in subpopulations based on age, gender, and other factors. Fewer studies have examined changes in symptoms or health status over time—across the trimesters of pregnancy, for example. Excluding the relational/predictive studies on stress, social support and health status already considered in Chapters 3 and 5, only a few relational/predictive studies of health status in parent-infant nursing have been done. Seven studies consider the health effects of such interventions as birthing centers, early discharge, nutrition counseling, and adolescent prenatal education.

DESCRIPTIVE RESEARCH

Descriptions of Health Status

Griffith (1983) conducted a survey which included within it measurements of women's physiological and psychological symptom patterns. The convenience sample (N = 579) of women aged 25 to 65 completed a self-

Table 7–2
HEALTH STATUS PARENT-INFANT NURSING RESEARCH

DESCRIPTIVE
Health Status/Symptom Patterns Identified
Abel & von Unwerth (1988), pregnant women
Alley (1984), pregnant women
Brown (1988), expectant couples
Clinton (1986), expectant fathers
Dilorio (1985), pregnant teens
Fawcett & York (1986), expectant couples
Griffith (1983), women aged 25 to 65
Strickland (1987), expectant fathers
Health Status/Symptom Patterns
Shelton & Gill (1989), childbearing in prison
Differences in Health Status/Symptom Patterns
Bernstein et al. (1988), previously infertile vs. never infertile parents
Brown (1987), homemaking vs. employed pregnant women
Fawcett & York (1986), gender and stage of pregnancy groups
Gennaro (1988), mothers of term vs. preterm infants
Halfar (1985), four maternal age groups
Holz, Cooney, & Marchese (1989), two maternal age groups
Mercer, Hackley, & Bostrom (1984), three maternal age groups
Stein (1983), two maternal age groups
Tulman & Fawcett (1988), vaginal vs. cesarean birth mothers
Changes in Health Status/Symptoms over Time
Brooten et al. (1988), mothers of preterm infants
Ferketich & Mercer (1989), fathers
Strickland (1987), expectant fathers
RELATIONSHIPS AMONG VARIABLES/PREDICTIVE MODELS
Brown et al. (1989), contextual factors and prematurity
Clinton (1986), couvade predictors
Gennaro (1986), problem solving and anxiety
Hodnett & Abel (1986), psychological predictors of labor
Longobucco & Freston (1989), couvade predictors
Strickland (1987), couvade predictors
Williams & Williams (1989), malnutrition and child development
INTERVENTION TO ENHANCE HEALTH STATUS OR DECREASE SYMPTOMS
Brooten et al. (1986), early discharge
Hutti & Johnson (1988), birthing room
Littlefield & Adams (1987), birthing center
Norr et al. (1989), early discharge
Scupholme & Kamons (1987), birth center
Slager-Earnest, Hoffman, & Beckmann (1987), adolescent program
Smoke & Grace (1988), adolescent program
Sweeney et al. (1985), nutrition program

report questionnaire. Overall, women between 25 and 34, the prime child-bearing years, experienced more physical and emotional symptoms than older-age groups. Among women between 25 and 34, the following physical symptoms predominated: restless/fidgety (48 percent), sinus trouble (34 percent), backache (34 percent), and trouble sleeping (34 percent). Over half of 25- to 34-year-old women reported experiencing the following emotional symptoms: frequently nervous/tense, anxious or easily upset, sudden mood changes, feel fat and overweight, and feel sad or depressed.

In another study of symptom patterns, DiIorio (1985) examined the phenomenon of nausea and vomiting of pregnancy (NVP) among 78 pregnant adolescents. In this sample, 56 percent of teens reported NVP. It most often occurred in early morning, lasted 2 to 4 hours, and was restricted in duration to 3 months or less. Teenagers most often used lying down as a relief measure for NVP. In this sample, NVP was positively associated with desire for the pregnancy. Alley (1984) also studied nausea in pregnant women. Medical charts were used to identify women who had experienced prenatal nausea and vomiting. Of these, 39 completed questionnaires and interviews about their symptoms. Most women stated that nausea and vomiting occurred in the morning. Most women's symptoms began in the first 2 months of pregnancy. Episodes lasted less than 1 hour for 16 women and 1 to 4 hours for 12 women. Symptoms occurred for less than 4 weeks for some women, but for others they lasted more than 13 weeks. Daily routines of most women were altered to some extent by the symptoms. Preparing meals and odors aggravated the symptoms in over half the women.

In a study of couvade syndrome, Clinton (1986) followed 81 fathers across their partners' pregnancies and postpartum recoveries. The majority of fathers reported at least one couvade symptom per month. Mean numbers of symptoms across the three trimesters of pregnancy were as follows: 9.4, 12.4, and 11.8, respectively. During postpartum, the mean number of symptoms was 7.1. Considering all four data collection points, the most frequently reported couvade symptoms included headache, irritability, restlessness, backache, colds, and nervousness. Similarly, Stickland (1987) reported that somatic symptoms occurred in 59 percent of fathers in early pregnancy, 64 percent at midpregnancy, and 71 percent in late pregnancy. Psychological symptoms were reported by less than half of the sample at early, mid-, and late pregnancy. Most frequent symptoms were backache, difficulty sleeping, irritability, increased appetite, fatigue, and restlessness.

In a cross-sectional sample of mothers and fathers in early and late pregnancy and postpartum, Fawcett and York (1986) surveyed symptom occurrence in 70 couples. Women's most frequently reported symptoms in early pregnancy were feeling tired, increased urination, less active than usual, feeling bloated, increase in appetite, sensitivity to odors, nausea and/or vomiting, feeling anxious, and feeling depressed. Women's most frequent symptoms in late pregnancy included increased urination, feeling tired, indigestion, backache, less active than usual, feeling clumsy/awkward, nausea and/or vomiting, increased appetite, sensitivity to odors, difficulty breathing, and feeling anxious. Among postpartal women, the most frequent symptoms were feeling tired, constipation, feeling anxious, and feeling depressed. Among expectant fathers the most frequent symptoms in early pregnancy were increased appetite and feeling better than usual, and the most frequent symptoms in late pregnancy were craving certain foods and feeling better than usual. During the postpartum period, fathers' most frequent symptoms were feeling tired, less active than usual, feeling anxious, and feeling better than usual.

In a related study, Brown (1988) studied health responses of first-time expectant mothers and fathers (313 couples). Health responses included both somatic and psychological symptoms as well as aspects of well-being. For both men and women well-being responses had higher mean scores than symptom responses. At least 70 percent of women reported they often or always felt pleased and proud, very interested in life, in good spirits, and emotionally stable. Similarly, at least 70 percent of fathers reported they often or always felt stable, pleased and proud, in good spirits, very interested in life, and in control of thoughts, feelings, and behavior. Of note, well-being responses were, overall, negatively related to symptoms.

To assess reproductive tract infections in pregnant women in a low-risk, low-income, nurse-midwifery service, Abel and von Unwerth (1988) studied 117 women at 34 weeks of gestation. Tests for gonorrhea and chlamydia were performed at a routine antepartal clinic visit. Incidence rates for chlamydia and gonorrhea were respectively 22.5 and 1.8 percent. Nineteen of 25 (76 percent) chlamydia-positive women were clinically asymptomatic at the time of testing.

Health Status Experiences and Patterns

Shelton and Gill (1989) conducted an ethnographic study of childbearing of female prisoners. They conducted antenatal and postnatal interviews and reviewed medical records of 26 female inmates. They concluded that all women viewed being pregnant in prison as a negative experience. Most women believed they did not receive good perinatal care. Separation from infants after delivery produced great psychological distress in women. Of the 26 inmates studied, 20 had perinatal complications. The most frequent complication was infection of the reproductive tract.

Differences between Subpopulations in Health Status

In an investigation of differences between three maternal-age groups (15 to 19, 20 to 29, and 30 to 42), Mercer, Hackley, and Bostrom (1984) compared 294 new mothers and their infants over a 12-month period. Maternal health, measured by several indicators, did not differ for the three groups at

4 or 12 months postpartum. At 1 month postpartum, the teenage group reported better health and at 8 months less positive health than the other two maternal-age groups. Infants of the three groups did not differ on health status at birth except that infants of teenage mothers weighed less at birth than infants of older mothers. At 1 month postnatally, infants of teenagers had poorer health than those of the other two groups; at 4 months postnatally, infants of teenagers and mothers 20 to 29 had less favorable health than infants of mothers 30 to 42. There were no differences in infant health among groups at 8 and 12 months. Also, at 1 and 8 months infants of teenage mothers had greater weight increments than infants of older mothers.

To determine if nulliparas over 30 years old have more frequent labor dysfunction, Halfar (1985) contrasted women in four different age groups. Convenience, nonprobability samples of nulliparous women aged 20 to 24, 25 to 29, 30 to 34, and 35 to 40 were selected from labor logs at two hospitals. Examination of labor curves was used to identify three labor dysfunctions: prolonged latent phase, protraction disorders, and arrest disorders. Statistical comparisons showed women aged 30 to 40 had a higher proportion of labor dysfunction than those aged 20 to 29.

In a related study, Stein (1983) conducted a review of nurse-midwifery records to test if women 35 years or older have less positive pregnancy outcomes than younger women. Of 188 women over age 35, 36 transferred to a physician for medical management. Of women over 35 delivered by the nurse-midwifery service, 87.5 percent delivered spontaneously; this percentage compares favorably with that for women less than 35 years, 90.2 percent. Women over 35 had four preterm births (2.6 percent) and four (2.6 percent) small-for-gestational age infants.

In a third study of childbearing and age, Holz, Cooney, and Marchese (1989) compared birth outcomes of younger and older primiparous women. Data from medical records of mothers aged 25 to 34 (n = 201) and 35 to 44 (n = 27) were compared. The two groups did not differ on the following: Apgar scores, type of delivery, length of second stage of labor, or infant birth weight. Older mothers were transferred to the hospital during labor for medical management more frequently than younger mothers.

Bernstein, Mattox, and Kellner (1988) compared previously infertile and never infertile parents on psychological symptoms after each group had successfully delivered healthy infants. The two groups did not differ on total symptoms. On one symptom, depression, differences were found between previously infertile and never infertile mothers; depression was greater among the previously infertile women.

Using a cross-sectional design, Fawcett and York (1986) studied differences in antepartal and postpartal symptoms associated with gender and stage of childbearing. Subjects were married couples: 23 in early pregnancy, 24 in late pregnancy, and 23 in postpartum. The three groups did not differ in age, education, or parity. For women, physical symptoms differed significantly among the three groups: The highest levels were reported by the group in late pregnancy and the lowest levels by the postpartal group. No differences in psychological symptoms or a measure of depression occurred. For men, no differences were found among the three groups on physical or psychological symptoms or depression. When women's and men's symptoms and levels of depression were compared, women consistently had higher levels than men.

In another study, Tulman and Fawcett (1988) compared mothers' return of functional ability after vaginal or cesarean birth. Seventy women who had given birth to full-term infants within the preceding 5 years were surveyed. A greater proportion of vaginal-birth mothers reported regaining their usual energy by 6 weeks after delivery compared to cesarean-birth mothers. Similarly, there were significant differences between groups in assuming infant care and resuming selected household tasks and selected social/community activities. All significant differences favored vaginal-birth mothers. No differences in resuming occupational activities were found.

Gennaro (1988) compared anxiety and depression levels among mothers of term (n = 41) and preterm infants (n = 41). At 1 week postpartum and the next 6 weeks thereafter, mothers completed anxiety and depression measures. In the first postpartum week, mothers of preterm infants had significantly higher depression and anxiety than mothers of term infants. Additional analyses across the 7 weeks of the study, however, failed to show any differences between the two groups on anxiety and depression.

Brown (1987) compared homemaking and employed pregnant women on health status and symptoms. There were low but significant correlations between employment and overall health, somatic symptoms, and psychological/behavioral symptoms. Employed women reported better health, but also more fatigue, leg cramps, and feelings of stress, than homemakers.

Changes in Health Status over Time

To determine what changes in new fathers' health status occur, Ferketich and Mercer (1989) followed fathers from pregnancy to 8 months postpartum. Physical symptoms were reported by 48 percent during pregnancy, 23 percent at 1 month, and 40 percent at 8 months. Psychological symptoms (anxiety and depression) did not increase significantly over time. Levels of perceived health status, however, declined significantly with levels during pregnancy and early postpartum significantly higher than at 8 months postpartum. In a related study of couvade symptoms, Strickland (1987) examined changes in expectant fathers' symptoms in early, mid-, and late pregnancy. Significant increases were found for total and somatic symptoms, but not for psychological symptoms. The interaction of fathers' race and stage of pregnancy was also significant, with black fathers' symptoms decreasing and white fathers' symptoms increasing as pregnancy progressed.

Brooten et al. (1988) examined psychological stress responses of mothers of preterm infants (N = 47) over time. Depression, anxiety, and hostility were measured in the week of infant discharge and when infants were 9 months old (adjusted gestational age). In comparing discharge and 9-month data, mothers' anxiety and depression were significantly higher at discharge. Scores for hostility were not significantly different.

RELATIONAL/PREDICTIVE RESEARCH

To identify risk factors associated with occurrence of couvade syndrome, Clinton (1986) conducted a longitudinal study of 81 expectant fathers from pregnancy to postpartum. Six couvade risk factors were identified in regression analyses: affective involvement in pregnancy, number of children, income, recent health, stress level, and minority status. A number of factors were not predictive of couvade: age, education, pregnancy planning, pregnancy complications, and behavioral involvement in the pregnancy. In another study of couvade, Strickland (1987) measured symptoms and affect (anxiety, depression, and hostility) in 91 fathers at early, mid-, and late pregnancy. Three biographic variables were associated with level of symptoms: planning of pregnancy, social class, and race. Higher numbers of symptoms were associated with unplanned pregnancies, working class status, and black racial group. When controlling for those factors, only anxiety (not depression or hostility) added to predicting total symptoms. In a third study, Longobucco and Freston (1989) studied couvade syndrome in 64 expectant fathers. The aim of their study was to investigate the relation between couvade symptoms and degree of fathers' role preparation. As predicted, presence of couvade was correlated with role preparation.

Gennaro (1986) studied correlates of state anxiety of mothers of preterm infants in the neonatal intensive care unit. Forty mothers were tested during the first week after their infants' admission. Of three correlates of anxiety—past-pregnancy outcomes, infant's physical condition, and maternal problem-solving ability—only problem-solving ability was associated with anxiety. Mothers with higher problem-solving ability reported greater state anxiety.

To study the effects of birth setting and psychological variables on length of labor, Hodnett and Abel (1986) conducted a prospective study of women intending home (n = 80) and hospital births (n = 80). Mothers having subsequent cesarean births were not included in the data analyzed. Anxiety (trait and state in third trimester), arousal seeking, and expected control in labor served as psychological predictors. There were no differences in labor length associated with home versus hospital births. For the total sample, three variables explained 13 percent of the variance in length of latent phase labor: third-trimester anxiety, birth environment, and parity. For the entire sample, over 20 percent of the variance in total labor length was predicted by three variables: parity, arousal seeking, and birth environment. When analyzed by subgroups, there were no significant predictors of length of latent phase labor in primiparas, nor were there any predictors of total labor length for hospital subgroups. In the remaining subgroups, length of labor (latent and total) was predicted by combinations of third trimester anxiety, trait anxiety, expected control, and arousal seeking.

In a study of mild malnutrition and child development, Williams and Williams (1989) studied 340 Filipino children below the 10th percentile for weight. Children's development was assessed with the Metro-Manila Developmental Screening Test. Children were between 2 weeks and 6 years of age. Malnourished children had approximately three times more questionable/abnormal developmental levels compared to the normative sample. The gross motor area was most affected. Five clusters of variables predicted delayed development: child's situation, health, socioeconomic status, mother, and age.

Finally, to determine contextual factors associated with extreme prematurity, Brown et al. (1989) conducted a study of families of very low birth weight infants. Seventy-two families and 79 infants were studied. Mothers of infants were predominantly black and unmarried and had more than one child. Infants' mean birth weight was 1168 g, and mean gestational age was 30 weeks. Infants' hospital stays averaged 52 days at an average cost of $56,341 for hospital fees and $6803 for physicians' fees. The majority of infants' families lived in the inner city, had annual incomes below $7500, and relied on public transportation or the police for transportation. In the 18 months after initial hospital discharge, 24 percent of the infants were rehospitalized and 79 percent had one or more visits to the emergency room with an average of four visits per infant.

INTERVENTION RESEARCH

Two studies addressed the effects of early discharge on maternal or infant status in low-income families. In the first study, Norr, Nacion, and Abramson (1989) examined the health impact of three different discharge patterns with a sample of low-risk, low-income mothers and infants. The three discharge conditions were as follows: (1) early discharge with separation (n = 94)—mother discharged at 24 to 47 hours and infant discharged after 48 hours, (2) conventional discharge (n = 115)—both mother and infant discharged at 48 to 72 hours, and (3) simultaneous early discharge (n =124)—both mother and infant discharged at 24 to 47 hours with home visitation within 3 days after discharge. Maternal and infant status were measured in the second postpartum week. There were no significant differences among the three discharge groups in the frequency of maternal or infant physical health problems. Significant group differences were found for maternal concerns and maternal attachment. Mothers in the simultaneous early discharge group had higher maternal attachment than the early discharge with separation group and lower maternal concerns than the conventional discharge group.

The second early discharge study focused on very low birth weight infants (Brooten et al., 1986). Group assignment was random. The control-group infants (36 mothers and 40 infants) were discharged when they were feeding well, were clinically well, and weighed approximately 2200 g. No home follow-up care occurred for the control group. The early-discharge infants (36 mothers and 39 infants) were discharged before weighing 2200 g if they met selected clinical and family criteria. Prior to discharge, parents of early-discharge infants had weekly contact with a master's degree nurse and had to demonstrate infant care skills. After early discharge, nurse follow-up in the home occurred within 1 week of discharge and at 1, 9, 12, and 18 months. On average, early-discharge infants went home 11.2 days earlier and weighed 200 g less than control-group infants. At 18-month follow-up, the two groups did not differ on the following: number of hospitalizations, number of acute care visits, or developmental level. There was a significant difference in hospital costs that favored the early-discharge group.

Three studies investigated outcomes of alternative birthing environments. First, Scupholme and Kamons (1987) tested whether two groups of women (those voluntarily selecting a birthing center and those assigned to the center because of hospital overcrowding) differed in outcomes. Each group consisted of 148 women matched for parity, age, race, financial status, and education. There were no significant group differences in length of labor, use of analgesia, meconium presence, intrapartum transfer, number of spontaneous deliveries, Apgar scores, birth weights, or transfer for neonatal problems.

In the second study, Hutti and Johnson (1988) compared infant outcomes associated with the use of a traditional delivery room (n = 272) versus an in-hospital birthing room (n = 89). Using retrospective review of medical records, infant Apgar scores were gathered and compared. There were no significant differences in 1- and 5-minute Apgar scores for infants in the two birthing environments.

Third, Littlefield and Adams (1987) examined the effects of alternative perinatal care. In addition to complications, they assessed health locus of control and patient satisfaction. Mothers self-selected either conventional care (n = 78) or alternative care, that is, a birthing center (n = 21), for childbirth. The two groups were similar in social characteristics except for the alternative care group being older and containing proportionately more multiparas than the conventional care group. Mothers in alternative care rated their sense of participation during labor and delivery higher and satisfaction with the delivery environment and experience greater and developed fewer complications than the conventional group. Admission criteria for alternative care, however, may have influenced the frequency of complications in that group. The alternative care group did not show any gains in health locus of control compared to the conventional care group.

Three other interventions, two in teenage prenatal programs and one in nutrition, also focused on assessing health outcomes. First, Slager-Earnest, Hoffman, and Beckmann (1987) evaluated the effects of a special prenatal education program for adolescents by comparing 50 program attenders with 50 nonattenders. The program consisted of seven classes covering pregnancy information and preparation for childbirth and parenting with special focus on issues of pregnant adolescents. Both obstetric and postnatal complications were fewer for program attenders than for nonattenders. Attenders and nonattenders were subsequently divided into 13- to 15- and 16- to 18-year age subgroups for further analysis. At both age levels, findings were still significant, and again attendees, regardless of age, had fewer obstetric and postnatal complications than attenders.

In another adolescent study, Smoke and Grace (1988) evaluated the effectiveness of a prenatal care and education program on knowledge and health outcomes. Two groups of adolescents were compared: the control group receiving prenatal care from the city health department (n = 46) and the experimental group receiving prenatal care from an adolescent service at a university hospital (n = 70). The experimental group also received nine class sessions focused on prenatal education and child care. Adolescents self-selected their sites for prenatal care. The two groups differed on race, education, and length of gestation at their first prenatal visit. Although both groups had equivalent knowledge of pregnancy and child care at the pretest, the experimental group had greater knowledge at posttest. The groups also differed on maternal and fetal complications and amount of medication used in labor, but not on incidence of low birth weight.

To measure the effects of a special nutrition counseling program, Sweeney et al. (1985) assigned pregnant clinic patients to either a control (n = 25) or experimental group (n = 18). The nutrition program took place during the latter half of pregnancy and included an individualized nutrition prescription for protein and calories and nutritional counseling. Women in the experimental group ingested significantly more protein, but not calories, than those in the control group. When pregnancy outcomes were compared, there were no significant group differences in any of the following: maternal weight gain, maternal complications, infant birth weight, and infant gestational age at birth.

FUTURE RESEARCH DIRECTIONS

Reviewing the instruments and measures used to assess health status in parent-infant nursing research, it is clear that investigators have been preoccupied with symptoms and morbidity. Key affective symptoms have been anxiety and depression. Investigators have studied such attributes of "positive" health as self-esteem and well-being far less often. Indeed, of descriptive surveys, Brown's (1988) research stands out as one of the few studies to give attention to wellness-oriented aspects of health. Perhaps because pregnancy and childbearing are assumed to be normal and healthy, studying positive health and well-being seems redundant. As a result, however, more is known about symptoms and morbidity than about well-being. To begin to redress the imbalance, nurses need a greater assortment of instruments suited to expectant and new parents that measure more positive dimensions of health. First, however, parent-infant nurse researchers must move conceptually beyond the clinical model of health (Chapter 6).

Intervention studies related to health status of parents and infants vary greatly in their methodological rigor. Some studies are impressive in their rigor; an example is Brooten et al. (1986). Other studies primarily consist of evaluations of practice innovations of particular local interest. Publication, however, necessarily makes the latter accessible nationally and beyond. To advance the science of parent-infant nursing and not mislead clinicians who read journals to improve their practice, it is essential that interventions be well designed, well executed, and well written. To maintain high standards critical to clinical work, investigators conducting interventions should actively seek out critique and consultation from colleagues knowledgeable in statistics, design, and measurement before beginning clinical intervention studies. Further, well-designed intervention tests with positive effects on one setting still need corroboration at other sites to establish the robustness of their effects. In this line, Anderson (1989) has called for multisite, controlled clinical trials for interventions, such as self-regulatory care, to enhance maternal and infant health and well-being.

REFERENCES

Aaronson, L. S., & Macnee, C. L. (1989). The relationship between weight gain and nutrition in pregnancy. *Nursing Research, 38,* 223–227.

Abel, E., & von Unwerth, L. (1988). Asymptomatic chlamydia during pregnancy. *Research in Nursing & Health, 11,* 359–365.

Alley, N. M. (1984). Morning sickness: The client's perspective. *Journal of Obstetric, Gynecologic, and Neonatal Nursing, 13,* 185–189.

Anderson, C. J. (1981). Enhancing reciprocity between mother and neonate. *Nursing Research, 30,* 89–93.

Anderson, G. C. (1989). Risk in mother-infant separation postbirth. *Image, 21,* 196–199.

Apgar, V. (1966). The newborn (Apgar) scoring system. *Pediatric Clinics of North America, 13,* 645–650.

Avant, K. C. (1981). Anxiety as a potential factor affecting maternal attachment. *Journal of Obstetric, Gnyecologic, and Neonatal Nursing, 10,* 416–419.

Barnard, K. E., Hammond, M. A., Sumner,

G. A., Kang, R., Johnson-Crowley, N., Snyder, C., Spietz, A., Blackburn, S., Brandt, P., & Magyary, D. (1987). Helping parents with preterm infants: Field test of a protocol. *Early Child Development and Care, 27,* 255-290.

Barnard, K. E., Magyary, D., Sumner, G., Booth, C. L., Mitchell, S. K., & Spieker, S. (1988). Prevention of parenting alterations for women with low social support. *Psychiatry, 51*(3), 248-253.

Beck, A. T., Ward, C. H., Mendelson, M., Mock, J., & Erbaugh, J. (1961). An inventory for measuring depression. *Archives of General Psychiatry, 4,* 561-571.

Bee, H. L., Barnard, K. E., Eyres, S. J., Gray, C. A., Hammond, M. A., Spietz, A. L., Snyder, C., & Clark, B. (1982). Prediction of IQ and language skill from perinatal status, child performance, family characteristics, and mother-infant interaction. *Child Development, 53,* 1134-1156.

Bernstein, J., Mattox, J. H., & Kellner, R. (1988). Psychological status of previously infertile couples after a successful pregnancy. *Journal of Obstetric, Gynecologic, and Neonatal Nursing, 17,* 404-408.

Blank, D. M. (1986). Relating mothers' anxiety and perception to infant satiety, anxiety, and feeding behavior. *Nursing Research, 35,* 347-351.

Bonachick, P. (1984). Progressive relaxation training in cardiac rehabilitation: Effect on psychological variables. *Nursing Research, 33,* 283-287.

Booth, C. L., Barnard, K. E., Mitchell, S. K., & Spieker, S. J. (1987). Successful intervention with multi-problem mothers: Effects on the mother-infant relationship. *Infant Mental Health Journal, 8,* 288-306.

Booth, C. L., Mitchell, S. K., Barnard, K. E., & Spieker, S. J. (1989). Development of maternal social skills in multiproblem families: Effects on the mother-child relationship. *Developmental Psychology, 25,* 403-412.

Bradburn, N. M. (1969). *The structure of psychological well-being.* Chicago: Aldine.

Brooten, D., Gennaro, S., Brown, L. P., Butts, P., Gibbons, A. L., Bakewell-Sachs, S., & Kumar, S. P. (1988). Anxiety, depression, and hostility in mothers of preterm infants. *Nursing Research, 37,* 213-216.

Brooten, D., Kumar, S., Brown, L. P., Butts, P., Finkler, S. A., Bakewell-Sachs, S., Gibbons, A., & Delivoria-Papadopoulos, M. (1986). A randomized clinical trial of early hospital discharge and home follow-up of very-low-birth-weight infants. *New England Journal of Medicine, 315,* 934-939.

Brouse, A. J. (1988). Easing the transition to the maternal role. *Journal of Advanced Nursing, 13,* 167-172.

Brouse, S. H. (1985). Effect of gender role identity on patterns of feminine and self-concept scores from late pregnancy to early postpartum. *Advances in Nursing Science, 7*(3), 32-48.

Brown, L. P., Brooten, D., Kumar, S., Butts, P., Finkler, S., Bakewell-Sachs, S., Gibbons, A., & Delivoria-Papadapoulos, M. (1989). A sociodemographic profile of families of low birth weight infants. *Western Journal of Nursing Research, 11,* 520-532.

Brown, M. A. (1986). Social support, stress, and health: A comparison of expectant mothers and fathers. *Nursing Research, 35,* 72-76.

Brown, M. A. (1987). Employment during pregnancy: Influences on women's health and social support. *Health Care of Women International, 8*(2-3), 151-167.

Brown, M. A. (1988). A comparison of health responses in expectant mothers and fathers. *Western Journal of Nursing Research, 10,* 527-549.

Brown, M. M. (1979). Parental concerns about infant behavioral organization from term to 4 months. In G. C. Anderson, B. Raff, M. Duxbury, & P. Carroll (Eds.), *Newborn behavioral organization: Nursing research and implications.* New York: Alan R. Liss for the March of Dimes Birth Defects Foundation. *Birth Defects, Original Article Series, 15*(7), 27-42.

Caldeyro-Barcia, R., & Poseiro, J. (1959). Oxytocin and contractility of the pregnant human uterus. *Annals of the New York Academy of Science, 75,* 813-830.

Campbell, A., Converse, P. E., & Rodgers, W. L. (1976). *The quality of American life: Perceptions, evaluations and satisfactions.* New York: Russell Sage Foundation.

Clinton, J. F. (1986). Expectant fathers at risk

for couvade. *Nursing Research, 35,* 290-295.

Consolvo, C. A. (1986). Relieving parental anxiety in the care-by-parent unit. *Journal of Obstetric, Gynecologic, and Neonatal Nursing, 15,* 154-159.

Coopersmith, S. (1967). *The antecedents of self-esteem.* New York: Freeman.

Cox, B. E., & Smith, E. C. (1982). The mother's self-esteem after a cesarean delivery. *MCN, The American Journal of Maternal/Child Nursing, 7,* 309-314.

Cranley, M. S. (1981). Roots of attachment: The relationship of parents with their unborn. In R. P. Lederman, B. S. Raff, & P. Carroll (Eds.), *Perinatal parental behavior: Nursing research and implications for newborn health.* New York: Liss. March of Dimes Birth Defects Foundation. *Birth Defects, Original Article Series, 17*(6), 59-83.

Curry, M. A. (1982). Maternal attachment behavior and the mother's self-concept: The effect of early skin-to-skin contact. *Nursing Research, 31,* 73-78.

Curry, M. A. (1983). Variables related to adaptation to motherhood in "normal" primiparous women. *Journal of Obstetric, Gynecologic, and Neonatal Nursing, 12,* 115-121.

Davies, A. R., & Ware, J. E. (1981). *Measuring health perceptions in the health insurance experiment.* Santa Monica, CA: Rand.

Davis, T., & Jensen, L. (1988). Identifying depression in medical patients. *Image, 20,* 191-195.

Derogatis, L. (1975a). *Affects balance scale.* Baltimore, MD: Clinical Psychometric Research.

Derogatis, L. (1975b). *Brief symptom inventory.* Available from L. Derogatis, 28 Wine Spring Lane, Baltimore, MD 21204.

Derogatis, L. R. (1977). *SCL-90-R: Administration, scoring and procedures manual-I.* Baltimore, MD: Clinical Psychometric Research.

DiIorio, C. (1985). First trimester nausea in pregnant teenagers: Incidence, characteristics, intervention. *Nursing Research, 34,* 372-374.

Dorinsky, N. L. (1984). Brief reports: The effects of a regular aerobic exercise program on selected measures of the stress response. *Health Care for Women International, 5,* 459-462.

Dubowitz, L. M. S., Dubowitz, V., & Goldberg, C. (1970). Clinical assessment of gestational age in the newborn infant. *Pediatrics, 77,* 1-10.

Engel, N. S. (1984). On the vicissitudes of health appraisal. *Advances in Nursing Science, 7*(1), 12-23.

Engstrom, J. L., & Chen, E. H. (1984). Prediction of birth weight by the use of extrauterine measurements during labor. *Research in Nursing and Health, 7,* 314-323.

Fawcett, J., Tulman, L., & Myers, S. T. (1988). Development of the inventory of functional status after childbirth. *Journal of Nurse-Midwifery, 33,* 252-260.

Fawcett, J., & York, R. (1986). Spouses' physical and psychological symptoms during pregnancy and the postpartum. *Nursing Research, 35,* 144-148.

Fehring, R. J. (1983). Effects of biofeedback-aided relaxation on the psychological stress symptoms of college students. *Nursing Research, 32,* 362-366.

Ferketich, S. L., & Mercer, R. T. (1989). Men's health status during pregnancy and early fatherhood. *Research in Nursing & Health, 12,* 137-148.

Fitts, W. H. (1965). *Tennessee self concept scale: Manual.* Nashville, TN: Counselor Recordings and Tests.

Friedman, E. A. (1978). *Labor: Clinical evaluation and management.* New York: Appleton-Century-Crofts.

Gaffney, K. F. (1986). Maternal-fetal attachment in relation to self-concept and anxiety. *Maternal-Child Nursing Journal, 15,* 91-101.

Gennaro, S. (1986). Anxiety and problem-solving ability in mothers of premature infants. *Journal of Obstetric, Gynecologic, and Neonatal Nursing, 15,* 160-164.

Gennaro, S. (1988). Postpartal anxiety and depression in mothers of term and preterm infants. *Nursing Research, 37,* 82-85.

Gibby, N. W. (1988). Relationship between fetal movement charting and anxiety in low-risk pregnant women. *Journal of Nurse-Midwifery, 33,* 185-188.

Glazer, G. L. (1980). Anxiety levels and concerns among pregnant women. *Research in Nursing and Health, 3,* 107-113.

Glazer, G. L., & Abraham, I. (1987). Obstetrical complications checklist: Description, factor analysis, and reliability. *Health Care for Women International, 8,* 305-316.

Gotlib, I. H., Whiffen, V. E., Mount, J. H., Milne, K., & Cordy, N. I. (1989). Prevalence rates and demographic characteristics associated with depression in pregnancy and the postpartum. *Journal of Consulting and Clinical Psychology, 57,* 269-274.

Griffith, J. W. (1983). Women's stress responses and coping patterns according to age groups: 2. *Issues in Health Care of Women, 6,* 327-340.

Halfar, M. M. (1985). Frequency of labor dysfunction in nulliparas over the age of thirty. *Journal of Nurse-Midwifery, 30,* 333-339.

Hangsleben, K. L. (1983). Transition to fatherhood: An exploratory study. *Journal of Obstetric, Gynecologic, and Neonatal Nursing, 12,* 265-270.

Hepworth, J. T., Bell, L., Feller, C., Hanson, D., Sands, D., & Muhlenkamp, A. (1987). Gynecologic age: Prediction in adolescent female research. *Nursing Research, 36,* 392-394.

Hobel, C. J., Hyvarinen, M. A., Okada, D. M., & Oh, W. (1973). Prenatal and intrapartum high-risk screening. *American Journal of Obstetrics and Gynecology, 117,* 1-9.

Hodnett, E. D., & Abel, S. M. (1986). Person-environment interaction as a determinant of labor length variables. *Health Care for Women International, 7,* 341-356.

Hodnett, E. D., & Osborn, R. W. (1989). Effects of continuous intrapartum professional support on childbirth outcomes. *Research in Nursing and Health, 12,* 289-297.

Holz, K., Cooney, C., & Marchese, T. (1989). Outcomes of mature primiparas in an out-of-hospital birth center. *Journal of Nurse-Midwifery, 34,* 185-189.

Humenick, S. S., & Bugen, L. A. (1981). Correlates of parent-infant interaction: An exploratory study. In R. P. Lederman, B. S. Raff, & P. Carroll (Eds.), *Perinatal parental behavior: Nursing research and implications for newborn health.* New York: Liss. March of Dimes Birth Defects Foundation. *Birth Defects, Original Article Series, 17*(6), 181-199.

Hutti, M. H., & Johnson, J. B. (1988). Newborn apgar scores of babies born in birthing rooms vs. traditional delivery rooms. *Applied Nursing Research, 1*(2), 68-71.

Kavanaugh, K., Meier, P. P., & Engstrom, J. L. (1989). Reliability of weighing procedures for preterm infants. *Nursing Research, 38,* 178-179.

Kearney, M., & Cronenwett, L. R. (1989). Perceived perinatal complications and childbirth satisfaction. *Applied Nursing Research, 2,* 140-142.

Kemp, V. H., & Page, C. (1987). Maternal self-esteem and prenatal attachment in high-risk pregnancy. *Maternal-Child Nursing Journal, 16,* 195-206.

Kirgis, C. A., Woolsey, D. B., & Sullivan, J. J. (1977). Predicting infant Apgar scores. *Nursing Research, 26,* 439-442.

Koniak-Griffin, D. (1988). The relationship between social support, self-esteem, and maternal-fetal attachment in adolescents. *Research in Nursing and Health, 11,* 269-278.

Lederman, E., Lederman, R. P., Work, B. A., & McCann, D. S. (1981). Maternal psychological and physiologic correlates of fetal-newborn health status. *American Journal of Obstetrics and Gynecology, 139,* 956-958.

Lederman, R. P., Lederman, E., Work, B. A., & McCann, D. S. (1978). The relationship of maternal anxiety, plasma catecholamines, and plasma cortisol to progress in labor. *American Journal of Obstetrics and Gynecology, 132,* 495-500.

Lederman, R. P., Lederman, E., Work, B. A., & McCann, D. S. (1979). Relationship of psychological factors in pregnancy to progress in labor. *Nursing Research, 28,* 94-97.

Lederman, R. P., Lederman, E., Work, B. A., & McCann, D. S. (1985). Anxiety and epinephrine in multiparous women in labor: Relationship to duration of labor and fetal heart rate pattern. *American Journal of Obstetrics and Gynecology, 153,* 870-877.

Lee, G. (1982). Relationship of self-concept during late pregnancy to neonatal perception and parenting profile. *Journal of Obstetric, Gynecologic, and Neonatal Nursing, 11,* 186–190.

Littlefield, V. M., & Adams, B. N. (1987). Patient participation in alternative perinatal care: Impact on satisfaction and health locus of control. *Research in Nursing & Health, 10,* 139–148.

Littman, B., & Parmelee, A. (1974a). *Manual for obstetrical complications.* Los Angeles: UCLA, Department of Pediatrics.

Littman, B., & Parmelee, A. (1974b). *Manual for postnatal complications.* Los Angeles: UCLA, Department of Pediatrics.

Longobucco, D. C., & Freston, M. S. (1989). Relation of somatic symptoms to degree of paternal-role preparation of first-time expectant fathers. *Journal of Obstetric, Gynecologic, and Neonatal Nursing, 18,* 482–488.

Lubin, B. (1967). *Manual for the depression adjective check lists.* San Diego, CA: Educational and Industrial Testing Service.

Marshall, V. A. (1989). A comparison of two obstetric risk assessment tools. *Journal of Nurse-Midwifery, 34,* 3–7.

McDowell, I., & Newell, C. (1987). *Measuring health: A guide to rating scales and questionnaires.* New York: Oxford.

McNair, D., Lorr, M., & Droppleman, L. F. (1971). *Profile of mood states.* San Diego, CA: Educational and Industrial Testing Service.

Meleis, A. I., & Swendsen, L. A. (1978). Role supplementation: An empirical test of a nursing intervention. *Nursing Research, 27,* 11–18.

Mercer, R. T. (1986a). Predictors of maternal role attainment at one year postbirth. *Western Journal of Nursing Research, 8,* 9–25.

Mercer, R. T. (1986b). The relationship of developmental variables to maternal behavior. *Research in Nursing & Health, 9,* 25–33.

Mercer, R. T., & Ferketich, S. L. (1988). Stress and social support as predictors of anxiety and depression during pregnancy. *Advances in Nursing Science, 10*(2), 26–39.

Mercer, R. T., Ferketich, S. L., DeJoseph, J., May, K. A., & Sollid, D. (1988a). Effect of stress on family functioning during pregnancy. *Nursing Research, 37,* 268–275.

Mercer, R. T., Ferketich, S., May, K., DeJoseph, J., & Sollid, D. (1988b). Further exploration of maternal and paternal fetal attachment. *Research in Nursing & Health, 11,* 83–95.

Mercer, R. T., Hackley, K. C., & Bostrom, A. G. (1983). Relationship of psychosocial and perinatal variables to perception of childbirth. *Nursing Research, 32,* 202–207.

Mercer, R. T., Hackley, K. C., & Bostrom, A. (1984). Adolescent motherhood. *Journal of Adolescent Health Care, 5*(1), 7–13.

Mitchell, S. K., Bee, H. L., Hammond, M. A., & Barnard, K. E. (1985). Prediction of school and behavior problems in children followed from birth to age eight. In W. K. Frankenburg, R. N. Emde, & J. W. Sullivan (Eds.), *Early identification of children at risk* (pp. 117–132). New York: Plenum.

Muhlenkamp, A. F., & Joyner, J. A. (1986). Arthritic patients' self-reported affective states and their caregivers' perceptions. *Nursing Research, 35,* 24–27.

Nichols, F. H. (1989). The use of an assessment tool to measure postpartum adaptation. (Abstract) *MCN, The American Journal of Maternal/Child Nursing, 14,* 273.

Norbeck, J. S., & Anderson, N. J. (1989a). Life stress, social support, and anxiety in mid- and late-pregnancy among low income women. *Research in Nursing and Health, 12,* 281–287.

Norbeck, J. S., & Anderson, N. J. (1989b). Psychosocial predictors of pregnancy outcomes in low-income black, hispanic, and white women. *Nursing Research, 38,* 204–209.

Norbeck, J. S., & Tilden, V. P. (1983). Life stress, social support, and emotional disequilibrium in complications of pregnancy: A prospective, multivariate study. *Journal of Health and Social Behavior, 24,* 30–46.

Norr, K. F., Nacion, K. W., & Abramson, R. (1989). Early discharge with home follow-up: Impacts on low-income mothers and infants. *Journal of Obstetric, Gynecologic, and Neonatal Nursing, 18,* 133–141.

Northouse, L. L., & Swain, M. A. (1987). Adjustment of patients and husbands to the initial impact of breast cancer. *Nursing Research, 36,* 221-225.

Nuckolls, K. B., Cassel, J., & Kaplan, B. (1972). Psychosocial assets, life crisis, and the prognosis of pregnancy. *American Journal of Epidemiology, 95,* 431-441.

Radloff, L. (1977). The CES-D scale: A self-report depression scale for research in the general population. *Journal of Applied Psychological Measurement, 1,* 385-401.

Reed, P. G. (1986). Religiousness among terminally ill and healthy adults. *Research in Nursing and Health, 9,* 35-41.

Riesch, S. K. (1984). Occupational commitment and the quality of maternal infant interaction. *Research in Nursing and Health, 7,* 295-503.

Roberts, F. B. (1983). Infant behavior and the transition to parenthood. *Nursing Research, 32,* 213-217.

Rosenberg, M. (1965). *Society and the adolescent self-image.* Princeton, NJ: Princeton University Press.

Rosenberg, M. (1979). *Conceiving the self.* New York: Basic Books.

Schodt, C. M. (1989). Parental-fetal attachment and couvade: A study of patterns of human-environment integrality. *Nursing Science Quarterly, 2*(2), 88-97.

Schraeder, B. D. (1986). Developmental progress in very low birth weight infants during the first year of life. *Nursing Research, 35,* 237-242.

Schraeder, B. D., Rappaport, J., & Courtwright, L. (1987). Preschool development of very low birthweight infants. *Image, 19,* 174-177.

Schroeder-Zwelling, E., & Hock, E. (1986). Maternal anxiety and sensitive mothering behavior in diabetic and nondiabetic women. *Research in Nursing and Health, 9,* 249-255.

Scupholme, A., & Kamons, A. S. (1987). Are outcomes compromised when mothers are assigned to birth centers for care? *Journal of Nurse-Midwifery, 32,* 211-215.

Shelton, B. J., & Gill, D. G. (1989). Childbearing in prison: A behavioral analysis. *Journal of Obstetric, Gynecologic, and Neonatal Nursing, 18,* 301-308.

Sibley, L., Ruhling, R. O., Cameron-Foster, J., Christensen, C., & Bolen, T. (1981). Swimming and physical fitness during pregnancy. *Journal of Nurse-Midwifery, 26,* 3-12.

Slager-Earnest, S. E., Hoffman, S. J., & Beckmann, C. J. A. (1987). Effects of a specialized prenatal adolescent program on maternal and infant outcomes. *Journal of Obstetric, Gynecologic, and Neonatal Nursing, 16,* 422-429.

Smith, J. A. (1981). The idea of health: A philosophical inquiry. *Advances in Nursing Science, 3*(3), 43-50.

Smith, J. A. (1983). *The idea of health.* New York: Teachers College Press.

Smoke, J., & Grace, M. C. (1988). Effectiveness of prenatal care and education for pregnant adolescents: Nurse-midwifery intervention and team approach. *Journal of Nurse-Midwifery, 33,* 178-184.

Spielberger, C. D., Gorsuch, R. L., & Lushene, R. E. (1970). *Manual for the state-trait anxiety inventory.* Palo Alto, CA: Consulting Psychologists Press.

Spielberger, C. D., Gorsuch, R. L., Lushene, R., Vagg, P. R., & Jacobs, G. A. (1983). *Manual for the state-trait anxiety inventory.* Palo Alto, CA: Consulting Psychologists Press.

Stein, A. (1983). Pregnancy in gravidas over age 35 years. *Journal of Nurse-Midwifery, 28*(1), 17-20.

Strickland, O. L. (1987). The occurrence of symptoms in expectant fathers. *Nursing Research, 36,* 184-189.

Sweeney, C., Smith, H., Foster, J. C., Place, J. C., Specht, J., Kochenour, N. K., & Prater, B. M. (1985). Effects of a nutrition intervention program during pregnancy. *Journal of Nurse-Midwifery, 30,* 149-158.

Taffel, S. M. (1986). Association between maternal weight gain and outcome of pregnancy. *Journal of Nurse-Midwifery, 31,* 78-81.

Taylor, J. A. (1953). A personality scale of manifest anxiety. *Journal of Personality and Social Psychology, 48,* 285-290.

Tilden, V. P. (1983). The relation of life stress and social support to emotional disequilibrium during pregnancy. *Research in Nursing and Health, 6,* 167-174.

Tilden, V. P. (1984). The relation of selected

psychosocial variables to single status of adult women during pregnancy. *Nursing Research, 33,* 102-107.

Trotter, C. W., Chang, P., & Thompson, T. (1982). Perinatal factors and the developmental outcome of preterm infants. *Journal of Obstetric, Gynecologic, and Neonatal Nursing, 11,* 83-89.

Tulman, L., & Fawcett, J. (1988). Return of functional ability after childbirth. *Nursing Research, 37,* 77-81.

Ventura, J. N. (1986). Parent coping, a replication. *Nursing Research, 35,* 77-80.

Wallace, A. M., Boyer, D. B., Dan, A., & Holm, K. (1986). Aerobic exercise, maternal self-esteem, and physical discomforts during pregnancy. *Journal of Nurse-Midwifery, 31,* 255-262.

Ware, J. E. (1976). Scales for measuring general health perceptions. *Health Services Research, 11*(4), 396-415.

Ware, J. E. (1984). Methodological considerations in the selection of health status assessment procedures. In N. K. Wenger, M. E. Mattson, C. D. Furberg, & J. Elinson (Eds.), *Assessment of quality of life in clinical trials of cardiovascular therapies* (pp. 87-111). New York: LeJacq.

Ware, J. E., Brook, R. H., Davies, A. R., & Lohr, K. N. (1981). Choosing measures of health status for individuals in general populations. *American Journal of Public Health, 71*(6), 620-625.

Watters, N. E., & Kristiansen, C. M. (1989). Evaluating hospital postnatal nursing care: Development of the instruments. *Research in Nursing & Health, 12,* 299-305.

Weaver, R. H., & Cranley, M. S. (1983). An exploration of paternal-fetal attachment behavior. *Nursing Research, 32,* 68-72.

White, M., & Dawson, C. (1981). The impact of the at-risk infant on family solidarity. In R. P. Lederman, B. S. Raff, & P. Carroll (Eds.), *Perinatal parental behavior: Nursing research and implications for newborn health.* New York: Liss. March of Dimes Birth Defects Foundation. *Birth Defects, Original Article Series, 17*(6), 253-284.

White-Traut, R. C., & Nelson, M. N. (1988). Maternally administered tactile, auditory, visual, and vestibular stimulation: Relationship to later interactions between mothers and premature infants. *Research in Nursing & Health, 11,* 31-39.

Williams, P. D., & Williams, A. R. (1989). Mild malnutrition and child development in the Philippines. *Western Journal of Nursing Research, 11,* 310-319.

Woods, N. F. (1981). The health diary as an instrument for nursing research: Problems and promise. *Western Journal of Nursing Research, 3,* 76-92.

Zuckerman, M., & Lubin, B. (1965). *Manual for the affect adjective check list.* San Diego, CA: Educational and Industrial Testing Service.

CHAPTER 8

Parent-Infant Nursing Research on Health Behaviors during Pregnancy and Early Parenting

DEFINITIONS AND DESCRIPTIONS OF HEALTH BEHAVIORS

DEFINING HEALTH BEHAVIORS

As with health status, most research undertaken by nurses has approached definition of health behaviors at the operational level. Therefore, the following working definition of health behaviors was used to guide the selection of research included in this chapter: (1) the various practices—

both positive and negative—and accompanying beliefs related specifically to promoting health and well-being and preventing disease or misfortune during pregnancy, childbirth, postpartum, and infancy, (2) health care patterns—both positive and negative—that influence general health during pregnant and nonpregnant states, and (3) decision making related to the extent and type of health care used and specific options selected, such as circumcision, breast feeding, and amniocentesis. Health care patterns related to general health were limited to parents during the childbearing and very early childrearing phases. Included within childbearing and associated practices were traditional scientific studies of health behaviors, as well as ethnographic studies of folk and population-specific health care practices, patterns, and beliefs.

THEORETICAL MODELS OF HEALTH BEHAVIORS

Several parent-infant investigators explicitly used theoretical models of health behaviors that served as a framework for model-testing studies. The health belief model (Chapter 6) and a modification of it were used in two studies (Kviz, Dawkins, & Ervin, 1985; Sweeney & Gulino, 1987). Also, Cox (Cox, Sullivan, & Roghmann, 1984; Cox & Roghmann, 1984) provided two reports of research using the interactional model of client health behavior (Cox, 1980, Chap. 6).

A third model guiding research about health behaviors was Rogers' (1983) decision-process model used by Sullivan and Jones (1986) to study adoption of breast feeding as an innovation. A fourth health behavior framework was presented in Hill and Humenick's (1989) model of determinants and indicators of insufficient milk supply among breast-feeding mothers. Among direct and indirect influences on milk supply, maternal breast-feeding behaviors served as one of three direct influences.

At a still higher level of analysis, several authors explicitly critiqued ethical and paradigmatic approaches to maternal and infant health care. Fry (1987) considered ethical dimensions of policy related to mandatory diagnostic screening of pregnant women for fetal pathology. In a related vein, Sandelowski (1988) identified conflicting paradigms at work in the application of reproductive technology, especially ultrasonography and amniocentesis, to maternal-fetal care.

MEASUREMENT

GENERAL STRATEGIES

Depending on the type of behavior of interest, a variety of means can be used to measure health behaviors. If overall or general health behaviors and beliefs are of interest, they can be captured most efficiently by questionnaires or structured interview items. If a particular health behavior or belief is of interest, then a measure suited to reliably and validly measuring it should be used. For example, a study of nutritional intake or alcohol consumption should not rely on one or two items in an overall survey; it is better measured by items which are specifically designed to measure the complexity of those behaviors accurately. If investigators are interested in the daily health behavior patterns of persons, other methods such as daily checklists or diaries may be most applicable. Finally, for some behaviors, such as seeking prenatal care, medical records may be of use to determine initiation and frequency of health care utilization.

SPECIFIC TOOLS

Table 8–1 contains measures, both general and specific, used in parent-infant nursing research to study health behaviors and health beliefs. A few of the measures are not pregnancy-specific; instead, they focus on behaviors and beliefs related to general health. Of studies focused on specific behaviors, the most frequent are operational measures—duration, amount, and perceptions—related to breast-feeding success. Although some studies of health behaviors are located in other chapters, for completeness their instrumentation is included in Table 8–1 as well.

SUMMARY OF RESEARCH

SCOPE OF HEALTH BEHAVIOR RESEARCH

Table 8–2 presents parent-infant research related to health behaviors. That research encompasses descriptive, relational-predictive, and intervention studies of a wide range of health behaviors during pregnancy and early parenting. (*Note:* Studies that deal with parental needs and concerns and information desired during pregnancy through postpartum are placed in Chapters 11 to 13. Also, studies that deal with social support and health behaviors are located in Chapter 5, on social support.)

In addition, nurse investigators have also studied health behaviors from a cultural perspective to provide insights into cultural belief systems and practices related to pregnancy, childbirth, postpartum, and infant care. Studies which investigate health behaviors from a cultural perspective are summarized in Table 8–3. The samples presented in Table 8–3 resided in Africa, Asia, and North America. Groups living in the United States included immigrants as well as US-born persons.

Table 8–1
MEASURES/TOOLS FOR THE CONCEPTS OF HEALTH BEHAVIORS AND BELIEFS

Tool	Source Described in	Studies Using Tool
GENERAL HEALTH BEHAVIOR AND BELIEF MEASURES		
Health-Promoting Lifestyle Profile: Six-subscale tool for health promotion	Walker, Sechrist, & Pender (1987)	Walker (1989a, 1989b)
Prenatal Support and Drinking Survey: Tool with support and drinking items	Coleman, Ryan, & Williamson (1989)	Coleman et al. (1989)
Health Behavior Questionnaire: Tool for health behavior during pregnancy	Albrecht & Rankin (1989)	Albrecht & Rankin (1989)
Dependent Care Agent Questionnaires: Thirty-nine-item scale of maternal child care practices	Moore & Gaffney (1989)	—
Personal Health Inventory: Twenty-four-item tool of health practices	Lewallen (1989)	Lewallen (1989)
Preventive Health Care Behavior Index: Ten-item scale	Parken (1978)	Parken (1978)
SPECIFIC HEALTH BEHAVIOR/BELIEF MEASURES		
Nutritional intake: Weighted score based on dietary recall; computer analysis of recall	Aaronson & Macnee (1989) Brooten et al. (1987)	Aaronson & Macnee (1989) Brooten et al. (1987)
Caffeine intake		Brooten et al. (1987) Aaronson (1989)
Alcohol consumption		Brooten et al. (1987) Aaronson (1989) Coleman et al. (1989) Stephens (1985)
Cigarette use		Brooten et al. (1987) Aaronson (1989)
Breast feeding: Frequency, duration, amount, reasons for selecting, etc.		Coreil & Murphy (1988) Janke (1988)

		Sullivan & Jones (1986)
		Morse & Bottorff (1989)
		Hellings (1985)
		Moon & Humenick (1989)
		Whitley (1978)
		Kaufman & Hall (1989)
		Sweeney & Gulino (1987)
		Yoos (1985)
		Hall (1978)
		Hill (1987)
		Wiles (1984)
		Evans et al. (1986)
Breastfeeding Knowledge Questionnaire: Thirty-two-item parallel forms scale	Hill (1987)	Hill (1987)
Breastfeeding Attitude Questionnaire: Eighteen-item scale of attitudes toward breast feeding	Baisch et al. (1989)	Baisch et al. (1989)
Prenatal care		Young et al. (1989)
Well-baby clinic visits		Kviz et al. (1985)
Provider selection		Brien et al. (1983)
Amniocentesis		Cox & Roghmann (1984)
		Cox et al. (1984)
		Davies & Doran (1982)
Circumcision		Lindeke et al. (1986)
Auto restraints		Arneson et al. (1986)
		Ford (1980)
		Goebel et al. (1984)
Charting fetal movements		Gibby (1988)

Table 8–2
RESEARCH RELATED TO HEALTH BEHAVIORS IN PREGNANCY AND EARLY PARENTING

DESCRIPTIVE
Health Behaviors Identified
Arneson et al. (1986), new mothers
Brien et al. (1983), expectant parents
Brooten et al. (1987), urban pregnant women
Christiano & Susser (1989), pregnant homeless women
Davies & Doran (1982), pregnant women 35 years or more
Ford (1980), new mothers
Harvey et al. (1989), lesbian mothers
Lindeke et al. (1986), new parents
Young et al. (1989), pregnant women who delay prenatal care
Health Behavior Patterns
Morse & Bottorff (1989), preparing to work and breast-feed
Differences in Health Behaviors
Baisch et al. (1989), adolescent vs. adult mothers
Yoos (1985), breast-feeding vs. bottle-feeding adolescents
RELATIONSHIPS AMONG VARIABLES/PREDICTIVE MODELS
General Health Behaviors
Lewallan (1989)
Nutrition
Aaronson & Macnee (1989)
Taffel (1986)
Breast Feeding
Aberman & Kirchhoff (1985)
Coreil & Murphy (1988)
Hellings (1985)
Janke (1988)
Moon & Humenick (1989)
Sullivan & Jones (1986)
Whitley (1978)
Provider Communication
Kishi (1983)
Testing and Applying Health Behavior Models
Cox & Roghmann (1984)
Cox et al. (1984)
Kviz et al. (1985)
Sweeney & Gulino (1987)

Table 8–2
(Continued)

*INTERVENTION TO MODIFY HEALTH BEHAVIORS**
Exercise
Dougherty et al. (1989)
Sibley et al. (1981)
Wallace et al. (1986)
Breast Feeding
Evans et al. (1986)
Hall (1978)
Hill (1987)
Wiles (1984)
Other Behaviors
Gibby (1988)
Goebel et al. (1984)

*Interventions aimed at teaching parenting skills are presented in the chapters in the section on parental role development.

DESCRIPTIVE RESEARCH

Descriptions of Health Behavior and Beliefs

Descriptive studies of health behaviors and beliefs cover a variety of topics such as seeking delayed prenatal care, provider selection, and the use of automobile restraints. To delineate women's reasons for delaying prenatal care, Young, McMahon, Bowman, and Thompson (1989) identified a cohort of women initiating prenatal care during the third trimester of pregnancy. Ninety percent of the cohort were unmarried, and 90 percent were unemployed. Reasons for delayed prenatal care were gathered during home interviews conducted by public health nurses. Women reported several high-risk behaviors: smoking, closely spaced pregnancies, and low maternal weight gain. Reasons for delayed prenatal care varied with women's ages and races. Overall, reasons for delay related to problems with pregnancy acceptance, utilization of prenatal care, financial matters, and family responsibilities.

In a health behavior survey of 308 women at their first prenatal visit, Brooten et al. (1987) gathered data on nutritional intake and caffeine, cigarette, and alcohol use. Women represented a predominantly black, urban population. Average nutritional intake for the sample was deficient in calories, calcium, and iron. Rates of use of cigarettes, alcohol, and caffeine within the sample were 40, 13, and over 30 percent, respectively.

Table 8–3
CULTURAL PERSPECTIVES ON HEALTH AND HEALTH PRACTICES

Citation: Group/Population	Method of Study	Study Outcomes
Scott & Stern (1985): Northern Louisiana black women	Grounded theory	A. Reports common health beliefs in sample. B. Proposes ethno-market theory: three factors that influence health care practices are (1) the respect-fear process, (2) testing of new ideas, and (3) cultural interaction
Zepeda (1982): Southern California Spanish-speaking women	Survey based on two interviews	Reports maternal-infant care practices in sample
Wadd (1983): Vietnamese families living in Utah	One-time interviews	Reports postpartum health practices in sample
Stern, Tilden, & Maxwell (1980): Pilipino-American [sic] women and men; health-care providers (all in San Francisco area)	Field research methods	A. Reviews Pilipino [sic] childbearing customs, beliefs, and practices. B. Proposes three sources of stress associated with Western obstetric care: (1) conflicting customs, beliefs, and practices, (2) differences in interpersonal style, and (3) language barriers.
Edwards (1989): Mende society of Sierra Leone	Methodological comments on program effectiveness research related to traditional birth attendants	A. Reviews child care beliefs and customs Mende society. B. Describes modifications in study design, measurement, data collection, and scheduling based on sociocultural awareness.

Edwards (1987): Women in Bo and Pujehun districts of Sierra Leone	Survey by interview	Reports comparative data on infant mortality, assistance of untrained attendants for delivery, and attendance at antenatal clinics in two samples.
Alade (1989): Adolescents in town of Ile-Ife in Oyo state, Nigeria	Survey using unspecified type of instruments	Reports contraceptive awareness of this sample of pregnant adolescents
Lee (1986): Pregnant and postpartal Hmong women from Laos in a refugee camp in northern Thailand	Survey conducted by interview using Hmong translators	Reports beliefs and health practices related to maternal-infant health in this sample
Choi (1986): Korean-born women living in Los Angeles area	Questionnaire and observations	A. Reviews traditional Korean childbearing beliefs and practices. B. Reports attitudes, beliefs, and practices related to childbearing and infant care in this sample.
Cohen (1982): Midwives and other women of Rio Tinto (black Carib village) in Honduras	Field work including participant observation, unscheduled interviews, and survey	Reports beliefs and practices related to childbearing and infant care in sample.
DeSantis (1986): Haitian-born women living in southern Florida	Interviews in home (mostly open-ended items)	A. Reviews infant feeding beliefs and practices. B. Reports beliefs and practices related to infant feeding in sample
Bushnell (1981): Native American women in an Indian Health Service Clinic area	Field research methods and survey by interview	Reports childbearing beliefs of sample
Kruger & Maetzold (1983): American women from a Midwest community	Survey with content analysis of responses	Reports knowledge of traditional (folk) practices during pregnancy in sample

Table 8–3
CULTURAL PERSPECTIVES ON HEALTH AND HEALTH PRACTICES *(Continued)*

Citation: Group/Population	Method of Study	Study Outcomes
Lin (1986): Chinese adolescent mothers in Taiwan	Review of literature and knowledge of Chinese culture to plan program	Reports implementation of home-visitation program (to be evaluated) modified to the cultural context of Taiwanese teenage mothers
Mercer & Stainton (1984): Sixty-six Calgary (Canadian) and 294 San Francisco (US) first-time mothers	Passive observation using questionnaires and records	For both groups, found that cesarean birth mothers had less positive birth experiences than vaginal birth mothers
Harris (1985): Lay parents and health professions in northern Louisiana	Grounded theory	Reports on three key categories related to circumcision decisions: (1) circumcision reasoning, (2) cultural decision-making, and (3) cultural franchising
Parken (1978): Eighty-one Puerto Rican women living on the U.S. mainland	Interviews in Spanish	A. Reviews sex role beliefs B. Describes relations of modesty and male domination to use of preventive health behaviors

Christiano and Susser (1989), using participant observation, studied 23 pregnant women living in a New York hotel for the homeless. Seven were self-identified drug users. Of 23, three women had not yet heard of AIDS. Of 20 who knew of AIDS, 16 had no knowledge of preventive measures. Only three knew AIDS could be transmitted from mother to fetus. Many women believed that if they had only one sexual partner at a time, they were protected against transmission of AIDS. Women who were prostitutes were least likely to use condoms. None of the women read a newsletter about AIDS distributed throughout the hotel.

Brien, Haverfield, and Shanteau (1983) investigated processes that parents who attended Lamaze classes used in selecting an obstetrician. Twenty-two couples ranked the importance of obstetrician characteristics before and after childbirth. Before childbirth, obstetricians' communication patterns were a primary concern. Few changes occurred on postdelivery evaluations. Overall, there was high agreement between husbands' and wives' rankings of importance of characteristics.

Harvey, Carr, and Bernheine (1989) used a self-report questionnaire to gather information about health care experiences of 35 mothers who were self-identified lesbians. Most of the women had conceived through physician-assisted donor insemination. All the women had initiated prenatal care by 16 weeks, with 89 percent attending childbirth preparation classes, 80 percent breast feeding for at least 6 months, and 49 percent selecting midwives for maternity care.

Two studies focused on the use of auto-restraining devices to reduce injury during accidents. In a 1980 study by Ford, 66 mothers were surveyed after hospital discharge about use of auto-restraining devices for infants. Twenty-nine percent owned and properly used infant auto restraints, and 18 percent did not own such a device. Few variables were related to proper device use except for father's education and mother's accident history. In a related study, Arneson et al. (1986) interviewed 87 women in the hospital postpartum unit and 2 months later about auto seat belt use before and during pregnancy and after delivery. Seat belt use progressively increased from before to during pregnancy to after delivery (20 to 28 to 40 percent, respectively, for always using seat belts). Mothers who used seat belts stated they did so for protection and because of habit. Of mothers who used seat belts routinely, about one-third did so improperly. Only two demographic variables were related to seat belt use: mother's education and age.

Davies and Doran (1982) interviewed a sample of 74 women aged 35 years or more about decisions related to amniocentesis. The health belief model (Becker and Maiman, 1975) served as the basis for interviews. Sixty-six of 74 women underwent amniocentesis, with one fetus diagnosed as having a genetic disorder. The principal reason for seeking genetic counseling was concern about the effects of maternal age on fetal normality. Reassurance that Down's syndrome was not present was the principal benefit derived from amniocentesis. Most women perceived their risk of carrying a fetus with Down's syndrome to be low; 84 percent had decided to have a therapeutic abortion if a genetic disorder was diagnosed, and 53 percent stated the decision for abortion would be difficult.

Lindeke, Inverson, and Fisch (1986) surveyed 204 parents of male newborns regarding circumcision decision making. Parents who elected circumcision differed from those who did not on two characteristics: whether the father was circumcised and the mother's education. Hygiene was the predominant reason given for circumcision among parents electing it. Among parents foregoing circumcision, the majority saw it as unnecessary.

Health Behavior Patterns

Morse and Bottorff (1989) conducted a study focused on decision making related to breast feeding and employment. Using a longitudinal, qualitative design, 61 Canadian mothers were contacted three times from pregnancy to 1 year postpartum. The core variable, "playing it by ear," reflected women's suspended decisions and potential contingency plans in the face of lack of control over many factors. Other components of preparing to work while breast feeding involved themes of preparing for the worst, timing it right, and gearing up.

Differences in Health Behaviors and Beliefs

Yoos (1985) compared reasons given for feeding method selected by adolescent mothers. Breast-feeders overwhelmingly identified reasons related to benefiting the infant. Bottle-feeders, in contrast, listed reasons, such as convenience and not being tied down, that were reflective of self-oriented benefits. Although statistical comparisons were not presented, bottle-feeders were younger than breast-feeders.

In a related study, Baisch, Fox, Whitten, and Pajewski (1989) conducted a comparative study of low-income adolescent and adult women's breast-feeding attitudes and practices. Two samples of adolescents (n = 127 from a comprehensive teenager program and n = 60 from a limited teenager program) and adult women (n = 87) completed a prenatal questionnaire on breast-feeding attitudes. Actual breast feeding was assessed during postpartum. Significant main effects were found for group and race: teenagers in the limited teenager program had the least-positive attitudes toward breast feeding; whites had the most positive attitudes. Breast-feeding attitudes differed according to planned and actual feeding method. There was a significant association between group and actual feeding method, with adolescent mothers in the limited program having the lowest rate of breast feeding.

RELATIONAL/PREDICTIVE RESEARCH

Factors Related to General Health Behaviors

To determine the relations between health locus of control and general health practices among pregnant women, Lewallen (1989) studied 51 women during pregnancy. Three components of health locus of control were measured: internal health locus of control, powerful others, and chance. Higher health practices were related positively to internal health locus of control, were related negatively to powerful others, and were unrelated to chance.

Studies of Nutrition in Pregnancy

Several studies have examined nutrition during pregnancy. Taffel (1986) analyzed data from the 1980 National Natality and Fetal Mortality Surveys to determine the association between nutrition and pregnancy outcomes. Maternal weight gain served as a proxy measure for nutrition. Low maternal weight gain was associated with the following: high prepregnancy weight, black, aged 35 or more, teenaged, less than 9 years of education, low income, and smoking during pregnancy. After controlling for confounding factors, women who gained less than 21 lb were 2.3 times more likely to deliver a low-birth-weight infant and 1.5 times more likely to have a fetal death than women with greater weight gains.

In another study aimed at determining the relations among maternal nutrition, maternal weight gain, and pregnancy outcomes, Aaronson and Macnee (1989) followed over 500 predominantly white and middle-class women. Data were gathered from questionnaires, interviews, and medical records. Maternal weight gain during pregnancy was more highly related to edema and gestational length than nutrition ($r = .08$). Income was not related to nutrition, but education was. Further, weight gain was related to infant birth weight, but nutrition was not.

Breast-Feeding Phenomena and Predictors

Moon and Humenick (1989) studied 54 women to determine if feeding practices were related to breast engorgement. Mothers kept records of engorgement and feedings while in the hospital. Engorgement was significantly related to early initiation of feeding, number of feedings (among primiparas), duration of feedings (negative relationship), and supplementation (negative relationship). Thus, engorgement was more extensive if feedings were initiated early, were of frequent occurrence and short duration, and if supplementation was less extensive.

Aberman and Kirchhoff (1985) studied breast-feeding decision making among low-income mothers. Over 50 percent had made their decision about feeding method during the first trimester. Convenience was the primary reason given by bottle-feeders, and benefit to baby's health was influential among breast-feeders. Thirty percent chose to breast-feed. Final decisions were affected by such external factors as books and relatives. Over half of mothers indicated that a nurse had not talked to them about infant feeding.

In a related study, Sullivan and Jones (1986) applied Rogers' (1983) model of innovation-decision process to a secondary analysis of data on breast feeding among 181 black mothers. Breast feeding was viewed as the innovation; the stages in the decision process included knowledge, persuasion, decision/implementation, and confirmation. Mothers adopting breast feeding differed from rejectors on several characteristics including having been breast-fed themselves and type of health professional with whom infant feeding was discussed. Other factors influencing the decision process were age, plans to return to work or school, and complications.

A number of studies have aimed at identifying predictors of successful breast feeding. Whitley (1978) did a 1-year follow-up of 34 breast-feeding mothers; 25 mothers had earlier attended one or more classes on breast feeding. Mothers varied on duration of breast feeding: 18 percent breast-fed for less than 6 weeks, 32 percent for 6 to 23 weeks, and 50 percent for 24 weeks or longer. Although statistical tests were not performed, longer duration of breast feeding appeared to be related to class attendance and fewer childbirth complications. Prenatal breast preparation (nipple rolling and breast massage with expression of colostrum) was not related to duration of breast feeding.

To determine predictors of successful breast feeding among 84 mothers, Hellings (1985) examined the role of four sets of factors: individual, sociocultural, family, and physiological. Successful breast feeding was defined as supplementing with less than 4 oz of formula each 24 hours when infants were 4 to 6 weeks old. Only one variable, maternal education, was correlated with success. In discriminant function analysis, predictors included such variables as feelings about pregnancy, education, and income.

In another study predicting breast-feeding success, Janke (1988) surveyed 215 women 6 weeks after childbirth. Contrary to expectation, cesarean birth and vaginal birth mothers did not differ in breast-feeding attrition rates. Among cesarean birth mothers, commitment to breast feeding was the only variable differentiating those who succeeded from those who did not. Among vaginal birth mothers, a number of variables were associated with success differences. Commitment to breast feeding was the one variable common to successful breast feeding regardless of delivery method.

Finally, Coreil and Murphy (1988) followed 44 breast-feeding mothers from pregnancy to 1 year postpartum to identify predictors of breast-feeding duration. Biological factors were unrelated to breast-feeding duration, but psychosocial and biobehavioral factors were. In regression analysis, two variables were identified as significant predictors of duration of breast feeding: prenatal intended duration of breast feeding and absence of formula supplementation.

Provider Communication

To test hypotheses about health care provider communication and client recall of health information, Kishi (1983) studied provider-client interaction during well-baby clinics. Sixty-eight mothers and 7 providers (4 pediatricians and 3 pediatric nurse practitioners) were observed, and interactions were coded according to Flanders' (1965) method. Contrary to predictions, only one of four hypotheses received partial support. When the amount of information provided was controlled, the ratio of client talk to provider talk was significantly related to mothers' recall of health information.

Models Predicting Health Behaviors

Two prospective studies tested the predictive utility of the health belief model (Chapter 6). First, Kviz, Dawkins, and Ervin (1985) used a prospective design to test components of the health belief model with 61 poor, black mothers. Interviews were conducted at 1 and 6 months postpartum to assess health beliefs about the variables: susceptibility, severity, benefits, and efficacy. The number of well-baby clinic visits and the number of infant immunizations served as target health behaviors. Contrary to expectations, health beliefs were not related significantly to the number of clinic visits. Health beliefs at 6 months, but not at 1 month, explained 30 percent of the variance in number of immunizations. Efficacy of immunizations was the most predictive belief.

Second, Sweeney and Gulino (1987) tested a modified version of the health belief model in predicting breast feeding at 6 weeks postpartum. In the modified model, variables were grouped into three higher-order categories: individual perceptions, modifying factors, and likelihood of action. Each category contained one or more variables predictive of breast feeding. Overall, model variables accounted for 13.33 percent of the variance in breast feeding at 6 weeks.

Two articles report testing the interaction model of client health behavior (Chapter 6). The model was used in explaining prenatal genetic screening, including genetic counseling and amniocentesis. Using data from an earlier, large-scale survey, Cox et al. (1984) analyzed responses of 203 new mothers over 34 years to predict the use of prenatal genetic diagnostic services. Analysis of data using structural equation modeling showed that 22 of 35 casual paths were significant. Important variables in explaining the use of prenatal services were insurance coverage, information sources, social support, and client-provider interaction. In a second report of the same study, Cox and Roghmann (1984) presented additional analyses of the data set. Overall, the individual and combined contributions of model variables accounted for 57.8 percent of the variance in the use of prenatal diagnostic services. Based on discriminant function analysis, persons who chose not to have an amniocentesis were more likely to (1) not be covered for amniocentesis by insurance, (2) be Catholic, (3) have less experience with birth defects, (4) have discussed amniocentesis with fewer people, (5) have more children, (6) have negative attitudes toward abortion, (7) be less knowledgeable about the test, (8) have less support for amniocentesis, (9) disagree with physician about amount of decisional control related to the test, and (10) want more decisional control related to abortion.

INTERVENTION RESEARCH

Exercise

Sibley, Ruhling, Cameron-Foster, Christensen, and Bolen (1981) examined the effect of aerobic swimming conditioning on maternal physical fitness and maternal and fetal circulation. Low-risk pregnant women were assigned randomly to the experimental group (n = 7) or control group (n = 6). Experimental subjects completed a 10-week conditioning program that consisted of 30 hours of swimming. Both groups were assessed for fitness by using respiratory gas analysis during treadmill tests before and after the conditioning program. Before and 1 and 5 minutes after each swimming bout, maternal blood pressure, pulse, and fetal heart rate were measured. The two groups did not differ significantly on oxygen consumption after 10 weeks of conditioning. In comparing mean baseline and postexercise cardiovascular values, there were significant increases in both maternal and fetal heart rates, but not in maternal blood pressure, at 5 minutes postexercise.

In a preexperimental study, Wallace, Boyer, Dan, and Holm (1986) examined relationships to aerobic exercise in exercising (n = 31) and nonexercising pregnant women (n = 22). Convenience samples were used; that is, investigators did not manipulate the independent variable themselves. Exercising women had higher self-esteem and fewer symptoms during pregnancy than nonexercising women. The two groups differed significantly in the following specific symptoms: shortness of breath, backache, headache, fatigue, and hot flashes.

Doughtery, Bishop, Abrams, Batich, and Gimotty (1989) examined the effects of perineal exercise and an intravaginal resistance device (IVRD) on pressure exerted by the circumvaginal muscles. Forty-five postpartum women were randomly assigned to protocol A—exercise with IVRD, protocol B—exercise without IVRD, or protocol C—IVRD without exercise. After 6 weeks of protocol use, there were no significant differences among groups in increased circumvaginal pressure.

Breast-Feeding Studies

Hill (1987) tested the effects of antenatal education about breast-feeding on breast-feeding success among low-income women. By random assignment, 31 women were entered into the experimental group (antenatal breast-feeding education) and 33 into the control group. The experimental group received one class on breast feeding. Women in the experimental group showed gains in knowledge after the class. They did not differ from the control group, however, in breast-feeding success at 6 weeks postpartum.

Hall (1978) reported outcomes from a three-group experimental study involving random assignment and postpartum breast-feeding education. The control group (n = 12) received routine postpartum care; the first experimental group (n = 13) viewed a slide-tape presentation and received a pamphlet; and the second experimental group (n = 15) received the same treatment as the first experimental group plus an average of 45 to 60 minutes of hospital visits and telephone follow-up by a nurse. At 6 weeks postpartum, 50 percent of the control group and first experimental group were successfully breast feeding compared to 80 percent of the second experimental group.

In a quasi-experimental design, Wiles (1984) compared the effectiveness of a prenatal breast-feeding education program using a control (n = 20) and experimental group (n = 20). At one month after delivery, 18 experimental mothers compared to 6 control mothers were totally breast-feeding. Also, experimental group mothers viewed their babies more positively at 1 month than controls.

Evans, Lyons, and Killien (1986) compared breast-feeding outcomes in two groups, one which received formula samples at hospital discharge (n = 55) and one which did not (n = 40). Mothers were randomly assigned to groups. At 6 to 7 weeks after delivery, the two groups did not differ significantly on breast-feeding outcomes. Differences for subgroups, for example, primiparas, were also not significant.

Other Intervention Studies

Goebel, Copps, and Sulayman (1984) reported on outcomes of a postpartum education program on use of infant car seats. Baseline data on frequency of infant car seat use at discharge were collected prior to beginning the program (n = 92), and then infant seat use was added to the hospital's postpartum education program. Subsequent observations were made on infant car seat use as mothers and infants were being discharged from the hospital (n = 90). There were significantly greater presence of car seats, placement of infants in car seats, and correct type of car seats. However, there was no significant difference when groups were compared on both proper use and correct type of seat.

Gibby (1988) evaluated the effects of fetal movement charting on maternal anxiety in a low-risk sample. Women were randomly assigned to control (n = 17) and experimental groups (n = 16). The experimental group monitored and recorded fetal movements on a daily basis. The two groups did not differ on anxiety before, during, or after the experimental period in which fetal movements were monitored.

FUTURE RESEARCH DIRECTIONS

Recent reviews of the effects of exercise during pregnancy testify to the growing interest in health behaviors of parents during pregnancy and beyond (Reich, 1987; Wallace & Engstrom, 1987). Indeed, health-promotive behaviors involving exercise, nutrition, and breast feeding have been a major focus of parent-infant nursing investigations. That research has also covered preventive and risk-detecting behaviors such as prenatal care, immunizations, auto restraints, and amniocentesis. Compared to health status, however, measuring health behaviors during pregnancy and early parenting is just beginning. To advance the study of health behaviors during this critical period of development, new instrumentation and protocols are needed to measure relevant health behaviors and beliefs. In addition, intervention studies in the future would benefit from increased sample sizes and stronger research designs.

Both descriptive and interventive studies should be replicated across diverse clinical populations to clarify issues of generalizability. Research already conducted from a cultural perspective demonstrates the complexity of understanding and intervening with specific ethnic groups. Introducing advances in health care is often complicated by incompatibility with existing beliefs and new desired health behaviors. Sensitivity to the dynamics of change is essential when behavioral innovations are introduced (Rogers, 1983).

REFERENCES

Aaronson, L. S. (1989). Perceived and received support: Effects on health behavior during pregnancy. *Nursing Research, 38,* 4–9.

Aaronson, L. S., & Macnee, C. L. (1989). The relationship between weight gain and nutrition in pregnancy. *Nursing Research, 38,* 223–227.

Aberman, S., & Kirchhoff, K. T. (1985). Infant-feeding practices: Mothers decision making. *Journal of Obstetric, Gynecologic, and Neonatal Nursing, 14,* 394–398.

Alade, M. O. (1989). Teenage pregnancy in Ile-Ife, western Nigeria. *Western Journal of Nursing Research, 11,* 609–613.

Albrecht, S. A., & Rankin, M. (1989). Anxiety levels, health behaviors, and support systems of pregnant women. *Maternal-Child Nursing Journal, 18,* 49-60.

Arneson, S., Beltz, E., Hahnemann, B., Smith, R., Triplett, J., & Witt, V. (1986). Automobile seat belt practices of pregnant women. *Journal of Obstetric, Gynecologic, and Neonatal Nursing, 15,* 339-344.

Baisch, M. J., Fox, R. A., Whitten, E., & Pajewski, N. (1989). Comparison of breastfeeding attitudes and practices: Low-income adolescents and adult women. *Maternal-Child Nursing Journal, 18,* 61-71.

Becker, M. H., & Maiman, L. (1975). Sociobehavioral determinants of compliance with health and medical care recommendations. *Medical Care, 13,* 10-24.

Brien, M., Haverfield, N., & Shanteau, J. (1983). How lamaze-prepared expectant parents select obstetricians. *Research in Nursing and Health, 6,* 143-150.

Brooten, D., Peters, M. A., Glatts, M., Gaffney, S. E., Knapp, M., Cohen, S., & Jordan, C. (1987). A survey of nutrition, caffeine, cigarette and alcohol intake in early pregnancy in an urban clinic population. *Journal of Nurse-Midwifery, 32,* 85-90.

Bushnell, J. M. (1981). Northwest coast American Indians' beliefs about childbirth. *Issues in Health Care of Women, 3,* 249-261.

Choi, E. C. (1986). Unique aspects of Korean-American mothers. *Journal of Obstetric, Gynecologic, and Neonatal Nursing, 15,* 394-400.

Christiano, A., & Susser, I. (1989). Knowledge and perceptions of HIV infection among homeless pregnant women. *Journal of Nurse-Midwifery, 34,* 318-322.

Cohen, F. S. (1982). Childbirth belief and practice in a Garifuna (Black Carib) village on the north coast of Honduras. *Western Journal of Nursing Research, 4,* 193-208.

Coleman, M., Ryan, R., & Williamson, J. (1989). Social support and the alcohol consumption patterns of pregnant women. *Applied Nursing Research, 2,* 154-160.

Coreil, J., & Murphy, J. E. (1988). Maternal commitment, lactation practices, and breastfeeding duration. *Journal of Obstetric, Gynecologic, and Neonatal Nursing, 17,* 273-278.

Cox, C. L. (1980). An interaction model of client health behavior: Theoretical prescription for nursing. *Advances in Nursing Science, 5,*(1), 41-56.

Cox, C. L., & Roghmann, K. J. (1984). Empirical test of the interaction model of client health behavior. *Research in Nursing and Health, 7,* 275-285.

Cox, C. L., Sullivan, J. A., & Roghmann, K. J. (1984). A conceptual explanation of risk-reduction behavior and intervention development. *Nursing Research, 33,* 168-173.

Davies, B. L. & Doran, T. A. (1982). Factors in a woman's decision to undergo genetic amniocentesis for advanced maternal age. *Nursing Research, 31,* 56-59.

DeSantis, L. (1986). Infant feeding practices of Haitian mothers in south Florida: Cultural beliefs and acculturation. *Maternal-Child Nursing Journal, 15,* 77-89.

Dougherty, M. C., Bishop, K. R., Abrams, R. M., Batich, C. D., & Gimotty, P. A. (1989). The effect of exercise on the circumvaginal muscles in postpartum women. *Journal of Nurse-Midwifery, 34,* 8-14.

Edwards, N. C. (1987). Traditional birth attendants in Sierra Leone: Key providers of maternal and child health care in West Africa. *Western Journal of Nursing Research, 9,* 335-347.

Edwards, N. C. (1989). Traditional Mende society in Sierra Leone: A sociocultural basis for a quantitative research study. *Health Care for Women International, 10,* 1-14.

Evans, C. J., Lyons, N. B., & Killien, M. G. (1986). The effect of infant formula samples on breastfeeding practice. *Journal of Obstetric, Gynecologic, and Neonatal Nursing, 15,* 401-405.

Flanders, N. A. (1965). *Teacher influence, pupil attitudes, and achievement.* (U.S. Office of Education Cooperative Research Monograph, No. 12). Washington, D.C.: GPO.

Ford, A. H. (1980). Use of automobile restraining devices for infants. *Nursing Research, 29,* 281-284.

Fry, S. T. (1987). The ethical dimension of

policy for prenatal diagnostic technologies. *Advances in Nursing Science, 9*(3), 44–55.

Gibby, N. W. (1988). Relationship between fetal movement charting and anxiety in low-risk pregnant women. *Journal of Nurse-Midwifery, 33,* 185–188.

Goebel, B., Copps, T. J. & Sulayman, R. F. (1984). Infant car seat usage: Effectiveness of a postpartum educational program. *Journal of Obstetric, Gynecologic, and Neonatal Nursing, 13,* 33–35.

Hall, J. M. (1978). Influencing breastfeeding success. *Journal of Obstetric, Gynecologic, and Neonatal Nursing, 7,* 28–32.

Harris, C. C. (1985). The cultural decision-making model: Focus-circumcision. *Health Care for Women International, 6*(1–3), 25–43.

Harvey, S. M., Carr, C., & Bernheine, S. (1989). Lesbian mothers: Health care experiences. *Journal of Nurse-Midwifery, 34,* 115–119.

Hellings, P. (1985). A discriminant model to predict breast-feeding success. *Western Journal of Nursing Research, 7,* 471–478.

Hill, P. D. (1987). Effects of education on breastfeeding success. *Maternal-Child Nursing Journal, 16,* 145–156.

Hill, P. D., & Humenick, S. S. (1989). Insufficient milk supply. *Image, 21,* 145–148.

Janke, J. R. (1988). Breastfeeding duration following cesarean and vaginal births. *Journal of Nurse-Midwifery, 33,* 159–164.

Kaufman, K. J., & Hall, L. A. (1989). Influences of the social network on choice and duration on breast-feeding in mothers of preterm infants. *Research in Nursing and Health, 12,* 149–159.

Kishi, K. I. (1983). Communication patterns of health teaching and information recall. *Nursing Research, 32,* 230–235.

Kruger, S., & Maetzold, L. D. (1983). Practices of tradition for pregnancy. *Maternal-Child Nursing Journal, 12,* 135–139.

Kviz, F. J., Dawkins, C. E., & Ervin, N. E. (1985). Mothers' health beliefs and use of well-baby services among a high-risk population. *Research in Nursing & Health, 8,* 381–387.

Lee, P. A. (1986). Health beliefs of pregnant and postpartum Hmong women. *Western Journal of Nursing Research, 8,* 83–93.

Lewallen, L. P. (1989). Health beliefs and health practices of pregnant women. *Journal of Obstetric, Gynecologic, and Neonatal Nursing, 18,* 245–246.

Lin, R. F. (1986). A project for facilitating maternal adaptation with Chinese adolescent mothers in Taiwan. *Health Care for Women International, 7,* 311–327.

Lindeke, L., Iverson, S., & Fisch, R. (1986). Neonatal circumcision: A social and medical dilemma. *Maternal-Child Nursing Journal, 15,* 31–37.

Mercer, R. T., & Stainton, M. C. (1984). Perceptions of the birth experience: A cross-cultural comparison. *Health Care for Women International, 5*(1–3), 29–47.

Moon, J. L., & Humenick, S. S. (1989). Breast engorgement: Contributing variables and variables amenable to nursing intervention. *Journal of Obstetric, Gynecologic, and Neonatal Nursing, 18,* 309–315.

Moore, J. B., & Gaffney, K. F. (1989). Development of an instrument to measure mothers' performance of self-care activities for children. *Advances in Nursing Science, 12*(1), 76–84.

Morse, J. M., & Bottorff, J. L. (1989). Intending to breastfeed and work. *Journal of Obstetric, Gynecologic, and Neonatal Nursing, 18,* 493–500.

Parken, M. (1978). Culture and preventive health care. *Journal of Obstetric, Gynecologic, and Neonatal Nursing, 7,* 40–46.

Reich, C. L. (1987). Exercise in pregnancy: A review for nurse practitioners. *Health Care for Women International, 8,* 349–360.

Rogers, E. M. (1983). *Diffusion of innovations.* New York: Free Press.

Sandelowski, M. (1988). A case of conflicting paradigms: Nursing and reproductive technology. *Advances in Nursing Science, 10*(3), 35–45.

Scott, M. D. S., & Stern, P. N. (1985). The ethno-market theory: Factors influencing childbearing health practices of northern Louisiana black women. *Health Care for Women International, 6*(1–3), 45–60.

Sibley, L., Ruhling, R. O., Cameron-Foster, J., Christensen, C., & Bolen, T. (1981). Swimming and physical fitness during pregnancy. *Journal of Nurse-Midwifery, 26,* 3–12.

Stephens, C. J. (1985). Identifying social support components in prenatal populations: A multivariate analysis on alcohol consumption. *Health Care for Women International, 6,* 285–294.

Stern, P. N., Tilden, V. P., & Maxwell, E. K. (1980). Culturally-induced stress during childbearing: The Pilipino-American experience. *Issues in Health Care of Women, 2,* 67–81.

Sullivan J., & Jones, L. C. (1986). Breastfeeding adoption by low-income black women. *Health Care for Women International, 7,* 295–309.

Sweeney, M. A., & Gulino, C. (1987). The health belief model as an explanation for breast-feeding practices in a Hispanic population. *Advances in Nursing Science, 9*(4), 35–50.

Taffel, S. M. (1986). Association between maternal weight gain and outcome of pregnancy. *Journal of Nurse-Midwifery, 31,* 78–81.

Wadd, L. (1983). Vietnamese postpartum practices: Implications for nursing in the hospital setting. *Journal of Obstetric, Gynecologic, and Neonatal Nursing, 12,* 252–258.

Walker, L. O. (1989a). A longitudinal analysis of stress process among mothers of infants. *Nursing Research, 38,* 339–343.

Walker, L. O. (1989b). Stress process among mothers of infants: Preliminary model testing. *Nursing Research, 38,* 10–16.

Walker, S. N., Sechrist, K. R., & Pender, N. J. (1987). The health-promoting lifestyle profile: Development and psychometric characteristics. *Nursing Research, 36,* 76–81.

Wallace, A. M., Boyer, D. B., Dan, A., & Holm, K. (1986). Aerobic exercise, maternal self-esteem, and physical discomforts during pregnancy. *Journal of Nurse-Midwifery, 31,* 255–262.

Wallace, A. M., & Engstrom, J. L. (1987). The effects of aerobic exercise on the pregnant woman, fetus, and pregnancy outcome: A review. *Journal of Nurse-Midwifery, 32,* 277–290.

Whitley, N. (1978). Preparation for breastfeeding: A one-year followup of 34 nursing mothers. *Journal of Obstetric, Gynecologic, and Neonatal Nursing, 7,* 44–48.

Wiles, L. S. (1984). The effect of prenatal breastfeeding education on breastfeeding success and maternal perception of the infant. *Journal of Obstetric, Gynecologic, and Neonatal Nursing, 13,* 253–357.

Yoos, L. (1985). Developmental issues and the choice of feeding method of adolescent mothers. *Journal of Obstetric, Gynecologic, and Neonatal Nursing, 14,* 68–72.

Young, C., McMahon, J. E., Bowman, V., & Thompson, D. (1989). Maternal reasons for delayed prenatal care. *Nursing Research, 38,* 242–243.

Zepeda, M. (1982). Selected maternal-infant care practices of Spanish-speaking women. *Journal of Obstetric, Gynecologic, and Neonatal Nursing, 11,* 371–374.

PART FOUR

Parental Development

CHAPTER 9

The Paradigm of Parental Development

OVERVIEW OF THE PARADIGM

Parental development is the paradigm that has been studied most extensively in parent-infant nursing research. At its heart, it deals with the formation of the parent-infant relationship and emphasizes the parent's tie to the infant. Within its broad scope the parental development paradigm contains a family of related theoretical approaches: (1) transitions, (2) role attainment and identity, (3) attachment, and (4) loss and separation (Table 9–1). Each is considered separately in this chapter to facilitate understanding its particular attributes. Of the four theoretical approaches, only role attainment and identity was articulated by a nurse. Correspondingly, it has had the most widespread influence—both direct and indirect—on nursing research related to parental development.

Although each theoretical approach may have had somewhat distinct origins, there is considerable overlap and blending between them. For example, the role attainment and identity framework emphasizes subjective cognitive experiences of women during pregnancy and postpartum. In contrast, literature on transition emphasizes the psychosocial and behavioral changes triggered by adaptation to a new situation. Recent theorists such as Mercer (1981), however, have blended aspects of role attainment and transition in their writings. Similarly, attachment and role attainment and identity have distinct as well as overlapping concerns. Attachment focuses primarily on affective components of the parent-infant relation, whereas role attainment emphasizes the cognitive. Rubin, however, explicitly says that attachment and identity are "interdependent coordinates of the same process" (1984, p. 51).

Table 9–1
CHARACTERISTICS OF PARENTAL DEVELOPMENT THEORETICAL APPROACHES

Approach/ Framework	Specific to Parenthood	Origins	Key Focus
Transition	No	Crisis theory Sociology	Reorganization triggered by a significant external or internal event or process with accompanying psychosocial and behavioral manifestations of disorganization and upset
Role attainment and identity	Yes	Psychoanalytic theory Sociology Clinical observations	Cognitive aspects of subjective experience related to pregnancy, childbirth, and motherhood; related alterations in the self system
Attachment	Yes*	Observations of maternal behavior in animals	Early contact between parents and infant set in motion the formation of a strong parental bond to the infant; early version of the theory emphasized the idea of a sensitive period in which contact was necessary for maternal attachment to the infant
Loss and separation	No†	Observations of acute grief in humans	Loss or prolonged separation lead to a mourning process

*Parental bonding theory applies specifically to parenthood; infant attachment theory relates specifically to early childhood but has implications for later developmental periods.
†Although loss and separation are not specific, there are unique aspects in a parent-infant context.

Further, although the primary focus of this chapter is on parental role development, the scope of two frameworks, that is, attachment and loss and separation, extend beyond the parent to include the infant as well. Because of major developmental differences between adults and infants, attachment and loss and separation are covered from both parental and infant vantage points.

THEORETICAL APPROACHES TO PARENTAL DEVELOPMENT

TRANSITIONS

Conceptual Considerations

Of the frameworks used to study parental development, the broadest in scope is that of transitions. The transition framework is not limited to periods of change triggered by such entrances and exits from the family as parenthood (Hrobsky, 1977), widowhood, and divorce. Rather, transitions can be classified in a number of different ways and include chronological or life span transitions, transitions in social roles, and transitions in specific areas of one's life, such as geographic, economic, and physical changes (Golan, 1981, pp. 12–14).

Golan has described transition as "the leaving of an old familiar world and the entry into an unknown new one, the passing from one relatively stable state into an interval of strangeness and uncertainty on the way to a new stable state" (1981, p. 3). That passage may be accompanied by upsets in cognitive, emotional, and behavioral aspects of daily functioning. Although transitions may be normal events (such as marriage), and although they usually are completed by reorganizing and adapting to the new situation, the transitional period may be marked by upheavals in most aspects of daily functioning. In nursing, "transition" has been proposed as a useful framework for elaborating the nursing metaparadigm (Chick & Meleis, 1986).

The term "transition" is sometimes used synonymously with the concepts of "crisis," "situational crisis," and "maturational crisis." It is beyond the scope of this chapter to trace the development of each of these terms and their uses, but readers may wish to consider Crummette's (1975) and Golan's (1981) discussions of this topic. In essence, early work on the transition to parenthood emanated from a crisis theory framework (LeMasters, 1957). Subsequent research and theoretical considerations (Rossi, 1968) led to viewing parenthood not in a crisis framework but rather as a developmental stage. Terminology consequently shifted from crisis to transition (Golan, 1981, pp. 80–81).

The process of transition is usually triggered by some external or internal event—marriage, birth, death, a move, or illness. The event alters relations between persons and their environments. At a psychological level there may be some resistance to the change or grief about the passing of a previous situation. In time, persons reorganize their views, feelings, and behaviors to fit the constraints of new situations. In transitions involving interpersonal changes, not only behaviors, but the nature of relationships to others may also change.

Golan (1981) has divided the parenthood transition into four phases: deciding to have a child, pregnancy, birth, and the first postpartal adjustment. Rossi (1968) proposed four alternative role cycle stages for the transition to parenthood: anticipatory (i.e., pregnancy), honeymoon, plateau, and disengagement-termination.

Because the transition to parenthood represents a shift in role from nonparenting adult to parent, it has focused on the birth of the first child and has given little consideration to the births of subsequent children. In that regard, transition theory is more restrictive in focus than parental development theories that consider the unique relationship between each parent and child, for example, role attainment and attachment. Because of its consideration of cognitive, affective, and behavioral responses to change, however, the transition framework overlaps and encompasses aspects of role attainment and identity as well as stress models. Finally, in contrast to more individual-focused frameworks, for example, role attainment and identity, transition lends itself well to viewing pregnancy and childbirth from a family perspective.

Methodological Considerations

The ambiguity of the term "transition," denoting an event, immediate reactions to that event, and adaptations to the event, has been reflected in research about transitions. Initial research about the transition to parenthood sought to establish the magnitude of upset engendered by parenthood. More recent approaches emphasize adaptive tasks necessary to successful completion of transitions (Felner, Farber, & Primavera, 1983) and understanding of transitional mechanisms (Connell & Furman, 1984). Further, unlike stressful life event models, which predict the occurrence of pathology or dysfunction, transition models predict not sequelae (e.g., illness) but rather types or levels of adaptation to a transitional event. Thus, transitions research enlightens us about outcomes primarily in terms of level of functioning within the context of a new life situation. For that reason, transition frameworks are potentially more congruent with the study of positive health outcomes, such as well-being, than are stress models (Felner et al., 1983).

ROLE ATTAINMENT AND IDENTITY

Conceptual Consideration

Role attainment and identity as a theoretical approach to parental development is based on Rubin's description of maternal role attainment (1967a, 1967b) and her related expositions, extensions, and modifications of that approach (1967c, 1968, 1970, 1972, 1975, 1977, 1983, 1984). Although

Rubin's earliest writings focused on postpartal experiences (e.g., taking-in and taking-hold) and maternal touch (1961a, 1961b, 1963), her description of maternal role attainment moved the origins of motherhood to the antenatal period.

Rubin's theoretical work has been framed almost exclusively from the perspective of the mother. Although Rubin mentioned briefly the father's experience, she saw his experience as unlike the mother's: "The man becoming father does not have the abundant stimuli, the immediacy of involvement, and the felt experience of the fantasies of a woman becoming a mother" (1984, p. 46). Thus, this review of Rubin's theoretical writings on role attainment and identity will necessarily be limited to the maternal perspective. That in no way diminishes the importance of theorizing about fatherhood.

Table 9-2 presents key statements from Rubin's exposition (1967a, 1967b) of maternal role attainment. In that work, Rubin described two fundamental phenomena involved in becoming a mother: (1) acquisition of the maternal role (role taking) and (2) identification of the partner, that is, infant (1967a, 1967b). With respect to acquisition of the maternal role, she began with a view of "human conduct as the product of the interaction of self and role" (1967a, p. 237). Based on content analysis of antepartal and postpartal interviews of women, Rubin (1967a, 1967b) described five operations, initiated during pregnancy, by which the maternal role is attained: (1) mimicry—copying behavior in dress, speech, and gesture, (2) role playing—trial actions undertaken as if in the role; (3) fantasy—self-generated, internal productions related to the aspired role, (4) introjection-projection-rejection—three-step process of search for a model, assessment of its fit with the subject's situation, and a judgment about acceptance or rejection of the modeled behavior, and (5) grief work—foregoing former roles no longer compatible with the new goal of anticipated motherhood. Finally, a maternal identity, a firm and clear sense of self in the maternal role, marks the completion of the role attainment process.

Rubin (1970) subsequently proposed that pregnancy brings with it alterations in cognitive style. The pregnant woman "is different in what she perceives, in how she interprets situations that are present or pending, and in how she responds in established interpersonal relationships" (Rubin, 1970, p. 502). Broadly, during pregnancy, women pass through developmental stages in response to basic questions about (1) "time [of the pregnancy] within life space" and (2) "a personal sense of identity" (1970, p. 502). Specifically, much of a woman's cognitive content of "pregnancy work" involves progression through four developmental tasks: "(1) seeking safe passage for herself and her child through pregnancy, labor, and delivery; (2) ensuring the acceptance of the child she bears by significant persons in her family; (3) binding-in to the unknown child; and (4) learning to give of herself" (Rubin, 1975, p. 145).

Table 9–2
KEY STATEMENTS IN RUBIN'S 1967 DESCRIPTION OF MATERNAL ROLE ATTAINMENT

Assumptions

1. "The childbearing period was assumed to be a preparatory period in maternal role acquisition." (1967b, p. 345.)

The Self System

2. "As object of what and how much is taken in [related to the maternal role], the self system also serves to determine what it will admit by selective perceptions and by an ordering and reordering of motivations for tentative priorities. Three comprehensive but not necessarily independent categories of the self system . . . [are]: the ideal image, the self image, and the body image." (1967a, p. 240).
3. Ideal image is "those qualities, traits, attitudes, and achievements that each subject found desirable for maternal behavior." (1967a, p. 240.)
4. Self image is "the representation of the consistent 'myself' for whom there was little or no sense of historical self but an accumulation and continuation of self into the here and now." (1967a, p. 240.)
5. Body image: "In maternal role taking, status achievement is contingent upon body accommodations, functions, and capacity. Every change in body is significant: loss of functional control lowers self esteem and raises the risks of role failure." (1967a, p. 240.)

Processes and Operations

6. "Despite the preponderance of literature that suggests that doll-play in childhood helps form the maternal role in the little girl, this historical fact had no place in the forming of maternal role in adult women." (1967b, p. 343.)
7. "The taking-in of the maternal role is a quiet, continuous process, but not a passive one." (1967a, p. 240.)
8. "Five distinct operations of taking-in of the maternal role were elicited [from interviews of mothers]. Mimicry and role-play were found to be early, tentative forms of taking-on the role. Fantasy and a circular process of introjection-projection-rejection were found to be later and more discriminating processes of taking-in of the role. Grief work . . . was found to be a letting-go of former roles incompatible with the new role. Grief work appeared as a catalyst for other role-taking operations." (1967b, p. 345.)
9. "Grief work by the multiparas in relation to their other child(ren) represented primarily the process of separating out from the exclusiveness of the former attachments, usually with the former 'baby'." (1967b, p. 344.)
10. "Identity is the end point or goal . . . of role-taking. . . . When the subjects had a sense of being in their roles, a sense of comfort about where they had been and where they were going, then role achievement could be said to exist." (1967a, p. 243.)

Models and Referrants

11. "Mother [of the pregnant woman] was a major prototype and was the most significant contributor of subject's set of anticipations in becoming a mother." (1967b, p. 343.)
12. "Subjects, particularly primiparas, used husbands not as a referrant but as support and reinforcement." (1976b, p. 342.)
13. "With increasing age and parity, the multiparas tend to use the preceding generation less and her own child(ren) more for self-appraisal in role-taking." (1967b, p. 346.)

Although birth brings a continuation of a relationship forged during pregnancy, it also requires a shift from a relationship experienced in fantasy to one now known in reality. Rubin describes "locating the child" through repeated observations and comparisons with significant others as aiding the transition from fantasy to reality (1972). The birth event shifts the binding-in process begun in pregnancy from a symbiotic one to one marked by (1) "an identification of the infant as an objective human entity with its own form, appearance, and behavior," and (2) "a claiming of her infant in a social context," and (3) "a polarization of selves in the postpartal period" (Rubin, 1977, p. 68).

In 1984 Rubin provided an updated exposition of her theoretical views. That work focused on "the subjective maternal experience" (p. vii). Of note, the term "maternal role attainment" was eliminated and the terms "maternal identity" and "maternal experience" were presented as defining labels for the new Rubin rubric. The new rubric continued to emphasize the importance of maternal identity: "With each childbearing experience there is an incorporation into a woman's self system of a new personality dimension" (1984, p. 38). Rubin revised her point of view of the process, however, by stating that the outcome of incorporating a new dimension "is more than a sentimental attachment and *more than a role* that is stepped into and out of again" [emphasis added] (1984, p. 38). Further, she states: "Becoming a mother is unlike taking a role where self and relationships with others remain constant, unchanged" (1984, p. 52). This revision emphasized maternal identity as an enduring yet evolving dimension of the mother's self-system. Beyond some changes in terminology, there is much continuity between Rubin's earlier and later work.

As earlier, in her 1984 book Rubin rejects instinct and childhood doll play as explanations for maternal behavior (pp. 1–2). Instead, she emphasizes the explanatory value of looking "for the origins of maternal behavior in the phenomenological and subjective experience of a woman becoming a mother" (1984, p. 3). The subjective dimensions of motherhood occur within the self-system. Rubin focuses on three components of the self: ideal self, self-image, and body image (pp. 12–24). Body image entails both body boundaries and functional properties, particularly of internal body parts.

In place of maternal role attainment and operations related to it, Rubin's 1984 work emphasizes incorporation of a maternal identity distinct to each childbearing experience. The importance of an ideal image of self is stressed: "Incorporation of the maternal identity into the self system is by way of the idealized image of self as mother of this child" (1984, p. 39). The maternal identity is developed by replication (includes mimicry and role play), fantasy (includes imaging, loosening bonds with others, and grief work), and dedifferentiation (includes introjection, projection, and acceptance or rejection) (1984, pp. 38–51). As in her earlier work, Rubin reiterates that maternal tasks of safe passage, acceptance by others, binding-in to the child, and giving of self are linked to preparing the woman and her family for the forthcoming child.

Rubin (1984) identifies significant body image dimensions of childbearing: growth in size, body boundaries, postural model, and pain, especially during childbirth. She also provides expositions of the following: time and space in childbearing, the puerperium, and identification of the child. Compared to her earlier work, Rubin (1984) gives added, but not extensive, attention to fatherhood and to the intrapartal experience.

Finally, other nurses have elaborated on ideas proposed by Rubin. Rees (1980) developed a theoretical model of identification with the mothering role, and Mercer proposed a theoretical framework for studying factors that influence the maternal role (1981). Wismont and Reame (1989) adapted Rubin's tasks of pregnancy for the lesbian childbearing experience, and Richardson (1982) provided an elaboration of Rubin's ideas within the context of research on relationships during pregnancy. Further, Richardson (1984) proposed a care framework based on women's body boundary experience in childbirth, and Burritt and Fawcett (1980) reviewed research and related literature on body experience during pregnancy. Rubin's general theory of clinical nursing was analyzed from a philosophical perspective by Schafer (1987), who also interpreted Rubin's ideas about maternal identity and maternal experience as a special case of the theory of clinical nursing. In a more critical approach, Gay, Edgil, and Douglas (1988) both summarized Rubin's work and questioned its validity in the current social and technological milieu.

Methodological Considerations

Because of the widespread influence of Rubin's theoretical work within nursing, it is essential that its empirical validity be corroborated by others. The complex nature of Rubin's ideas and their grounding in largely qualitative thematic observations make empirical testing difficult. Such testing would require clear definitions, both theoretical and operational, of key terms in her conceptual system. Articulating such definitions, though not impossible, is made more difficult by the phenomenological approach that Rubin adopted in both studying and presenting maternal experience. Potential methods of testing hypotheses about thematic material, or hypotheses about relationships between thematic material and actual maternal nurturant behavior, could be done by using such techniques as content analysis. Its use is contingent, however, on a well-developed and well-defined classification system.

Although Rubin's theoretical work provides insights into the psychological processes that explain the origins of maternal behavior, extrapolating from those insights to how best to assess and enhance maternal identity is less clear. It would be of great benefit if key elements in maternal identity could be efficiently assessed. Development of frameworks for intervention that test alternative ways to support formation of maternal identity is much needed also.

Rubin's work touches on but does not give a full account of the psychological experiences of women during childbirth. Further study of the intrapartal period—issues related to body boundaries, time, pain—would be helpful in understanding the full cycle of maternal experience. Because Rubin did not study fathers extensively, it is not clear to what extent her theoretical work fits the paternal experience. Investigation of that question would demarcate the boundaries of her work.

ATTACHMENT

Parental Perspectives: Conceptual and Methodological Considerations

Unlike literature on child development, which has stressed the infant's tie to its mother or caregiver (Bowlby, 1969; Sroufe, 1983), nursing literature has emphasized parental attachment—parents' ties to the fetus and infant (Tulman, 1981; Gay, 1981; Mercer, 1983; Gaffney, 1988). Although a nurse wrote about the early acquaintance process between mother and infant (Kennedy, 1973), it was the work of two physicians on maternal attachment that most profoundly influenced nurses (Klaus et al., 1972; Klaus & Kennell, 1976). Indeed, Tulman (1981) proposed that, in nursing literature, the concept of maternal attachment had become synonymous with Klaus and Kennell's theoretical writing on bonding (1976).

Klaus and Kennell began their research by noting that among animals, such as cows, goats, and sheep, "There is a special period immediately after delivery in the adult animal. If the animal mother is separated from her young during this period, deviant behavior may result" (Klaus et al., 1972, p. 460.)

In their research with 28 mothers of full-term infants, they sought to test if "there is a period shortly after birth that is uniquely important for mother-to-infant attachment in the human being" (Klaus et al., 1972, p. 460). Specifically, mothers in the experimental group were given extended contact with their newborns (1 hour of contact with the baby during the first 3 hours after delivery and 5 extra hours of contact each afternoon for 3 days in addition to the routine contact provided the control group). Mothers in the control group saw their babies only briefly at birth and at 6 to 12 hours afterward and then had 20- to 30-minute visits every 4 hours for feeding. Subsequently, group differences were noted; for example, there were more eye-to-eye contacts between mothers and infants in the experimental group than between those in the control group.

Based on their own and others' research, Klaus and Kennell (1976) proposed the existence of a phenomenon of human parent-infant bonding. One of the key principles of their exposition of that phenomenon was that:

> *There is a sensitive period in the first minutes and hours of life during which it is necessary that the mother and father have close contact with their neonate for later development to be optimal. (Klaus & Kennell, 1976, p. 14.)*

Thus, more than proposing that an emotional tie develops between parent and infant, Klaus and Kennell proposed that there was a vital period shortly after birth during which parent-infant contact must occur for optimal development.

In a subsequent revision of their theory of bonding, Klaus and Kennell (1982) moderated their initial claims and acknowledged that: "The human is highly adaptable, and there are many fail-safe routes to attachment" (p. 55). Still, the idea that early contact is necessary for "bonding" or parental attachment to occur is difficult to extinguish in the minds of many parents and nurses. Several important critical reviews of Klaus and Kennell's writings have provided balance to their original ideas (Tulman, 1981; Lamb & Hwang, 1982; Lamb, 1982; Goldberg, 1983; Palkovitz, 1985).

Methodological considerations in the study of parental attachment relate to alternative views of the origins of attachment and measurement of its indicators. Although Klaus and Kennell's view of attachment or bonding is not the only one, it is the one that has dominated in nursing. Tulman (1981) proposed three alternative views of the origins of maternal attachment that may be pertinent to nursing: (1) predelivery experience, (2) perception of the infant, and (3) mother-infant interaction. As another alternative, Gay (1981) integrated the concepts of acquaintance and attachment with a conceptual framework of the bonding process. Disenchantment with Klaus and Kennell's view of bonding should not lead nurses to reject the broader idea of the importance of the parental tie to the infant.

Among others, Goldberg (1983) had noted that there is little agreement about how to operationally define attachment or bonding. Attachment—as an emotional tie to the infant—is by its nature not directly observable. Instead, its presence is inferred on the basis of observation of discrete behaviors. Lacking is careful work that demonstrates the relationship of discrete behaviors to internal emotional feelings of parents toward their infants (Goldberg, 1983).

Infant Perspectives: Conceptual and Methodological Considerations

"Infant attachment" refers to the infant's tie, which develops in the second half of the first year, to the parent or primary caregiver. Attachment theory as articulated by Bowlby (1958, 1969) was proposed to explain "the empirical fact that within 12 months the infant has developed a strong libidinal tie to a mother figure" (Bowlby, 1958, p. 350). Contrary to secondary drive theories, in attachment theory the infant's tie to its parent or caregiver is viewed as a system of behavior "with its own dynamics distinct from the behavior and dynamics of either feeding or sex" (Bowlby, 1982, p. 668). The tie to an attachment figure is most likely to be manifest when the infant is ill, tired, or frightened (Bowlby, 1982). The function of the attachment behavioral system, comprised of such behaviors as clinging, following, crying, and smiling, is to protect the infant.

Recent expositions and interpretations of infant attachment theory emphasize the underlying behavioral control system, not discrete behaviors (Sroufe & Waters, 1977; Bowlby, 1982). Thus, it is the overall system of attachment behaviors as they relate to an attachment figure, particularly in times of distress, and not the occurrence of specific behaviors, such as frequent smiling, that represents the construct of attachment. In addition, although the goal of the attachment behavioral system is to maintain proximity to the attachment figure, the subjective goal from the infant's perspective is to feel secure (Bretherton, 1985). Through patterns of interaction with attachment figures, theorists propose that infants form internal working models of themselves and others in their world (Bretherton, 1985). It is hypothesized that these models are carried over to other later relationships.

Attachment relationships have usually been classified as secure, avoidant, or resistant. In secure attachments, infants use parents or caregivers as bases for exploring the environment and seek them when in distress. Infants with avoidant attachments use strategies to avoid contact with the parent under conditions of distress (i.e., do not approach or avoid eye contact). Infants with resistant attachment seek contact with the parent when in distress but also express anger. Ainsworth, Blehar, Waters, and Wall (1978) reported that these attachment patterns at 1 year were correlated with earlier patterns of mother sensitivity and responsivity in interaction with the infant.

Because infant attachment represents a behavioral system focused on specific attachment figures, measurement of attachment has emphasized observation of infants' behavior in relation to their parents or caregivers. As of this date, the "strange-situation procedure" is the standardized and widely accepted method for assessing infant attachment (Ainsworth et al., 1978). In that procedure the infant's attachment behavioral system is elicited by exposing the infant to progressively more stressful social situations induced by brief separations from the attachment figure and introduction of a stranger. Based on complex classification rules, infants are judged to have secure (B), avoidant (A), or resistant (C) attachments to a specific parent or caregiver. It is essential that investigators planning to use the strange-situation procedure obtain training from scientists who have themselves been trained by Ainsworth or her colleagues.

LOSS AND SEPARATION

Parental Perspectives: Conceptual and Methodological Considerations

As a consequence of the emotional investment in a pregnancy and fetus, parental experiences of perinatal loss may result in acute grief responses. Because separation of parent and infant also may lead to emotional responses, it is viewed as pertinent to the consideration of loss. Parental loss may result from spontaneous abortion or fetal or infant death. In addition, Steele (1987) indicates that parental loss may also occur with the birth of a critically ill infant. Loss in the form of grief work also was described by Rubin (1967a) as part of the maternal role-taking process. Parental experiences of loss and separation may also occur in the course of illness, political and military changes, and adoptive placement of an infant.

The experiences of loss and prolonged separation can result in profound human reactions. Lindemann's (1944) classic study outlined acute grief responses of adults to loss. Characteristic behaviors in acute grief included somatic distress, preoccupation with the deceased's image, guilt, hostility, and loss of behavior patterns. Successful adaptation to loss involved completing grief work comprised of (1) freeing oneself from bonds to the deceased, (2) readjusting to a world in which the deceased is absent, and (3) forming new relationships (Lindemann, 1944). Among others, Engel (1964) described the phases in the grief experience; they included shock and disbelief, developing awareness of the loss, restitution, resolving the loss, idealization, and, finally, healing. Murphy (1983), however, argues that there is insufficient evidence of a stage model of grief.

Three models of parental responses to loss have been developed by nurses. First, Swanson-Kaufmann (1986) described the six phenomenological experiences of women who had miscarriages. The experiences were: coming to know, losing and gaining, sharing the loss, getting through it, going public, and trying again. Second, based on clinical observations of parents, Steele (1987) proposed four phases in parental adaptation to the birth of a critically ill infant: giving in, letting go, hanging on, and taking hold. Third, Horan (1982), by contrast, used existing literature to propose an attributional model of parents' responses to an infant with a birth defect.

In a review of grief literature, Hutti (1984) identified the need to determine by qualitative methods if parental experiences of perinatal loss indeed conform to prevailing ideas of adult grief. Studies of perinatal loss, such as the study of Swanson-Kauffman (1986), have begun to fulfill that need. In addition, studies of parental grief need to take note of the role that parental gender may play in differential severity and length of women's and men's grief responses to miscarriage, stillbirth, and infant death (Steele, 1987, p. 15).

Infant Perspectives: Conceptual and Methodological Considerations

The responses of infants and young children to loss and separation were initially observed by such investigators as Spitz and Wolf (1946), who described the phenomenon as "anaclitic depression." Bowlby, among others, related mourning responses to loss of or separation from the caregiving figure, usually the mother:

> *Once the child has formed a tie to a mother-figure, which has ordinarily occurred in the middle of the first year, its rupture leads to separation anxiety and grief and sets in train processes of mourning. (1961, p. 317.)*

Based on actual observations of young children's responses to separation, Bowlby and Robertson proposed a stage model of their mourning process which included protest, despair, and detachment (Bowlby, 1961, 1973, 1982). Protest manifests itself in crying and acute distress; despair is evidenced in sadness and withdrawal; and detachment is shown by shallow acceptance of other caregivers and indifference to the attachment figure. These responses were graphically displayed in Robertson's (1952) film "A Two-Year-Old Goes to Hospital." While Bowlby (1961) noted similarities between adult and childhood grief, he noted the potentially damaging effects of mourning on the developing young child.

Much has been learned about the damaging effects of separation and loss, particularly on infants over 6 months of age, and factors that mitigate those effects (Bowlby, 1951/1966; Ainsworth, 1962/1969; Rutter, 1979). Still, it is important for researchers to examine infants' responses to new caregiving arrangements arising from social or technological change. There is no substitute for careful observation of infants' affective and behavioral responses to caregiving environments to inform us about their effects on infants.

REFERENCES

Ainsworth, M. (1962/1969). The effects of maternal deprivation: A review of findings and controversy in the context of research strategy. In *Deprivation of maternal care* (pp. 289-357). New York: Schocken.

Ainsworth, M. D. S., Blehar, M. C., Waters, E., & Wall, S. (1978). *Patterns of attachment: A psychological study of the strange situation.* Hillsdale, NJ: Erlbaum.

Bowlby, J. (1951/1966). *Maternal care and mental health.* New York: Schocken.

Bowlby, J. (1958). The nature of the child's tie to his mother. *International Journal of Psycho-Analysis, 39,* 350-373.

Bowlby, J. (1961). Process of mourning. *International Journal of Psycho-Analysis, 42,* 317-340.

Bowlby, J. (1969). *Attachment and loss,* Vol. 1, *Attachment.* New York: Basic Books.

Bowlby, J. (1973). *Attachment and loss,* Vol. 2, *Separation.* New York: Basic Books.

Bowlby, J. (1982). Attachment and loss: Retrospect and prospect. *American Journal of Orthopsychiatry, 52,* 664-678.

Bretherton, I. (1985). Attachment theory: Retrospect and prospect. In E. Bretherton & E. Waters (Eds.), *Growing points of attachment theory and research* (pp. 3-35). *Monographs of the Society for Research in Child Development. 50*(1-2), Serial No. 209.

Burritt, J., & Fawcett, J. (1980). Body experience during pregnancy. *Issues in Health Care of Women, 2*(3-4), 1-10.

Chick, N., & Meleis, A. I. (1986). Transitions: A nursing concern. In P. L. Chinn (Ed.), *Nursing research methodology: Issues and implementation* (pp. 237-257). Rockville, MD: Aspen.

Connell, J. P., & Furman, W. (1984). The study of transitions: Conceptual and methodological issues. In R. N. Emde & R. I. Harmon (Eds.), *Continuities and discontinuities in development* (pp. 153-173). New York: Plenum.

Crummette, B. D. (1975). Transitions in motherhood. *Maternal-Child Nursing Journal, 4,* 65-73.

Engel, G. L. (1964). Grief and grieving. *American Journal of Nursing, 64*(9), 93-98.

Felner, R. D., Farber, S. S., & Primavera, J. (1983). Transitions and stressful life events: A model for primary prevention. In R. D. Felner, L. A. Jason, J. N. Moritsugu, & S. S. Farber (Eds.), *Preventive psychology* (pp. 199-215). Elmsford, NY: Pergamon.

Gaffney, K. F. (1988). Prenatal maternal attachment. *Image, 20,* 106-109.

Gay, J. (1981). A conceptual framework of bonding. *Journal of Obstetric, Gynecologic, and Neonatal Nursing, 10,* 440-444.

Gay, J. T., Edgil, A. E., & Douglas, A. B. (1988). Reva Rubin revisited. *Journal of Obstetric, Gynecologic, and Neonatal Nursing, 17,* 394-399.

Golan, N. (1981). *Passing through transitions: A guide for practitioners.* New York: The Free Press.

Goldberg, S. (1983). Parent-infant bonding: Another look. *Child Development, 54,* 1355-1382.

Horan, M. L. (1982). Parental reaction to the birth of an infant with a defect: An attributional approach. *Advances in Nursing Science, 5*(1), 57-68.

Hrobsky, D. M. (1977). Transition to parenthood: A balancing of needs. *Nursing Clinics of North America, 12,* 457-468.

Hutti, M. H. (1984). An examination of perinatal death literature: Implications for nursing practice and research. *Health Care for Women International, 5,* 387-400.

Kennedy, J. C. (1973). The high-risk maternal-infant acquaintance process. *Nursing Clinics of North America, 8,* 549-556.

Klaus, M. H., Jerauld, R., Kreger, M. C., McAlpine, W., Steffa, M., & Kennell, J. H. (1972). Maternal attachment: Importance of the first post-partum days. *New England Journal of Medicine, 286,* 460-463.

Klaus, M. H., & Kennell, J. H. (1976). *Maternal-infant bonding.* St. Louis: Mosby.

Klaus, M. H., & Kennell, J. H. (1982). *Parent-infant bonding* (2nd ed.). St. Louis: Mosby.

Lamb, M. E. (1982). The bonding phenomenon: Misinterpretations and their implications. *Journal of Pediatrics, 101,* 555–557.

Lamb, M. E., & Hwang, C. (1982). Maternal attachment and mother-neonate bonding: A critical review. In M. E. Lamb & A. L. Brown (Eds.), *Advances in developmental psychology* (Vol. 2, pp. 1–39). Hillsdale, NJ: Erlbaum.

LeMasters, E. E. (1957). Parenthood as crisis. *Marriage and Family Living, 19,* 352–355.

Lindemann, E. (1944). Symptomatology and management of acute grief. *American Journal of Psychiatry, 101,* 141–148.

Mercer, R. T. (1981). A theoretical framework for studying factors that impact on the maternal role. *Nursing Research, 30,* 73–77.

Mercer, R. T. (1983). Parent-infant attachment. In L. J. Sonstegard, K. M. Kowalski, & B. Jennings (Eds.), *Women's health* (Vol. 2) *Childbearing* (pp. 17–42). New York: Grune & Stratton.

Murphy, S. A. (1983). Theoretical perspectives on bereavement. In P. L. Chinn (Ed.), *Advances in Nursing Theory Development* (pp. 191–206). Rockville, MD: Aspen.

Palkovitz, R. (1985). Fathers' birth attendance, early contact, and extended contact with their newborns: A critical review. *Child Development, 56,* 392–406.

Rees, B. L. (1980). Maternal identification and infant care: A theoretical perspective. *Western Journal of Nursing Research, 2,* 686–706.

Richardson, P. (1982). Significant relationships and their impact on childbearing: A review. *Maternal-Child Nursing Journal, 11,* 17–40.

Richardson, P. (1984). The body boundary experience of women in labor: A framework for care. *Maternal-Child Nursing Journal, 13,* 91–101.

Robertson, J. (1952). A two-year-old goes to hospital. New York University Film Library, New York. (Film).

Rossi, A. S. (1968). Transition to parenthood. *Journal of Marriage and the Family, 30*(1), 26–39.

Rubin, R. (1961a). Basic maternal behavior. *Nursing Outlook, 9,* 683–686.

Rubin, R. (1961b). Puerperal change. *Nursing Outlook, 9,* 753–755.

Rubin, R. (1963). Maternal touch. *Nursing Outlook, 11,* 828–831.

Rubin, R. (1967a). Attainment of the maternal role: 1. Processes. *Nursing Research, 16,* 237–245.

Rubin, R. (1967b). Attainment of the maternal role: 2. Models and referrants. *Nursing Research, 16,* 342–346.

Rubin, R. (1967c). The neomaternal period. In M. Duffey, E. H. Anderson, B. S. Bergersen, M. Lohr, & M. H. Rose (Eds.), *Current Concepts in Clinical Nursing: Vol 1.* (pp. 388–391). St. Louis: Mosby.

Rubin, R. (1968). Body image and self-esteem. *Nursing Outlook, 16,* 20–23.

Rubin, R. (1970). Cognitive style in pregnancy. *American Journal of Nursing, 70,* 502–508.

Rubin, R. (1972). Fantasy and object constancy in maternal relationships. *Maternal-Child Nursing Journal, 1,* 101–111.

Rubin, R. (1975). Maternal tasks of pregnancy. *Maternal-Child Nursing Journal, 4,* 143–153.

Rubin, R. (1977). Binding-in in the postpartum period. *Maternal-Child Nursing Journal, 6,* 67–75.

Rubin, R. (1983). Two psychological aspects of the postpartum period. In L. J. Sonstegard, K. M. Kowalski, & B. Jennings (Eds.), *Women's health: Vol 2. Childbearing* (pp. 245–254). New York: Grune & Stratton.

Rubin, R. (1984). *Maternal identity and the maternal experience.* New York: Springer.

Rutter, M. (1979). Maternal deprivation, 1972-1978: New findings, new concepts, new approaches. *Child Development, 50,* 283–305.

Schafer, P. J. (1987). Philosophical analysis of a theory of clinical nursing. *Maternal-Child Nursing Journal, 16,* 289–363.

Spitz, R. A., & Wolf, K. M. (1946). Anaclitic depression: An inquiry into the genesis of psychiatric conditions in early childhood. *Psychoanalytic Study of the Child, 2,* 313-342.

Sroufe, L. A. (1983). Infant-caregiver attachment and patterns of adaptation in preschool: The roots of maladaptation and competence. In M. Perlmutter (Ed.), *The Minnesota symposium on child psychology: Vol. 16. Development and policy concerning children with special needs* (pp. 41–83). Hillsdale, NJ: Erlbaum.

Sroufe, L. A., & Waters, E. (1977). Attachment as an organizational construct. *Child Development, 48,* 1184–1199.

Steele, K. H. (1987). Caring for parents of critically ill neonates during hospitalization: Strategies for health care professionals *Maternal-Child Nursing Journal, 16,* 13–27.

Swanson-Kaufmann, K. M. (1986). A combined qualitative methodology for nursing research. *Advances in Nursing Science, 8*(3), 58–69.

Tulman, L. J. (1981). Theories of maternal attachment. *Advances in Nursing Science, 3*(4), 7–14.

Wismont, J. M., & Reame, N. E. (1989). The lesbian childbearing experience: Assessing developmental tasks. *Image, 21,* 137–141.

CHAPTER 10

Parent-Infant Nursing Research on the Transition to Parenthood

DEFINITIONS AND DESCRIPTIONS OF THE TRANSITION TO PARENTHOOD

DEFINING THE TRANSITION TO PARENTHOOD

As indicated in Chapter 9, the transition to parenthood framework deals with the transition from nonparenting adult to parent. In addition to the transitional event of the infant's birth, the transition framework may include the anticipatory phase of pregnancy (Rossi, 1968). The transition to parenthood also includes the cognitive, emotional, and behavioral upsets and changes that may accompany any transition (Golan, 1981). Because the transition to parenthood involves adopting a new social role within the family context, it may involve changes in family relationships. Like the parental role attainment and identity framework, the transition to parenthood framework encompasses psychosocial aspects of becoming a parent. In selecting research articles for inclusion in this chapter, two operational definitions of transitions were used: (1) explicit reference to transition to parenthood and (2) focus on dimensions or changes in family roles or relationships during pregnancy and early parenthood.

The majority of studies in this chapter mentioned the transition to parenthood as a marker event of significance (Table 10–1). Actual definition of

Table 10–1
DEFINITIONS AND DESCRIPTIONS OF THE TRANSITION TO PARENTHOOD

"The transition to fatherhood is frequently a time of great change, stress, and even crisis for men experiencing parenthood for the first time." (Hangsleben, 1983, p. 265.)

"The period of transition to parenthood is a stressful one." (Broom, 1984, p. 224.)

"Transition to parenthood is considered a role transition of very great impact on the individual." (Roberts, 1983, p. 214.)

"The birth of the couple's first child has been viewed as a crisis event because it forces the reorganization of the family as a social system." (Majewski, 1986, p. 10.)

the concept of transition to parenthood as a theoretical concept, however, was incomplete in the research literature reviewed.

THEORETICAL MODELS OF THE TRANSITION TO PARENTHOOD

Roberts (1983) proposed a theoretical model to predict the transition to parenthood. Outcomes included the ease of transition to parenthood and perception of the infant. Infant obligatory behavior influenced outcomes directly as well as through the following: normative changes, perception of role competence, and self-esteem (Fig. 10–1). Other theoretical models applied to transition-to-parenthood research include role supplementation (Meleis & Swendsen, 1978), family developmental theory (Majewski, 1986; Dooher, 1980), and equity theory (Tomlinson, 1987).

MEASUREMENT

GENERAL STRATEGIES

Studies of the transition to parenthood have largely relied on self-report methods gathered by interview or questionnaire. Observational or physiological techniques have not been explored in transition research conducted by nurses. One noteworthy exception is a rating scale employed by Majewski (1986). The two concepts most frequently assessed by transition measures are marital relationships and ease/difficulty of transition.

SPECIFIC TOOLS

The tools cited here as indicators of the transition to parenthood reflect the broad psychosocial nature of transitions. Tools included in this chapter deal with the transition to parenthood experience, as well as such dimensions of the parenting role as child care (Table 10–2). Not included

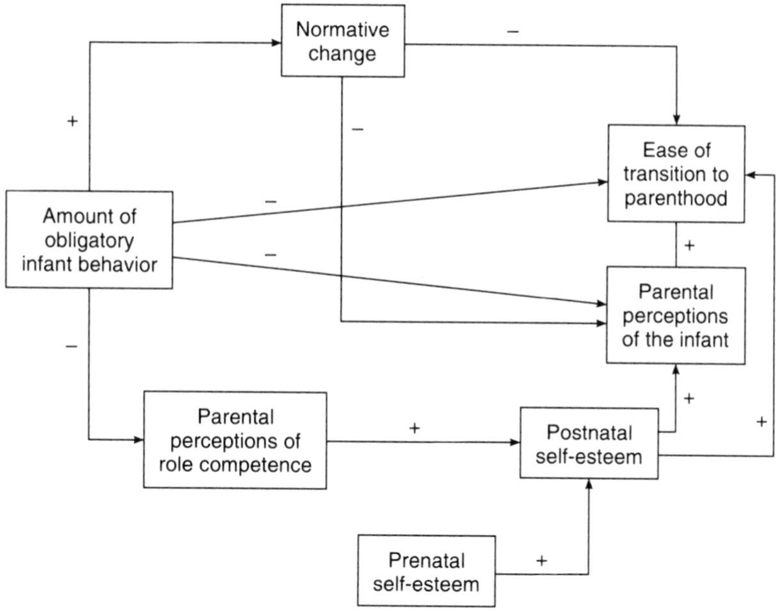

Figure 10–1

A model for infant behavior effects on transition to parenthood and parental perceptions of the infant. (Copyright 1986, American Journal of Nursing Company. Reprinted from *Nursing Research*, Nov/Dec, 1986, *35* (6). Used with permission. All rights reserved.)

here are measures of the marital relationship often employed as an index of transition smoothness. Tools related to dyadic or marital relationships are located in Chapter 5, on social support.

SUMMARY OF RESEARCH

SCOPE OF TRANSITION RESEARCH

Research reported in this chapter either explicitly mentioned the transition framework within the report or focused on roles or relationships within the marital dyad during pregnancy and postpartum.

Approximately half of the research on the transition to parenthood has been descriptive. In particular, gender differences in the transition experience have been examined in several studies. Of the correlational studies of the transition to parenthood, many examined relations among various proposed predictors, such as infant difficulty, attitudinal variables, or marital variables, and such outcomes as ease of transition or marital satisfaction. In addition, several intervention studies have focused on the transition to parenthood.

Table 10–2
MEASURES/TOOLS FOR THE CONCEPT OF TRANSITION

Tool	Source Described in	Studies Using Tool
Transition to the Maternal Role Scale: Seven-item observer-rated scale	Majewski (1986, 1987)	Majewski (1987) Majewski (1986)
Transition to Parenthood Concerns Scale: Eight-subscale tool	Imle & Atwood (1988)	—
Crisis Checklist: Twenty-three-item index of ease of transition	Hobbs (1965) Roberts (1983) (modification)	Roberts (1983) Dooher (1980) Mercer (1986)
What Being the Parent of a New Baby Is Like: Twenty-five items on revised tool	Pridham & Chang (1985, 1989)	Pridham & Chang (1989) Grace (1989)
Maternal Attitude Questionnaire: Tool measuring positive and negative aspects of motherhood	Miller (1981)	Meisenhelder & Meservey (1987)
Lifestyle Changes Inventory: Fifteen-item postnatal scale	Hangsleben (1983)	Hangsleben (1983)
Normative Change Index: Nine-item index of life-style changes	Roberts (1983)	Roberts (1983)
Role Conflict Scale: Scale for role conflict between major life roles	Holahan & Gilbert (1979)	Majewski (1986)
Postpartum Concerns: Thirty-five concerns used in card sort of importance ranking	Broom (1984)	Broom (1984)
Maternal concerns scale: Scale of concerns about infant care and life-style adjustment	Ellis & Hewat (1982)	Brouse (1988)

Baby Care Activities Inventory: Twelve-item scale of expected and actual activities	Hangsleben (1983)	Hangsleben (1983)
Father's Activity Questionnaire: Self-report diary of parenting activities	Tomlinson (1987)	Tomlinson (1987)
Child Care Activities Scale: Scale for parental involvement in 21 child care activities	Cronenwett, Sampselle, & Wilson (1988)	—
Parental Role Preference Scale: Twelve-item scale of ideal, spouse's view, and actual child care participation	Cronenwett et al. (1988)	—
Parental Caretaking Activities Questionnaire: Tool for amount of involvement in caretaking	Sawin as cited in Fortier (1988)	Fortier (1988)
Parent-Infant Interaction Scale: Self-report of anticipated amount of time in infant care	Humenick & Bugen (1987)	Humenick & Bugen (1987)
Projected Paternal Behavior Scale: Thirty-three item scale of child care behaviors.	Alter (1978) as cited in Fishbein (1984)	Fishbein (1984)

Generally, needs and concerns related to the parenting role and infant care are included in Chapters 11 to 13. Because of the overlap between aspects of the transition to parenthood and stress, coping, social support, and role attainment and identity, some research reports in one chapter may have relevance to topics covered in other chapters as well. This is particularly true of research in this chapter and Chapters 11 to 13, on the experiences of pregnancy, childbirth, and parenting (Table 10-3).

Table 10–3
TRANSITION TO PARENTHOOD RESEARCH

DESCRIPTIVE
Descriptions of the Transition
Meisenhelder & Meservey (1987), older mothers
Patterns (Sexual) during the Transition
Ellis (1980)
Guana-Trujillo & Higgins (1987)
Hames (1980)
Differences in the Transition
Dooher (1980), mothers vs. fathers
Hangsleben (1983), fathers' changes over time
Humenick & Bugen (1987), mothers' vs. fathers' changes over time
Majewski (1986), employed vs. nonemployed mothers
Rankin & Campbell (1983), mothers vs. fathers
Roberts (1983), mothers vs. fathers
Saunders & Robins (1987), first vs. third trimester couples
Tomlinson (1987), couples' changes over time
RELATIONSHIPS AMONG VARIABLES/PREDICTIVE MODELS
Maternal Transition
Majewski (1986)
Paternal Transition
Hangsleben (1983)
Couples' Transition
Broom (1984)
Lenz et al. (1985)
Roberts (1983)
Tomlinson (1987)
INTERVENTIONS DURING TRANSITION
Brouse (1988), teaching infant behaviors and liabilities
Dooher (1980), Lamaze childbirth
Meleis & Swendsen (1978), role supplementation

DESCRIPTIVE RESEARCH

Descriptions of the Transition to Parenthood

Meisenhelder and Meservey (1987) conducted a study of the transition to parenthood among women 29 years and older to describe their characteristics and satisfaction with motherhood. Sixty-eight women completed the study questionnaires. All women were white, married, and middle to upper social class. Primary reasons for delaying childbearing were the need for time to develop the marriage, develop a career, and set up financial base/husband's career. Women were about evenly divided across employment levels of full time, part time, and unemployed. Compared to a standardization sample, this sample had a higher mean maternal satisfaction but greater variance in satisfaction. Specifically, the sample viewed the positive aspects of motherhood less positively than the standardization sample but was also more tolerant of the negative aspects of motherhood. Few demographic or contextual variables were related to maternal satisfaction.

Patterns during the Transition to Parenthood

Descriptive studies of the transition to parenthood have primarily focused on sexual changes in the couple's relationship during pregnancy and childbirth. Viewing pregnancy as a maturational crisis that triggers changes in sexuality, Ellis (1980) conducted a pilot study among 15 expectant couples. Based on a survey questionnaire, some of the study findings included: (1) Both husbands and wives reported a decline in enjoyment of sexual intercourse during pregnancy. (2) Men in particular expressed a sexual interest in persons other than their mates. (3) Desired sources of information about sexual activity during pregnancy were books, prenatal instructors, and physicians. (4) During pregnancy, women had a greater need to be told they were loved.

In a study of sexual needs, interests, and changes after childbirth, Hames (1980) surveyed 42 first-time parents. Questionnaire responses indicated the following: (1) Most women acquired information about changes related to sexuality from classes and reading. (2) The majority indicated that breast changes and vaginal bleeding had no effect on sexuality for them. (3) Sixty-two percent resumed sexual relations prior to 6 weeks after childbirth. (4) More women than men reported problems or worries related to resuming sexual intercourse. (5) Over half of the women feared sexual intercourse after childbirth.

Guana-Trujillo and Higgins (1987) conducted a retrospective survey about sexuality during pregnancy and postpartum. Fifty-two women at health clinics or a day care center responded to a survey questionnaire. Responses indicated that the majority refrained from sexual relations for at least some of the time during pregnancy, usually the third trimester. Most women resumed intercourse 2 to 8 weeks after childbirth. Most women reported that counseling about sexuality during pregnancy and postpartum was insufficient. Women did not always comply with health-care providers' prohibition of intercourse.

Differences in the Transition Experiences

To assess the transition to parenthood during pregnancy, Saunders and Robins (1987) compared two sets of couples experiencing their first pregnancy. One set was in the first trimester (n = 48), and the other set was in the third trimester (n = 52). Three indicators of marital strain showed no differences between couples in early and late pregnancy: ambivalence, amount of time together, and marital satisfaction. Differences were found on the following: (1) Greater love was reported by both men and women in late versus early pregnancy. (2) Women reported more conflict in late versus early pregnancy. (3) Men reported engaging in more relationship-oriented communication in late versus early pregnancy. In addition, when effects of gender role attitudes on marital strain were examined, few significant differences were found.

In a related study, Rankin and Campbell (1983) studied perceived marital changes over the last 3 months in 192 couples during the last trimester of pregnancy. In comparing first-time versus second-time parents, no significant differences in marital relationship changes were found for either men or women. For first-time parents, there was a trend for women to perceive relationship changes as more positive than did men.

In comparing mothers and fathers during the transition to parenthood, Roberts (1983) reported that fathers had greater ease of transition than mothers, whereas mothers reported more normative changes in lifestyle than fathers. In a related study of marital satisfaction before and after the transition to parenthood, Tomlinson (1987) reported that both first-time mothers and fathers showed declines in satisfaction from pregnancy to 12 weeks postpartum. Further, Dooher (1980) examined gender differences in degree of crisis during the transition to parenthood: Mothers' degree of crisis exceeded that of fathers'.

To examine gender differences in interaction, that is, involvement with the infant, Humenick and Bugen (1987) compared prenatal anticipations and postnatal actual involvement among 36 mothers and fathers. Mothers' actual time involvement exceeded expectations, whereas fathers' expectations exceeded actual involvement. Both differences were significant. In addition, both anticipated and actual involvement were greater for mothers than for fathers. In a related study of the transition to fatherhood, Hangsleben (1983) reported that fathers did fewer infant care activities than they had expected. In particular, fathers did less bathing of infants, babysitting, caring for infants during sickness, and infant feeding than they had expected.

In comparing mothers who were employed versus those who were not employed during the transition to motherhood, Majewski (1986) reported that the two groups did not differ in amount of role conflict in the areas of spouse, parent, and self. In comparing mothers who saw their employment as a job versus a career, no differences were found on four of six subscales; mothers with careers did report more conflict between worker and self roles and worker and spouse roles than mothers with jobs.

RELATIONAL/PREDICTIVE RESEARCH

Transition Studies of Mothers

Majewski (1986) examined influences during the transition to motherhood among 86 first-time mothers who varied with regard to employment. Their infants were from 5 to 18 months of age. As expected, more perceived role conflict was related to more difficulty in the transition to motherhood, whereas greater marital satisfaction was related to more ease of transition. Among employed mothers, however, attitudes toward employment were unrelated to ease of the transition to motherhood.

Transition Studies of Fathers

In a study of the transition to fatherhood, Hangsleben (1983) studied 53 first-time fathers using prenatal and postnatal questionnaires covering depression, child care activities, marital adjustment, and life-style changes. Prenatal depression was related to postnatal depression; the latter was also related to more life-style changes, preferring a son, and an unplanned pregnancy. Greater age and income were related to less expected child care, whereas greater actual child care involvement was related to more life-style changes. Better marital adjustment was related to younger age, less depression, and greater expectation for child care involvement.

Transition Studies of Couples

Broom (1984) studied 11 prenatal and 11 postnatal couples to assess consensus among couples during the transition to parenthood. Couples rank-ordered 35 concerns from most to least important. Rankings of prenatal and postnatal concerns were significantly related. Husbands' and wives' rankings were generally in agreement, but more agreement was perceived by husbands and wives than actually existed except for postpartum wives. However, husbands were more accurate in predicting wives' concerns than wives were in predicting husbands' concerns. Couples most often discussed the concerns ranked as most important.

To assess the effect of infant behavior on the transition to parenthood, Roberts (1983) proposed a theoretical model of influences during the transition. Mediating between infant behaviors and transition outcomes were normative changes, perception of role competence, and self-esteem. To test the model, 64 couples were studied during pregnancy and postpartum. For both mothers and fathers, infant behavior was related to normative changes, which in turn were related to ease of transition. Infant behaviors also were related to transition outcomes and perceptions of role competence. Post hoc analyses indicated that role competence also was related to transition outcomes.

Tomlinson (1987) studied 96 couples to determine predictors of marital satisfaction during the transition to parenthood. Sex role attitudes, marital equity, perceived father involvement, and infant temperament served as predictors. The control variable, prebirth marital satisfaction, accounted for the greatest amount of variance in postnatal marital satisfaction. Postbirth equity explained significant amounts of additional variance for both mothers and fathers.

In another study of couples during the parental transition, Lenz, Soeken, Rankin, and Fischman (1985) examined relationships among gender, sex-role attributes, and components of the marital relationship during postpartum. The sample of 147 women and 146 men were recruited during pregnancy and assessed for marital attributes at 4 months postpartum. Reports of positive overall marital and intimate changes were related to positive appraisal of marital quality. In regression analyses, gender and sex role attributes (except for femininity) were not significant predictors of any marital attributes. Femininity predicted overall marital change and marital quality.

INTERVENTION RESEARCH

Three intervention studies, all containing some educational dimensions, have attempted to enhance the transition to parenthood. Brouse (1988) tested the effects of teaching new mothers about infant behaviors and abilities on ease of transition to motherhood. The intervention, presented on the third postpartum day, provided information on infant states, behavioral and defensive abilities, and reflexes. Mothers (n = 16 in control group, n = 15 in experimental group) completed outcome measures on anxiety and maternal concerns about life-style adjustment and infant care at 3 weeks postpartum. There were no significant differences between groups on outcome measures.

Meleis and Swendsen (1978) tested an intervention based on role supplementation among couples experiencing the situational transition of becoming parents. Forty-six low-risk couples with a first pregnancy served as subjects in three groups: (1) control group (n = 36 couples); (2) FamCap group (n = 10 couples) involving an early discharge program with prenatal nursing assessment and prenatal preparation for discharge; and (3) experimental group (n = 12 couples) involving the role supplementation intervention. Included in role supplementation were the following theoretically based strategies: reference group, role modeling, and role rehearsal. None of the groups differed on prenatal attitudes, but groups did differ significantly on predelivery marriage role expectations. Contrary to expectation, couples in the FamCap groups experienced the greatest change in role perceptions postdelivery. There were no significant differences among groups on wives' predelivery or postdelivery anxiety, but husbands' anxiety was significantly higher within the experimental group prior to delivery although not after delivery. In addition, wives' postdelivery attitudes differed significantly toward infants but not toward themselves, with FamCap and experimental groups generally scoring more favorably.

Dooher (1980) tested whether Lamaze-prepared childbirth eased the transition to parenthood among 20 first-time parents. Couples in the control group (n = 10) and experimental group (n = 10) completed questionnaires at 3 weeks prior to delivery and at 3 to 4 weeks after delivery. The two groups differed on levels of stress predelivery with the higher levels in the experimental group. The two groups did not differ on predelivery marital adjustment, but they did differ after delivery. Differences favored the control group. With regard to degree of crisis experienced during the transition, there were no differences between groups.

FUTURE RESEARCH DIRECTIONS

Extent studies of the transition to parenthood inform nurses about gender differences and factors such as infant temperament, marital quality, and attitudes that affect ease of transition. Important as these findings may be, they shed little light on the specific adaptive tasks associated with the transition or the relation between role preparation, adaptive tasks, and transition outcomes. This limitation of transition research may reflect the difficulty of using a general transition framework for studying a specific developmental transition. Greater explication of the transition framework within early parenting would contribute to more substantive research in this area. (See Tilden's [1980] effort to explicate psychological development during the transitional event of pregnancy.) Further tests of hypotheses about the transition to parenthood also should be conducted with low-income families to overcome the middle-class bias in many past studies.

So far, measuring transition outcomes has relied primarily on marital quality or ease of transition. Indeed, marital attributes have been the most frequently used indicators for exploring the transition to parenthood (Rankin & Campbell, 1983; Saunders & Robins, 1987; Majewski, 1986;

Tomlinson, 1987; Hangsleben, 1983; Dooher, 1980; Melies & Swendsen, 1978; Lenz et al., 1985). Other indicators relevant to the transition to parenthood, such as duration of the transition phase, should be considered. In addition, transition measures often are framed in terms of ease or difficulty. That captures only one dimension of the transition. Hypothetically, a transition might involve much effort, but it might also be seen as a positive challenge. Better sorting out of "effort invested" versus "turmoil" also reflects alternative views of the transition to parenthood: that of normative transition versus stressor.

Intervention research conducted in a transition-to-parenthood framework is scant. Most of the existing studies were conducted some time ago, and they reflect the exploratory nature of early research in a field. Future interventions aimed at enhancing the transition to parenthood would benefit from increased sample sizes, statistical control for pretreatment group differences, and use of random assignment.

REFERENCES

Broom, B. L. (1984). Consensus about the marital relationship during transition to parenthood. *Nursing Research, 33,* 223–228.

Brouse, A. J. (1988). Easing the transition to the maternal role. *Journal of Advanced Nursing, 13,* 167–172.

Cronenwett, L. R., Sampselle, C. M., & Wilson, W. R. (1988). The child care activities scale and parental role preference scale. *Research in Nursing & Health, 11,* 301–308.

Dooher, M. E. (1980). Lamaze method of childbirth. *Nursing Research, 29,* 220–224.

Ellis, D. J. (1980). Sexual needs and concerns of expectant parents. *Journal of Obstetric, Gynecologic, and Neonatal Nursing, 9,* 306–308.

Ellis, D. J., & Hewat, R. (1982). Assisting women with breastfeeding. In G. Zilm, A. Hilton, & M. Richmond (Eds.), *Nursing research: A base for practice, service and education* (pp. 258–268). Vancouver, British Columbia: University of British Columbia.

Fishbein, E. G. (1984). Expectant father's stress—due to the mother's expectations? *Journal of Obstetric, Gynecologic, and Neonatal Nursing, 13,* 325–328.

Fortier, J. C. (1988). The relationship of vaginal and cesarean birth to father-infant attachment. *Journal of Obstetric, Gynecologic, and Neonatal Nursing, 17,* 128–134.

Golan, N. (1981). *Passing through transitions: A guide for practitioners.* New York: The Free Press.

Grace, J. T. (1989). Development of maternal-fetal attachment during pregnancy. *Nursing Research, 38,* 228–232.

Guana-Trujillo, B., & Higgins, P. G. (1987). Sexual intercourse and pregnancy. *Health Care for Women International, 8,* 339–348.

Hames, C. T. (1980). Sexual needs and interests of postpartum couples. *Journal of Obstetric, Gynecologic, and Neonatal Nursing, 9,* 313–315.

Hangsleben, K. L. (1983). Transition to fatherhood: An exploratory study. *Journal of Obstetric, Gynecologic, and Neonatal Nursing, 12,* 265–270.

Hobbs, D. F. (1965). Parenthood as crisis: A third study. *Journal of Marriage and the Family, 27,* 367–372.

Holahan, C. K., & Gilbert, L. A. (1979). Interrole conflict for working women. *Journal of Applied Psychology, 64,* 86–90.

Humenick, S. S., & Bugen, L. A. (1987). Parenting roles: Expectation versus reality. *MCN, The American Journal of Maternal-Child Nursing, 12,* 36–39.

Imle, M. A., & Atwood, J. R. (1988). Retaining qualitative validity while gaining quantitative reliability and validity: Development of the transition to parenthood concerns scale. *Advances in Nursing Science, 11*(1), 61–75.

Lenz, E. R., Soeken, K. L., Ranking, E. A., & Fischman, S. H. (1985). Sex-role attributes, gender, and postpartal perceptions of the marital relationship. *Advances in Nursing Science, 7*(3), 49–62.

Majewski, J. L. (1987). Social support and the transition to the maternal role. *Health Care for Women International, 8,* 397–407.

Majewski, J. L. (1986). Conflicts, satisfactions, and attitudes during transition to the maternal role. *Nursing Research, 35,* 10–14.

Meisenhelder, J. B., & Meservey, P. M. (1987). Childbearing over thirty: Description and satisfaction with mothering. *Western Journal of Nursing Research, 9,* 527–541.

Meleis, A. I., & Swendsen, L. A. (1978). Role supplementation: An empirical test of a nursing intervention. *Nursing Research, 27,* 11–18.

Mercer, R. T. (1986). Predictors of maternal role attainment at one year postbirth. *Western Journal of Nursing Research, 8,* 9–25.

Miller, W. B. (1981). *The psychology of reproduction.* Springfield, VA: National Technical Information Service.

Pridham, K. F., & Chang, A. S. (1985). Parents' beliefs about themselves as parents of a new infant: Instrument development. *Research in Nursing and Health, 8,* 19–29.

Pridham, K. F., & Chang, A. S. (1989). What being the parent of a new baby is like: Revision of an instrument. *Research in Nursing and Health, 12,* 323–329.

Rankin, E. A. D., & Campbell, N. D. (1983). Perception of relationship changes during the third trimester of pregnancy. *Issues in Health Care of Women, 6,* 351–359.

Roberts, F. B. (1983). Infant behavior and the transition to parenthood. *Nursing Research, 32,* 213–217.

Rossi, A. S. (1968). Transition to parenthood. *Journal of Marriage and the Family, 30*(1), 26–39.

Saunders, R. B., & Robins, E. (1987). Changes in the marital relationship during the first pregnancy. *Health Care for Women International, 8,* 361-377.

Tilden, V. P. (1980). A developmental conceptual framework for the maturational crisis of pregnancy. *Western Journal of Nursing Research, 2,* 667–685.

Tomlinson, P. S. (1987). Spousal differences in marital satisfaction during transition to parenthood. *Nursing Research, 36,* 239–243.

CHAPTER 11

Parent-Infant Nursing Research on the Experience of Pregnancy

DEFINITIONS AND DESCRIPTIONS OF THE EXPERIENCE OF PREGNANCY

This chapter contains parent-infant nursing research on the experience of pregnancy, particularly the cognitive and affective components. Much of that research stems from Rubin's maternal role attainment and identity framework. Because of their long history, Rubin's writings (1967a, 1967b, 1984) have had both direct and indirect effects on how pregnancy has been viewed by nurse investigators. (See Chapter 9 for a review of Rubin's theoretical work.) Some investigators explicitly cite Rubin's work; others represent her point of view implicitly by the types of variables studied and research questions asked. As a result, in this chapter the experience of pregnancy is broadly defined so that studies that explicitly or implicitly reflect the role attainment and identity framework are included. Although Rubin gave only limited consideration to the paternal experience (Rubin, 1984, p. 46), fathers' experiences during their partners' pregnancies are included here.

DEFINING THE EXPERIENCE OF PREGNANCY

Following Rubin (1975), many studies that are reported in this chapter explicitly mentioned that women's experience of pregnancy is more than one of changing physical adaptations. It was defined as including adaptations in identity and interpersonal relationships and maturation of the maternal personality (e.g., Richardson, 1981, 1983). When conceptual definitions of the experience of pregnancy were presented in studies, most often they related to body image (e.g., Strang & Sullivan, 1985; Fawcett, 1989b) (Table 11–1). By contrast, because studies of expectant fathers during pregnancy have been less common, many studies of men adopted an exploratory stance without clear starting definitions of the phenomena of interest (e.g., May, 1980).

THEORETICAL MODELS OF THE EXPERIENCE OF PREGNANCY

Although a number of studies of the experience of pregnancy made reference to concepts and relations among concepts within Rubin's descriptive writings (e.g., Rubin, 1975), few theoretical models elaborating on the pregnancy experience were explicitly proposed or tested in the studies reviewed here. One exception was the program of research grounded in the framework of the family as an open system (Fawcett, 1989b).

MEASUREMENT

GENERAL STRATEGIES

Because the experience of pregnancy as defined by Rubin (1984) is essentially subjective, measurement of it is largely dependent on self-reports

Table 11–1
DEFINITIONS AND DESCRIPTIONS OF THE EXPERIENCE OF PREGNANCY

Definitions/Descriptions of Body Image and Related Concepts

Body image "is the composite of perceptions, attitudes, and feelings each individual has of his/her own body as it exists in space." (Strang & Sullivan, 1985, p. 332.)

Body image is composed of "two independent dimensions, body perception and body attitude." (Strang & Sullivan, 1985, p. 332.)

Body perception "refers to the direct mental experience of the physical appearance of the body, which encompasses surface depth and postural mental pictures." (Strang & Sullivan, 1985, p. 332.)

Body attitude "encompasses a broad spectrum of feelings, attitudes, and emotional reactions toward the body and represents the individuals' valuation of their bodies." (Strang & Sullivan, 1985, p. 332.)

by either interviews or questionnaires. Qualitative data derived from interviews can be analyzed in a number of ways, for example, content analysis or grounded theory, to mention only two. Given the theoretically rich descriptions of the pregnancy experience that already exist, however, it is an appropriate time to develop theoretically based coding schemes that can be used across studies. Application of extant coding schemes requires training and satisfactory interrater agreement across investigators to maximally benefit knowledge development.

SPECIFIC TOOLS

There are surprisingly few tools that are well-designed and consistently used to measure the dimensions of the experience of pregnancy. One promising exception is Lederman's (1984) Prenatal Self-Evaluation Questionnaire. Although a number of different tools have been used to study dimensions of the pregnancy experience, no tool has served as a common anchor across diverse studies. As a result, no clear comparability of measurement exists in the studies reviewed in this chapter. Table 11-2 presents measures of the experience of pregnancy used in studies cited in this chapter and other studies reviewed in this book.

SUMMARY OF RESEARCH

SCOPE OF RESEARCH ON THE EXPERIENCE OF PREGNANCY

This chapter includes studies, mostly descriptive, that focus on the experience of pregnancy as broadly outlined at the chapter outset (Table 11-3). Further, this section includes studies that began during pregnancy and continued into the postpartum period so that the continuity across periods can be presented. (*Note:* For studies of social support during pregnancy, see Chapter 5.)

DESCRIPTIVE RESEARCH

Descriptions of Aspects of the Experience of Pregnancy

To identify educational needs of pregnant teenagers aged 15 to 19, Copeland (1979) interviewed 15 teenagers. Eighty percent said their pregnancies were accidental. The educational needs identified by teenagers as important were self-oriented and dealt with understanding bodily

Table 11–2
MEASURES/TOOLS FOR THE CONCEPT OF EXPERIENCE OF PREGNANCY

Tool	Source Described in	Studies Using Tool
Prenatal Self-Evaluation Questionnaire: Seventy-nine-item scale	Lederman (1984)	Curry (1987) Shaw (1986)
Maternal Expectations and Childbearing Attitudes: Attitudes Toward Self During Pregnancy: Anxiety and attitude scale	Field (1981)	Shaw (1986)
Pregnancy Acceptance Questionnaire: Two-page scale	Porter & Demeuth (1979)	Porter & Demeuth (1979)
Readiness for pregnancy index: Feelings about pregnancy when discovered	Mercer, Ferketich, May, DeJoseph & Sollid (1988)	Mercer et al. (1988)
Maternal Attitude to Pregnancy Instrument: Forty-eight-item scale of pregnancy attitudes	Blau, Welkowitz, & Cohen (1964)	Hart (1980)
Feelings about pregnancy: Six-item index	Nuckolls, Cassel, & Kaplan (1972)	Mercer (1985a) Mercer (1985b)
Pregnancy Research Inventory: Eight subscale prenatal feelings inventory	Schaefer & Manheimer (1960)	Hellings (1985) Meleis & Swendsen (1978) McCraw & Abplanalp (1984)
Prenatal Assessment of Parenting Guide: Clinical assessment tool based on tasks of pregnancy	Josten (1981)	Josten (1982)
Rees Scales: Three summated rating scales for identification with the mothering role	Rees (1980)	Kemp & Page (1987)

Table 11–2
MEASURES/TOOLS FOR THE CONCEPT OF EXPERIENCE OF PREGNANCY *(Continued)*

Tool	Source Described in	Studies Using Tool
Imaginal Processes Inventory as adapted by Sherwen: Scale for tapping fantasies in pregnancy	Sherwen (1986)	Sherwen (1986)
Affectional Relationship Questionnaire, Phase I: Scale focused on affectional bond with fetus and involvement in pregnancy	Bills (1980)	Sherwen (1986)
Perception of Fetus: Ten items dealing with fetal growth and development	Heidrich & Cranley (1989)	Heidrich & Cranley (1989)
Body Attitude Scale: Semantic differential scale for global body attitude using 30 different body concepts	Kurtz (1969)	Drake et al. (1988) Fawcett et al. (1986)
Attitude to Body Image Scale (modified version of Body Cathexis Scale of Jourard & Secord, 1955): Ten-item scale	Strang & Sullivan (1985)	Strang & Sullivan (1985)
Identification Scale: Measure of the extent to which connotative meanings are shared by two people	Lazowick (1955)	Drake et al. (1988) Fawcett et al. (1986) Fawcett (1977)
Topographic Device: Fifty-inch sheet of vinyl marked with concentric circles used in estimating one's perceived body space, i.e., body perception	Fawcett & Frye (1980) Fawcett (1977)	Drake et al. (1988) Fawcett et al. (1986) Fawcett (1977)
Articulation of Body Concept Scale: Protocol for rating body articulation	Witkin, Dyk, Faterson, Goodenough, & Karp (1974)	Fawcett (1977)

Semantic Differential Scales: Eighteen paired adjectives for rating body image	Moore (1978)	Moore (1978)
Concerns Questionnaire: Sixty-two-item scale for eliciting maternal concerns during pregnancy	Glazer (1980)	Glazer (1980)
Interview schedule on concerns about learning infant care: Open-ended schedule	Bliss-Holtz (1988)	Bliss-Holtz (1988)
Knowledge test (parallel forms): Fifty-item tests about the care and characteristics of newborns (used prenatally)	Sullivan (1984)	Sullivan (1984)
Presonograph questionnaire: Fourteen items on maternal perception of fetus	Kohn et al. (1980)	Kohn et al. (1980)
Postsonograph questionnaire: Fifteen items on maternal perception of fetus	Kohn et al. (1980)	Kohn et al. (1980)

Table 11–3
PARENT-INFANT NURSING RESEARCH ON THE EXPERIENCE OF PREGNANCY

DESCRIPTIVE
Descriptions of the Experience of Pregnancy
Copeland (1979), pregnant adolescents
Glazer (1980), pregnant women
Richardson (1981, 1983), pregnant women
Patterns of the Experience of Pregnancy
Corbin (1987), pregnancy with chronic illness
May (1980), fathers' detachment/involvement in pregnancy
May (1982), phases in fathers' experience of pregnancy
Milne & Rich (1981), womens' experiences with ultrasonography
Winslow (1987), pregnancy in older women
Differences in the Experience of Pregnancy
Bliss-Holtz (1988), pregnant women in early, mid-, and late pregnancy
Moore (1978), pregnant women vs. contrast groups
Richardson (1987), women with preterm labor vs. normal pregnancies
Sherwen (1986), expectant fathers vs. contrast groups
Speraw (1987), adolescents in four ethnic groups
Strang & Sullivan (1985), pregnant women over time
RELATIONSHIPS AMONG VARIABLES/PREDICTIVE MODELS
Correlates of Fantasies, Pregnancy Tasks
Josten (1982)
Sherwen (1986)
Correlates of Self-Concept in Pregnancy
Brouse (1985)
Lee (1982)
Correlates of Body Image
Drake et al. (1988)
Fawcett (1977)
Fawcett et al. (1986)
INTERVENTION RESEARCH
Prenatal Education
Jones (1986)
McCraw & Abplanalp (1984)
Petrowski (1981)
Shaw (1986)
Sullivan (1984)
Other
Kohn et al. (1980)

changes during pregnancy and the labor and delivery experience. Also rated as important was learning about baby care and the effects of parental drug use on babies. The majority preferred to talk with other pregnant teenagers about feelings in pregnancy, which suggested that group discussion formats are desirable for teenaged parent education.

Glazer (1980) investigated concerns and anxiety in pregnancy. One hundred randomly selected prenatal patients completed questionnaires. Overall, the most prevalent concerns focused on childbirth, medical care, and self, but they varied somewhat by trimester. Items of greatest concern focused on the baby and childbirth. The number of concerns was significantly related to anxiety. Women with higher anxiety and number of concerns tended to be younger, have less education, have shorter relationships with partners, and be poorer than those with lower anxiety and number of concerns.

In a study of pregnant women's experiences of important relationships, Richardson (1981) repeatedly interviewed 14 women (5 primiparas and 9 multiparas) from at least the 14th week of gestation through the end of pregnancy. Using content analysis, relationships mentioned in interviews were coded in terms of whether they were perceived as changing or stable and satisfactory or unsatisfactory. Of relationships mentioned by women, 38 percent were with parent figures, 24 percent with peers, 18 percent with husbands, and 20 percent with womens' own or others' children. Overall, women perceived that a greater proportion of relationships were changing rather than remaining stable. From early to midpregnancy, an increasing proportion of all relationships were seen as changing. From mid- to late pregnancy, an increasing proportion of relationships with parent figures and husbands were seen as stable while relationships with children were seen as increasingly changing. Overall, women described the greatest proportion of relationships with parental figures, peers, husbands, and children as satisfactory. In the early pregnancy, however, a greater proportion of relationships with husbands were seen as unsatisfactory rather than satisfactory, and in late pregnancy a greater proportion of relationships with children were seen as unsatisfactory rather than satisfactory.

In an extension of the preceding study, Richardson (1983) examined further women's perceptions of changing relationships with children during pregnancy. The 14 women who served as subjects were identical, it appears, to those in the preceding study. Again, content analysis of interviews was used for data analysis. Perceived changes in important relationships were coded in terms of task performance (changes in usual functional patterns) and affective involvement (changes in attitudes and feelings within the mother-child dyad). Perceived relationships with children were mentioned in multiparas' interviews, but not in primiparas'. The changing relationships were more often seen as unsatisfactory (59 percent) rather than satisfactory (41 percent). A greater proportion of reported changes occurred in affective involvement (65 percent) than in task performance (35 percent). The three most frequently reported specific changes were related to affection displays, managing roles, and attitudes about the pregnancy or baby.

Qualitative Patterns of the Experience of Pregnancy

Winslow (1987) used grounded theory methods to study the pregnancy experience of 12 women who were 35 years or older. All the women were well educated, and all had planned their pregnancies. The core concept evolved from "learning experiences" to "pregnancy as a project." The pregnancy project was divided into four phases that reflected the following four concepts: (1) planned change, (2) control, (3) transition, and (4) uncertainty. Each concept was elaborated in subdimensions. For example, planned change was associated with five factors that contributed to the decision to conceive: (1) strong relationship with father of the baby, (2) delaying conception would further increase the risks of infertility and Down's syndrome, (3) sense of completeness about other areas of life, (4) desire to have a child, and (5) rejection of the alternative of childlessness.

In a qualitative study involving both cross-sectional and longitudinal designs, May (1980) interviewed 20 expectant couples to explore fathers' experiences of pregnancy. Using grounded theory methods, May proposed a typology of fathers' perceived relationships to their partners' pregnancies. Three levels of detachment/involvement composed that typology: observer styles, expressive styles, and instrumental styles. In the observer styles, men reported low emotional involvement in the pregnancies and saw themselves as bystanders. By contrast, in the expressive styles, men reported heavy emotional involvement and saw themselves as full partners. Instrumental styles were characterized by task-oriented involvement and managerial roles in relation to pregnancies.

In a further report of the preceding study, May (1982) described three phases in father involvement in pregnancy. Each phase marked a change in level of behavioral and emotional involvement. The phases included the announcement phase (period about when the pregnancy was confirmed); moratorium (period, following confirmation, when thoughts of pregnancy were avoided); and the focusing phase (period when pregnancy became real and important to men). During the moratorium, couple communication may be altered and tensions may rise as men and women approach pregnancy differently. At about 25 weeks' gestation men moved to the focusing phase, wherein they began to see themselves as fathers. This shift brought couples into more congruence with each other.

Completing developmental tasks of pregnancy (Rubin, 1975), particularly safe passage, is more complex for women with chronic illnesses. Corbin (1987) conducted a qualitative study of 20 chronically ill women during their pregnancies to describe their experiences. A process of protective governing was identified; by it, women attempted to control threats to their pregnancy outcomes. Three specific strategies were included in protective governing: assessing, balancing, and controlling. Assessing entailed defining the level of risk to the pregnancy and self; balancing involved weighing treatment or care options against risks and benefits; and controlling referred to shared care decisions made by women and health care providers to enhance pregnancy outcomes. Factors influencing women's ability to manage risks included knowledge, support, stability of illness, and perceived sense of control.

To assess cognitive and affective aspects of women's responses to ultrasonography, Milne and Rich (1981) conducted a cross-sectional study of 20 pregnant women. Immediately preceding the procedure, women evidenced anxiety about it and the information it would provide. During the procedure, women went through a process of personal recognition of fetal stimuli involving preset, pattern recognition, and synthesis. Responses to the imaging procedure included attention and affective responses to images recognized. Following the procedure, women continued to respond cognitively and affectively to the experience of imaging the fetus.

Differences in the Experience of Pregnancy

In a study of body image during pregnancy, Moore (1978) conducted a cross-sectional study of pregnant and nonpregnant women. Pregnant women viewed their body image less positively than the ideal, and as pregnancy progressed, body image became more negative. In ratings of pregnant women's bodies, more significant differences in adjective pairs was found for women than for men. Only 1 of 15 magazines read by pregnant women contained photographs of pregnant women.

Using a retrospective design, Strang and Sullivan (1985) examined differences in the body-attitude component of body image changes in response to childbearing. Postpartum data were gathered from 93 women at 2 and 6 weeks postpartum; retrospective data on body attitude during the prepregnant and pregnant state were gathered at the 2-week postpartum occasion. Body attitude became more negative both from prepregnancy to pregnancy and from prepregnancy to postpartum, but it was more positive in postpartum than during pregnancy. Body attitude did not change significantly between the two postpartum occasions. Multiparas showed more positive body attitudes than primiparas.

To determine whether pregnant women's wish to learn about infant care varied with the trimester of pregnancy, Bliss-Holtz (1988) interviewed 189 pregnant women (n = 63 for each trimester). Interviews were content-analyzed by thematic units. Desire to learn infant care was coded as either psychological (concerns about development of emotional ties to baby and general role learning) or pragmatic (concerns about specific infant care skills). There were significant differences in overall and pragmatic desire to learn infant care; in both cases, concerns were proportionately greater in late pregnancy than in early or midpregnancy. There was no significant difference in the proportion of the psychological component across the trimesters. However, concerns about learning infant care were a small portion (5 percent in late pregnancy) of the total concerns expressed by pregnant women.

Sherwen (1986) compared fantasy patterns of expectant fathers (n = 38) to those of expectant mothers (n = 38) and nonexpectant men (n = 40). Assessment of fantasies of expectant fathers and their partners occurred in the third trimester of pregnancy. Expectant fathers and nonexpectant men differed in only 1 of 10 fantasy dimensions: present-oriented daydreams. Expectant fathers and mothers differed in only 1 of 10 fantasy dimensions: nightdreaming frequency, with mothers scoring higher than fathers.

Speraw (1987) conducted a cross-cultural study of perceptions of pregnancy among white, black, Hispanic, and Pacific Asian pregnant adolescents. By use of an open-ended questionnaire, 59 adolescents in California and Hawaii were surveyed in school-based programs. Responses were analyzed qualitatively and by percentages. Distinct differences among groups emerged. Whites most often reacted negatively to the initial confirmation of the pregnancy. Blacks were most often positive about the timing of the pregnancy. In giving hypothetical reasons for the pregnancy, 50 percent of whites' responses were classified as "accidental" and 50 percent of Hispanics' were classified as "love." The pregnancy was unplanned for 100 percent of whites, 65 percent of blacks, 100 percent of Hispanics, and 80 percent of Pacific Asians. Hispanics most often anticipated the best part of motherhood to be caretaking. Whites most often anticipated the worst part of motherhood to be loss of freedom.

In a study of the relations between women's interpersonal relationships and preterm labor, Richardson (1987) compared two groups: 30 women hospitalized for preterm labor and 15 women with normal pregnancies. Women in the preterm labor group more often perceived important relationships with husbands and parental figures as unsatisfactory compared to the normal pregnancy group. For example, 66 percent of the preterm labor group perceived their relationships with husbands to be unsatisfactory compared to 27 percent of the normal pregnancy group. Satisfaction with peer relationships did not differ between the two groups.

RELATIONAL/PREDICTIVE RESEARCH

In an investigation of fantasy in the paternal role attainment process, Sherwen (1986) studied 38 expectant fathers. Two correlates of fathers' fantasy patterns were examined: sex role orientation and involvement in the pregnancy. Sex role orientation was associated with differences in fantasy patterns. Men with feminine versus masculine or androgynous orientations scored significantly higher on about half of the 10 fantasy dimensions studied. Also, involvement in the pregnancy was related to about half of the dimensions of fathers' fantasies.

In a longitudinal study from pregnancy to the infant's first year, Josten (1982) tested the predictive accuracy of an assessment based on Rubin's (1975) tasks of pregnancy. Fifty-two pregnant women were assessed during clinic visits by using a semistructured interview. Quality of maternal care was rated by independent raters. There was a significant association between prenatal assessments and later quality of maternal care. Modal age of inadequate care mothers was 17 years compared to 27 years for adequate care mothers.

Two studies examined the role of self-concept during pregnancy. First, Lee (1982) explored self-concept during pregnancy as a predictor of mothers' perceptions of the infant and parenting. A sample of 31 low-income women completed assessments during pregnancy and at 1 to 2 days and 4 to 6 weeks postpartum. Self-concept was related to maternal perceptions of the infant, but it was opposite from the predicted direction. Parenting scores were unrelated to maternal self-concept or perception of the infant.

Second, Brouse (1985) studied interrelationships among gender role identity, femininity, self-concept, and comfort in the mothering role over the course of late pregnancy and postpartum. Primiparas and multiparas did not differ with regard to increases in self-concept and femininity across testing occasions. Nor did women typed as high feminine compared to low feminine demonstrate greater increases in self-concept and femininity in a multivariate test. However, femininity was consistently correlated with self-concept across testing occasions for the whole sample. Contrary to expectation, self-concept was unrelated to comfort in the mothering role.

In a program of research based on the family as an open system, Fawcett (1989a, 1989b) completed a number of studies pertinent to body image during childbearing. In the first study (Fawcett, 1977), identification and changes in body image were studied in 50 married couples during and after pregnancy. As expected, changes in perceived body space across two points in pregnancy and two points in postpartum were statistically significant for both wives and husbands. Changes for wives followed a cubic trend; those for husbands conformed to a quadratic trend. Trend analysis indicated that the data curves for perceived body space of wives and husbands differed. Neither wives nor husbands, however, showed changes in body articulation from pregnancy to postpartum. Hypotheses about relations between couple identification and body image were not supported.

In an extension of the preceding study, Fawcett, Bliss-Holtz, Haas, Leventhal, and Rubin (1986) again assessed identification and body image in 54 couples. Assessment began at the third month of pregnancy and ended with the second month postpartum. In this sample, only wives perceived body space changed over the course of pregnancy and postpartum: wives perceived that body space increased progressively during pregnancy, dropped at 1 month postpartum, and then rose slightly at 2 months postpartum. Neither husbands nor wives showed changes in global body attitude. Also relations between identification and changes in body image were not significant.

In a further replication with a Canadian sample (N = 20 couples), Drake, Verhulst, Fawcett, and Barger (1988) again assessed body image and identification from pregnancy to postpartum. Again, wives but not husbands perceived that body space changed over the course of pregnancy and postpartum. Husbands' and wives' patterns of perceived body space were not similar. Global body attitude changed significantly for wives and approached significance for husbands; husbands' and wives' patterns were not similar, however. Couple identification was not related in the predicted manner to either perceived body space or global body attitude.

INTERVENTION RESEARCH

Five studies have used prenatal education in some form as an intervention to enhance antepartal or postpartal knowledge or outcomes. In the first study, Petrowski (1981) used a four-group design (control, antepartal education, postpartal education, and combined antepartal-postpartal education) to assess the effects of three components of instruction: timing, repetition, and readiness. Forty (10 per condition) inner city primigravidas were randomly assigned to conditions. Experimental groups received instruction antepartally, postpartally, or both via four audiocassettes. Instruction focused on cord care, burping, perineal care, rest, and activity. Outcomes were measured by a multiple-choice test administered in the home at 5 to 13 days postpartum. After controlling for education differences, there were no significant differences among groups.

In the second study, Shaw (1986) tested the efficacy of telephone audiotapes as a medium for delivering prenatal education. Twenty-five primigravidas were randomly assigned to the control (n = 15) or experimental conditions (n = 10). On pretests, the two groups did not differ in childbearing anxiety or identification with motherhood. The experimental group subsequently listened to 18 audiotapes on such topics as infant care and parenting skills prior to delivery. At 1 to 3 days after delivery, the two groups differed in one of two outcomes: the experimental group had less favorable scores on confidence about motherhood. At 4 to 6 weeks postpartum, the two groups differed in three of four outcomes: The experimental group was less satisfied with motherhood, perceived the average mother as having difficulty adjusting to motherhood, and had greater difficulty in making that adjustment than the control group.

In the third study, Sullivan (1984) tested the efficacy of an instructional program (linear self-instructional primary health education) aimed at teaching pregnant women about the care and characteristics of newborns. Ninety-nine women were randomly assigned to either the experimental or the control group. Pretests and posttests (parallel forms) about knowledge of newborn care and characteristics were used to measure program efficacy. The program consisted of four programmed instructional booklets with accompanying instructional slides. The interval between pretests and posttests was 5 days. Women were further blocked as high, medium, and low based on pretest knowledge scores. Results indicated significant main effects for groups, entry knowledge level, and the interaction of both. The experimental group scored significantly higher than the control group on the posttest, and the low-knowledge group benefited more than the medium- and high-knowledge groups from the instructional program.

Fourth, McCraw and Abplanalp (1984) tested the effects of Lamaze classes on maternal attitudes and feelings during pregnancy. Both the Lamaze group (n = 45) and the control group, which had no formal childbirth classes (n = 29) completed a prenatal attitude inventory that served as both the pretest and the posttest. Groups differed on four of five demographic variables. Thus, in a subsample (n = 14 in each group) that was drawn, the control and Lamaze groups were matched on demographic characteristics. After matching, no significant posttest differences in prenatal attitudes and feelings were found.

The fifth study was a meta-analytic investigation of the effects of childbirth education on the parent-infant relationship. Jones (1986) collected 27 published and unpublished studies of childbirth education, 1960 to 1981. The studies were examined for their effect sizes in relation to measures of the parent-infant relationship. Eighty percent of the effect sizes were positive, and an overall effect size of 0.38 for attitudinal and behavioral measures was found. Effects were more pronounced for middle-income than for low-income parents. Allegiance to childbirth education on the part of the investigators was associated with greater effect size.

The remaining interventive study examined the effects of ultrasonography on pregnant women's perception of their fetuses. Kohn, Nelson, and Weiner (1980) studied 100 women before and after viewing images of their fetuses. Although no significance tests were provided, the authors reported that changes occurred in perception of fetal anatomy, traits, and well-being. For example, changes in the percent of mothers reporting various perceptions of fetuses before and after ultrasonography were as follows: That the fetus is fully developed—from 60 to 71 percent; that the fetus can see and hear—from 18 to 31 percent; that the fetus is very active—from 45 to 62 percent; and that the fetus is happy in utero—from 66 to 80 percent.

FUTURE RESEARCH DIRECTIONS

Parent-infant nursing research on the experience of pregnancy is surprisingly less extensive than would be expected, given Rubin's (1967a, 1967b, 1975, 1984) emphasis on antenatal processes in role attainment and identity. Although several studies (e.g., Richardson, 1981, 1983; Sherwen, 1986; Josten, 1982; Bliss-Holtz, 1988) sought to augment or confirm ideas inherent in Rubin's framework, careful testing of propositions based on that work was rarely evident.

In part, the testing and extension of Rubin's work are probably hampered by two factors: (1) the need for a carefully done analysis of her work to identify testable propositions and (2) the need for a battery of suitable measurement methods, both qualitative and quantitative, to capture phenomena cited in her writings. With regard to the first need, many aspects of her work have been merely cited but have not been systematically analyzed. As a result, there has been an insufficient degree of scientific skepticism about her work. Although the work is based on an extensive number of observations (Rubin, 1984), it is traditional in science not to consider a hypothesis well established until independent replications have been completed. Rubin's theoretical work deserves more analytic attention and more extensive testing.

With regard to the second need, many studies presented in this chapter gathered data with newly developed instruments. The failure of these instruments to reappear in improved form in subsequent studies suggests that there were no instrument development programs; instead, the instruments were developed to meet the needs of one study. As a result, the field is lacking an array of methods by which to conduct well-designed studies of some of the nursing discipline's most extensively articulated clinical phenomena. Programs of research to develop sound instrumentation flowing from theoretical work on role attainment and identity during pregnancy are critical.

An additional measurement problem evident in a number of the studies reviewed in this chapter is the apparent idiosyncratic modification of existing instruments for a specific study. Typically, no rationale is given for the modifications made, and the implications of such modifications on tool reliability and validity go unrecognized by the investigators. Tool modifications may well be needed, but sound research also requires that modification be done in a scientifically responsible manner. It is critical that doctorally prepared nurses who guide student research or consult on clinical projects ensure that research completed by novices meets minimum standards for scientific investigation.

REFERENCES

Bills, B. (1980). Enhancement of paternal-newborn affectional bonds. *Journal of Nurse-Midwifery, 25,* 21-25.

Blau, A., Welkowitz, J., & Cohen, J. (1964). Maternal attitude to pregnancy instrument. *Archives of General Psychiatry, 10,* 325-330.

Bliss-Holtz, V. J. (1988). Primiparas' prenatal concern for learning infant care. *Nursing Research, 37,* 20-24.

Brouse, S. H. (1985). Effect of gender role identity on patterns of feminine and self-concept scores from late pregnancy to early postpartum. *Advances in Nursing Science, 7*(3), 32-48.

Copeland, D. Z. (1979). Unwed adolescent primigravidas identify subject matter for prenatal classes. *Journal of Obstetric, Gynecologic, and Neonatal Nursing, 8,* 248-253.

Corbin, J. M. (1987). Women's perceptions and management of a pregnancy complicated by chronic illness. *Health Care for Women International, 8,* 317-337.

Curry, M. A. (1987). Maternal behavior of hospitalized pregnant women. *Journal of Psychosomatic Obstetrics and Gynaecology, 7,* 165-182.

Drake, M. L., Verhulst, D., Fawcett, J., & Barger, D. F. (1988). Spouses' body image changes during and after pregnancy: A replication in Canada. *Image, 20,* 88-92.

Fawcett, J. (1977). The relationship between identification and patterns of change in spouses' body images during and after pregnancy. *International Journal of Nursing Studies, 14,* 199-213.

Fawcett, J. (1989a). Spouses' experiences during pregnancy and the postpartum. *Applied Nursing Research, 2,* 49-51.

Fawcett, J. (1989b). Spouses' experiences during pregnancy and the postpartum: A program of research and theory development. *Image, 21,* 149-152.

Fawcett, J., Bliss-Holtz, V. J., Haas, M. B., Leventhal, M., & Rubin, M. (1986). Spouses' body image changes during and after pregnancy: A replication and extension. *Nursing Research, 35,* 220-223.

Fawcett, J., & Frye, S. (1980). An exploratory study of body image dimensionality. *Nursing Research, 29,* 324-327.

Field, T. (1981). Early development of infants born to teenage mothers. In K. G. Scott, et al. (Eds.), *Teenage parents and their offspring* (pp. 145-175). New York: Grune & Stratton.

Glazer, G. (1980). Anxiety levels and concerns among pregnant women. *Research in Nursing and Health, 3,* 107-113.

Hart, G. (1980). Maternal attitudes in prepared and unprepared caesarean deliveries. *Journal of Obstetric, Gynecologic, and Neonatal Nursing, 9,* 243-245.

Heidrich, S. M., & Cranley, M. S. (1989). Effect of fetal movement, ultrasound scans, and amniocentesis on maternal-fetal attachment. *Nursing Research, 38,* 81-84.

Hellings, P. (1985). A discriminant model to predict breast-feeding success. *Western Journal of Nursing Research, 7,* 471-478.

Jones, L. C. (1986). A meta-analytic study of the effects of childbirth education on the parent-infant relationship. *Health Care for Women International, 7,* 357-370.

Josten, L. (1981) Prenatal assessment guide for illuminating possible problems with parenting. *MCN, The American Journal of Maternal Child Nursing, 5,* 113-117.

Josten, L. (1982). Contrast in prenatal preparation for mothering. *Maternal-Child Nursing Journal, 11,* 65-73.

Jourard, S., & Secord, P. (1955). Body cathexis and the ideal female figure. *Journal of Abnormal Social Psychology, 50,* 243-246.

Kemp, V. H., & Page, C. (1987). Maternal self-esteem and prenatal attachment in high-risk pregnancy. *Maternal-Child Nursing Journal, 16,* 195-206.

Kohn, C. L., Nelson, A., & Weiner, S. (1980). Gravidas' responses to realtime ultrasound fetal image. *Journal of Obstetric, Gynecologic, and Neonatal Nursing, 9,* 77-80.

Kurtz, R. M. (1969). Sex differences and variations in body attitudes. *Journal of Consulting and Clinical Psychology, 33,* 625-629.

Lazowick, L. M. (1955). On the nature of identification. *Journal of Abnormal and Social Psychology, 51,* 175-183.

Lederman, R. P. (1984). *Psychosocial adaptation in pregnancy: Assessment of seven dimensions of maternal development.* Englewood Cliffs, NJ: Prentice-Hall.

Lee, G. (1982). Relationship of self-concept during late pregnancy to neonatal perception and parenting profile. *Journal of Obstetric, Gynecologic, and Neonatal Nursing, 11,* 186-190.

May, K. A. (1980). A typology of detachment/involvement styles adopted during pregnancy by first-time expectant fathers. *Western Journal of Nursing Research, 2,* 445-461.

May, K. A. (1982). Three phases of father involvement in pregnancy. *Nursing Research, 31,* 337-342.

McCraw, R. K., & Abplanalp, J. M. (1984). Changes in maternal attitudes as a function of participation in childbirth preparation classes. *Health Care for Women International, 5,* 115-124.

Meleis, A. I., & Swendsen, L. A. (1978). Role supplementation: An empirical test of a nursing intervention. *Nursing Research, 27,* 11-18.

Mercer, R. T. (1985a). Relationship of the birth experience to later mothering behavior. *Journal of Nurse-Midwifery, 30,* 204-211.

Mercer, R. T. (1985b). The relationship of age and other variables to gratification in mothering. *Health Care for Women International, 6,* 295-308.

Mercer, R. T., Ferketich, S., May, K., DeJoseph, J., & Sollid, D. (1988). Further exploration of maternal and paternal fetal attachment. *Research in Nursing & Health, 11,* 83-95.

Milne, L. S., & Rich, O. J. (1981). Cognitive and affective aspects of the responses of pregnant women to sonography. *Maternal-Child Nursing Journal, 10,* 15-39.

Moore, D. S. (1978). The body image in pregnancy. *Journal of Nurse-Midwifery, 22,* 17-27.

Nuckolls, K. B., Cassel, J., & Kaplan, B. H. (1972). Psychosocial assets, life crisis, and the prognosis of pregnancy. *American Journal of Epidemiology, 95,* 431-441.

Petrowski, D. D. (1981). Effectiveness of prenatal and postnatal instruction in postpartum care. *Journal of Obstetric, Gynecologic, and Neonatal Nursing, 10,* 386-389.

Porter, L. S., & Demeuth, B. R. (1979). The impact of marital adjustment on pregnancy acceptance. *Maternal-Child Nursing Journal, 8,* 103-113.

Rees, B. L. (1980). Measuring identification with the mothering role. *Research in Nursing and Health, 3,* 49-56.

Richardson, P. (1981). Women's perceptions of their important dyadic relationships during pregnancy. *Maternal-Child Nursing Journal, 10,* 159-174.

Richardson, P. (1983). Women's perceptions of change in relationships shared with children during pregnancy. *Maternal-Child Nursing Journal, 12,* 75-88.

Richardson, P. (1987). Women's important relationships during pregnancy and the preterm labor event. *Western Journal of Nursing Research, 9,* 203-217.

Rubin, R. (1967a). Attainment of the maternal role. Part I. Processes. *Nursing Research, 16,* 237-245.

Rubin, R. (1967b). Attainment of the maternal role. Part II. Models and referrants. *Nursing Research, 16,* 342-346.

Rubin, R. (1975). Maternal tasks of pregnancy. *Maternal-Child Nursing Journal, 4,* 143-153.

Rubin, R. (1984). *Maternal identity and the maternal experience.* New York: Springer.

Schaefer, E., & Manheimer, H. (1960, April). Dimensions of perinatal adjustment. Paper presented at the meeting of the Eastern Psychological Association, New York, NY.

Shaw, H. S. W. (1986). Telephone audiotapes for parenting education: Do they really help? *MCN, The American Journal of Maternal/Child Nursing, 11,* 108-111.

Sherwen, L. N. (1986). Third trimester fantasies of first-time expectant fathers. *Maternal-Child Nursing Journal, 15,* 153-170.

Speraw, S. (1987). Adolescents' perceptions of pregnancy: A cross-cultural perspective. *Western Journal of Nursing Research, 9,* 180-202.

Strang, V. R., & Sullivan, P. L. (1985). Body image attitudes during pregnancy and the postpartum period. *Journal of Obstet-*

ric, Gynecologic, and Neonatal Nursing, 14, 332–337.

Sullivan, P. L. (1984). Designed instruction for pregnant women: Its effect on their learning. *Health Care for Women International, 5,* 1–27.

Winslow, W. (1987). First pregnancy after 35: What is the experience? *MCN, The American Journal of Maternal/Child Nursing, 12,* 92–96.

Witkin, H. A., Dyk, R. B., Faterson, H. F., Goodenough, D. R., & Karp, S. A. (1974). *Articulation of body concept (ABC) scale for evaluation of figure drawings.* Princeton, NJ: Educational Testing Service.

CHAPTER 12

Parent-Infant Nursing Research on the Experience of Childbirth

DEFINITIONS AND DESCRIPTIONS OF THE EXPERIENCE OF CHILDBIRTH

This chapter broadly defines the experience of childbirth as that which directly or indirectly reflects the maternal identity framework related to childbirth put forth by Rubin (1984). That framework explicates the maternal experience of childbirth with such concepts as body image and related dimensions of body boundaries; pain (pp. 70–85); and time and space (pp. 91–95). That broad framework incorporates psychological attitudes, perceptions, and reactions related to childbirth. As a result, topics covered in this chapter include studies of the temporal, tactile, and spatial dimensions of the labor and birth experience; studies of parents' reactions and responses to the birth experience, particularly that of cesarean birth; and correlates with and predictors of the birth experience. This chapter also covers the experiences of family members, particularly partners, related to childbirth and several interventions for cesarean birth parents. (*Note:* Studies of childbirth pain are presented in Chapters 3 and 4, on stress and coping.)

DEFINING THE EXPERIENCE OF CHILDBIRTH

Whether explicitly stated or not, most studies included in this chapter begin with the assumption that childbirth is not only a biological but a psychological process. Rich (1973), for example, writes of the "inner experience of the laboring woman" and "the inner process of labor" (p. 239). She defines part of that inner process in terms of temporal and spatial experiences. In another study, Berry (1983) has provided a series of definitions related to body image as a means of delineating aspects of the cesarean childbirth experience. Finally, Birch (1986) has provided definitions for therapeutic meanings and the effects of touch during childbirth. (See the definitions in Table 12–1.)

THEORETICAL MODELS OF THE EXPERIENCE OF CHILDBIRTH

Although several studies were initiated within clearly defined theoretical frameworks (e.g., Beck, 1983, used a living systems framework), most

Table 12–1
DEFINITIONS RELATED TO THE EXPERIENCE OF CHILDBIRTH

Body Image

"Body image is defined as the dynamic, fluctuating mental representation and perception of the physical self. Body image includes boundary, sensation, function, and appearance." (Berry, 1983, p. 369)

"Body boundary is the impression of the physical margin that separates self from nonself." (Berry, 1983, p. 369)

"Body sensation is the awareness of one's physical feelings." (Berry, 1983, p. 369)

"Body function is the impression of the ability to perform physical work in a manner for which one is specifically fitted." (Berry, 1983, p. 369)

"Body appearance is defined as the outward expression of the physical self." (Berry, 1983, p. 369)

Temporal and Spatial Aspects

Temporal experience "refers to an individual's experiential view of the relationships of past, present, and future as they flow in chronological time." (Rich, 1973, p. 240)

"Spatial experience refers to an individual's view of the psychosocial space surrounding his [sic] person." (Rich, 1973, p. 241)

Tactile Aspects

Therapeutic meaning of touch: "What the subject denotes from the experience of received touch." (Birch, 1986, p. 270)

Therapeutic effect of touch: "What the subject perceives as occurring because of the experience of being touched." (Birch, 1986, pp. 270–271)

studies did not adopt or present a well-articulated theoretical framework; instead, they cited a blend of theoretical work and research as the basis of the investigations. Thus, well-developed models of body image and other salient aspects of the experience of childbirth were not a driving force in the research reported in this chapter. That may be explained in part by the descriptive posture adopted in many of the studies presented.

MEASUREMENT

GENERAL STRATEGIES

Because the nursing view of childbirth emphasizes the subjective or experiential nature, methods of capturing the inner experience necessarily rely on some form of communication with the person being studied. Questionnaires and interviews during labor are logistically difficult, so when they are used, they are mostly retrospective accounts of childbirth. Alternative methods that can be applied during labor and delivery include naturalistic observations of nonverbal behavior and speech. If the latter are analyzed quantitatively, however, rigorous methods of data gathering and analysis are needed (Bakeman & Gottman, 1986).

SPECIFIC TOOLS

The predominant methods used in nursing to study the childbirth experience have been introspective questionnaires and interviews (Table 12-2). Other methods that have been applied include naturalistic observations of speech, hand, and other nonverbal behaviors, and time estimation protocols. Time estimation protocols can be applied during the childbirth process.

SUMMARY OF RESEARCH

SCOPE OF RESEARCH ON THE EXPERIENCE OF CHILDBIRTH

This chapter contains studies of women's experiences in childbirth (Table 12-3). In addition to perceptions of childbirth or cesarean birth, specific experiences of touch, time passage, and spatial dimensions also are considered, and behavioral responses of women during labor are included. Investigations concerned with the perceptions and experiences of fathers during childbirth are presented as well. Studies that view childbirth in terms of stress or coping are contained in Chapters 3 and 4. Additional studies of childbirth from a support perspective can be found in Chapter 5.

DESCRIPTIVE RESEARCH

Descriptions of the Experience of Childbirth

In a study of women's perceptions of labor, Butani and Hodnett (1980) interviewed 50 women 48 hours after they had given birth. Among those who expressed regret about their behavior during labor, losing control was the focus of the regret. Labor was different from expectations for over half of the women; differences from expectations centered around length, difficulty, and painfulness. With regard to time perception, 14 reported that time passed slowly, 29 that it passed quickly, and 7 had neutral perceptions of time. The two most positive aspects of the labor experience were seeing and touching the baby after birth and the supportive care received from others during labor.

Gabel (1982) interviewed 20 fathers who attended birth but were unprepared (had not had formal classes). Seventy percent reported they had negative expectations about birth; yet 90 percent indicated they had positive experiences when they actually attended birth. Positive aspects mentioned included witnessing birth (65 percent), being present at a key life event (55 percent), religious and family solidarity (40 percent), and fulfilling a desire to know (30 percent). In a related study of fathers' motives for attending birth, Palkovitz (1987) studied 37 couples expecting their first baby. Expectant fathers reported their reasons for birth attendance as follows: to support wife (38 percent), to meet expectations of father's role (14 percent), to satisfy curiosity (14 percent), to attend a special event (11 percent), for the marriage (8 percent), for themselves (8 percent), persuaded by friends (5 percent), and to bond with the baby (3 percent). Forty-one percent of fathers reported they felt pressure from spouses to attend birth, and 81 percent had received positive reports from other fathers who had attended their own children's births.

Descriptions of Spatial, Temporal Aspects of Childbirth

To understand the inner (psychological) process of labor, Rich (1973) studied verbal expression during labor as an indicator of inner experience. She specifically described spatial and temporal aspects of multigravidas' experiences from early labor to delivery. Using a "clinico-observational method" (p. 261), observations of speech behaviors were made while administering nursing care to 19 laboring women. Data were recorded within 24 hours of making observations and were subsequently subjected to content analysis. Data regarding women's verbal behavior were segmented according to phase and stage of labor. Categories for content analysis were based on three variables: (1) temporal dimension, (2) dynamic intensity (loudness), and (3) quantitative dimension. Using tense of speech produc-

Table 12–2
MEASURES/TOOLS FOR DIMENSIONS OF THE EXPERIENCE OF CHILDBIRTH

Tool	Source Described in	Studies Using Tool
ATTITUDES, PERCEPTIONS, AND REACTIONS TO CHILDBIRTH		
Battery of semantic differential scales for set of concepts pertinent to childbearing	Hott (1980)	Hott (1980)
Perception of Birth Scale: Twenty-nine-item scale of perceptions of birth experience	Marut & Mercer (1979)	Marut & Mercer (1979) Cranley et al. (1983) Mercer et al. (1983) Mercer (1985)
Cesarean Birth Experience Questionnaire: Open-ended items about birth experience	Fawcett & Burritt (1985)	Fawcett & Burritt (1985)
Interview related to the experience of childbirth	Norr et al. (1980)	Norr et al. (1980)
Feeling-tone instrument: Ten items pertinent to cesarean birth experience	Tcheng (1984)	Tcheng (1984)
Labor/delivery evaluation: Eight item semantic differential scale	Humenick & Bugen (1981)	Humenick & Bugen (1981)
Instrument for fathers' responses to childbirth: Twenty-nine-item scale	Cronenwett & Newmark (1974)	Cronenwett & Newmark (1974)
Questionnaire on fathers' need during childbirth: Fifty items	MacLaughlin & Taubenheim (1983)	MacLaughlin & Taubenheim (1983)
Decision Participation Scale: Fourteen items on perception of participation in birth-related decisions	Cranley et al. (1983)	Cranley et al. (1983)

Patient Participation & Satisfaction Questionnaire: Contains items on satisfaction with experience	Littlefield & Adams (1987)	Littlefield & Adams (1987)
SPECIFIC DIMENSIONS OF THE CHILDBIRTH EXPERIENCE		
Verbal estimation of time passage: Procedure to assess time passage	Beck (1983)	Beck (1983)
Speed of Time Passing Scale: Subjective measure of time passage	Isenberg (1978) as cited in Beck (1983)	Beck (1983)
Interview on touch in labor: Ten items, mostly open-ended	Penny (1979)	Penny (1979)
Interview on touch in labor: Extension of Penny (1979) interview schedule	Birch (1986)	Birch (1986)
Interaction Modes: Categories for coding women's visual, verbal, postural, and tactual behaviors in labor	Richardson (1979)	Richardson (1979)
Hand action coding scheme: Three dimensions of hand actions	VanMuiswinkel (1984)	VanMuiswinkel (1984)

Table 12–3
PARENT-INFANT NURSING RESEARCH ON THE EXPERIENCE OF CHILDBIRTH

DESCRIPTIVE
Descriptions of the Experience of Childbirth
Affonso & Stichler (1978), cesarean birth mothers
Beck (1983), mothers
Berry (1983), cesarean birth mother
Birch (1986), mothers
Butani & Hodnett (1980), mothers
Fawcett (1981), cesarean birth couples
Gabel (1982), fathers
May & Sollid (1984), cesarean birth fathers
Palkovitz (1987), fathers
Penny (1979), mothers
Rich (1973), mothers
Richardson (1979), mothers
VanMuiswinkel (1984), mothers
Patterns of the Experience of Childbirth
Tilden & Lipson (1981), cesarean birth
Differences in the Experience of Childbirth
Cox & Smith (1982), cesarean vs. vaginal birth mothers
Cranley et al. (1983), cesarean vs. vaginal birth mothers
Cronenwett & Newmark (1974), prepared vs. unprepared fathers; fathers who attended vs. did not attend birth
Hott (1980), couples who shared vs. did not share birth
MacLaughlin & Taubenheim (1983), prepared vs. unprepared fathers
Marut & Mercer (1979), cesarean vs. vaginal birth mothers
Mercer et al. (1983), cesarean vs. vaginal birth mothers
Norr et al. (1980), primiparas vs. multiparas
Tcheng (1984), primary vs. repeat cesarean mothers
RELATIONSHIPS AMONG VARIABLES/PREDICTIVE MODELS
Kearney & Cronenwett (1989), complications and satisfaction
Mercer (1985), birth perceptions and mothering
Mercer et al. (1983), predictors of birth perceptions
INTERVENTION RESEARCH
Fawcett & Burritt (1985), cesarean preparation
Fawcett & Henklein (1987), cesarean preparation
Hart (1980), cesarean preparation

tions as the focus of analysis, time perspective during overall labor was as follows: 16 percent far past, 4 percent immediate past, 72 percent present, 5 percent immediate future, and 3 percent far future. As labor advanced, percent of speech productions in all future and past categories decreased while those in the present increased.

With regard to dynamic intensity (loudness), Rich reported that vocalizations of normal tone predominated in all stages of labor. However, the use of whispered tones increased progressively during phases of first-stage labor. Loud or scream tones occurred almost exclusively during the third phase of first-stage labor and in second-stage labor. Proximity of interactants was not necessarily correlated with dynamic intensity of vocalizations. The quantitative dimension (density of verbalizations) was measured by women's level of verbal completeness of ideas. Categories ranged from sentence fragments to sentence elaborations. Although complete sentences predominated across labor phases and stages, sentence fragments increased and sentence elaborations decreased with advancing labor. Thus, the lowest density of speech occurred in second-stage labor.

In a related study, Beck (1983) used a living systems framework to test hypotheses about women's temporal experiences in latent and active phases of first-stage labor. Sixty women provided estimates of time passage by the use of two techniques: a subjective estimate and a verbal estimate of the duration of a fixed interval (40 seconds) of clock time. As predicted, verbal estimates of the fixed time interval were perceived as shorter (passed more quickly) during the active phase than during the latent phase of labor. When women who received and did not receive medication in labor were compared, those who received medication gave verbal estimates of time passing more quickly than those who received no medication. However, those who received medication also differed in age and gravidity, among other variables, from those who received no medication. No significant differences were associated with the other measure of time: subjective estimate.

Descriptions of Touch in Childbirth

Penny (1979) conducted an exploratory study of women's perceptions of touch during labor. One hundred fifty low-risk maternity patients were interviewed on their first postpartum day about their recollections of touch experiences in labor. The majority of the women rated their overall perception of touch as positive. Teenagers perceived touch less positively than women in their 20s and 30s. Touch was also perceived less positively by nonwhite and single women. Husbands were most often the source of positive touch experiences, and physicians were the source of most negative ones. Positive touch experiences most often centered on the hand; negative touch experiences involved the abdomen and pelvic areas. Overall, positive touch was interpreted by women as conveying concern or caring, and negative touch was usually associated with procedures that were painful.

In a further study of touch in labor, Birch (1986) examined the perceived therapeutic (helpful) value in postpartum interviews with 30 women. Positive touch experiences most often were received from husbands or nurse-midwives. The nature of the touch was described as rubbing, holding, pressure, or patting. The back and hands were the most frequent body areas receiving touch of therapeutic value. Touch was most often therapeutic during the transition phase of labor. The beneficial effects of touch changed with phases and stages of labor. Touch of therapeutic value was interpreted as conveying sympathy, participation, and encouragement. Overall, women reported that touch aided in coping with labor. Nontherapeutic touch experiences were most often described as being irritating or annoying.

Descriptions of Behavioral Responses in Childbirth

To clarify "the importance of others to the woman in labor" (p. 2), Richardson (1979) observed approach and avoidance behaviors of women in labor toward others. Using a coding scheme for visual, verbal, postural, and tactual behaviors, Richardson recorded behaviors of 24 women during first-stage labor. The number of behaviors occurring per contraction (including contraction and the interval until the next contraction) did not differ across early, mid-, or late phases of first-stage labor. The ratio of approach to avoidance behaviors remained about 3:1 across all three phases. The largest increase in a behavior was in requests for assistance (an approach behavior) during the late phase of first-stage labor.

VanMuiswinkel (1984) studied hand behaviors of women in labor; those of 30 women were observed and recorded by using a three-dimensional coding scheme covering hand actions, object of hand action, and purpose of hand action. Observations were made every 30 minutes and were of two kinds: during one contraction and during 1 minute between contractions. Behaviors were recorded as they occurred. The frequencies of types of hand actions were as follows: 28 percent grasping, 25 percent pressing, 16 percent rubbing, 11 percent nonmoving actions, 8 percent gesticulating, 5 percent holding, 4 percent playing, 2 percent pulsating, and 1 percent striking. The purpose of hand actions included: 54 percent comforting, 14 percent caretaking, 11 percent inactivating, 5 percent bracing, 5 percent containing, 4 percent augmenting, 2 percent informing, 2 percent orienting, and 3 percent other. The objects of hand actions were 61 percent self, 31 percent inanimate object, and 8 percent other.

VanMuiswinkel reported that the most frequently used hand action, grasping, was most often aimed at comfort and caretaking. Its use, however, was equally distributed across uterine contraction and uterine relaxation. When used for comfort, the self was the object most often grasped. Grasping for caretaking was almost totally directed at inanimate objects. Pressing hand actions were used mainly for comforting and occurred slightly more often between, rather than during, contractions. Rubbing hand actions, in contrast, occurred most often during and not between contractions. Rubbing actions were most often used to comfort the self.

Descriptions of Cesarean Birth Experiences

In an exploratory study of women's reactions to cesarean birth, Affonso and Stichler (1978) interviewed 105 women who had cesarean deliveries. Forty-one percent learned that a cesarean was needed less than 2 hours before it occurred. The following were identified by women as helpful with cesarean birth: explanations about cesarean birth (47 percent), support from husband and others (21 percent), and experience with a prior cesarean birth (21 percent). Before surgery, 48 percent reported having distorted body perceptions in the operating room. Feelings prior to surgery were fear (92 percent); dissatisfaction, anger, or depression (50 percent); or relief (30 percent). In turn, 70 percent reported feeling relief in the recovery room. In recalling the preparations for surgery, 50 percent stated that more explanations would have been helpful.

Berry (1983) further examined reactions to cesarean birth in a case study of body image following cesarean birth. She followed a 26-year-old primipara for 5 weeks after delivery through interviews and observations. Concerns about body boundary changes stemming from internal and external body intrusions dominated. Also of concern were body sensations, bodily functions, and appearance. As ideal and real body dimensions became more congruent, self-preoccupation decreased and the woman's attention shifted to her infant.

In an exploratory study of fathers' reactions to cesarean birth, May and Sollid (1984) interviewed 46 fathers whose wives had been delivered by unexpected cesarean birth. Fifty-two percent were present at birth; 48 percent were not. Fathers' reactions to the cesarean birth were relief (52 percent), acceptance (27 percent), moderate disappointment (10 percent), and strong disappointment or anger (11 percent). Negative reactions focused not on cesarean birth itself, but on hospital policies excluding fathers from cesarean births or staff behaviors toward fathers when cesarean birth occurred.

In a retrospective survey of 24 couples who experienced cesarean birth, Fawcett (1981) examined the responses according to four adaptive modes (Roy, 1976). In the physical-physiological mode, both mothers and fathers experienced fatigue and need for rest if long labor preceded cesarean birth. Also, mothers reported pain during labor and postpartum. In regard to the self-concept mode, women experienced disappointment about being unable to deliver vaginally as well as feelings of loss of control related to birth-related events. In the role function mode, both parents experienced some role failure. Finally, with regard to the interdependence mode, both parents expressed the need for being together and also for contact with their infant; further, parents expressed dissatisfaction with the lack of information provided by health professionals about cesarean birth.

Patterns of the Experience of Childbirth

In an effort to identify factors that affect women's reactions to cesarean birth, Tilden and Lipson (1981) conducted a qualitative study of groups and individual women. Participant observation was done on two cesarean support groups, and, in addition, interviews were conducted with 22 women who had experienced cesarean births. Four broad types of antecedent variables influenced reactions to cesarean birth: birth plans and expectations, women's relationships with their physicians and hospitals, time of learning that cesarean was needed, and women's perceptions of why the cesarean occurred. Further, concurrent variables, such as atmosphere in the operating room, and consequent variables, such as postoperative complications, also influenced women's reactions.

Differences in the Experience of Childbirth

To study the effect of parity on the obstetric and experiential aspects of childbirth, Norr, Block, Charles, and Meyering (1980) randomly selected low-risk married maternity clients at a large teaching hospital for a comparative study. One hundred eighteen primiparas and 131 multiparas were interviewed 1 to 3 days postpartum. Supplemental information was gathered via questionnaires and medical records. Although multiparas were more likely to worry about childbirth, they did less to prepare for it than primiparas. On 15 obstetric indicators, multiparas fared better than primiparas: They had shorter labor and fewer complications. On three measures of the subjective experience of childbirth (positive feelings, pain, and enjoyment), multiparas and primiparas did not differ after controls for childbirth preparation were applied. In addition, unprepared multiparas (no childbirth classes) were more likely to be alone during labor than unprepared primiparas. Antepartal and postpartal parity effects also were found; for example, unprepared primiparas selected rooming-in more often than unprepared multiparas.

In a comparative study of couples who planned to share delivery (have husband present at birth), Hott (1980) measured attitudes of men and women during pregnancy and 2 to 3 weeks postpartum. Attitude measures included three dimensions (activity, potency, and evaluation) of a number of concepts such as self, wife, ideal woman, or ideal mother. Of 47 couples, 34 shared delivery (Y/Y) and 13 did not (Y/N) because of labor complications. Comparison of the two groups showed that Y/N wives had less positive prenatal attitudes toward many concepts than Y/Y wives had; few differences were evident at postpartum. In prepost comparisons, however, both Y/Y wives and Y/N wives had increased activity scores for such concepts as self and ideal woman. Among men, Y/Y husbands increased in activity scores for self, whereas Y/N husbands showed no gains in any concept.

In an early study of fathers' experiences, Cronenwett and Newmark (1974) compared three groups of fathers: men who attended childbirth classes and birth (prepared attenders), men who did not attend classes but attended birth (unprepared attenders), and men who did not attend birth but may or may not have attended classes (nonattenders). Of six hypotheses about fathers' reactions shortly after childbirth, three were supported. Positive effects on the couple's relationship were found among both those attending classes and those attending birth. Neither attendance at birth nor attendance at classes had any effect on the father-child relationship. MacLaughlin and Taubenheim (1983) also conducted a study comparing prepared and unprepared fathers. They reported few differences, and their reported findings included little quantitative or statistical analysis.

Differences Associated with Cesarean Birth

Marut and Mercer (1979) compared perceptions of 20 cesarean birth mothers with those of 30 mothers who delivered vaginally. All mothers were primiparas, and all completed open-ended interviews as well as a childbirth perception questionnaire. As expected, cesarean birth mothers had less positive perceptions of their childbirth experiences than vaginal birth mothers. Differences were found in control and fear during childbirth, worry about the infant, and time delays in mother-infant contact. In addition, cesarean birth mothers delivered with regional anesthesia had more positive perceptions than those delivered with general anesthesia. Overall, cesarean birth mothers expressed greater hesitancy to name their babies than vaginal birth mothers. Further, data from interviews showed that cesarean birth mothers viewed their childbirth experience with a "sense of unreality" (p. 263).

In a replication of Marut and Mercer's study, Cranley, Hedahl, and Pegg (1983) further studied perceptions of birth experiences in women having vaginal births (n = 40), emergency cesarean births (n = 39), and planned cesarean births (n = 43). As hypothesized, women who had emergency cesarean births had less positive birth perceptions than women with vaginal or planned cesarean births. A positive perception of birth was associated with the presence of a significant other at delivery. Further, among women with cesarean births, those delivered with regional anesthesia had more positive birth perceptions than those delivered with general anesthesia. Participation in decisions related to birth was related to perceptions of birth only among planned cesarean birth mothers. Contrary to Marut and

Mercer's earlier findings, few mothers in any group delayed naming their infants. In a further comparison of childbirth perceptions, Mercer, Hackley, and Bostrom (1983) studied 294 women (56 cesarean births and 238 vaginal births). Again, vaginal birth mothers had more positive perceptions of childbirth than cesarean birth mothers.

In still another comparative study of women who have vaginal and cesarean births, Cox and Smith (1982) had mothers complete a measure of self-esteem approximately 1 month after childbirth. Mothers were similar with regard to demographic variables, although statistical tests for differences are not reported. As predicted, cesarean birth mothers had lower self-esteem than vaginal birth mothers.

Unlike the preceding studies, Tcheng (1984) compared emotional responses only in women (N = 50) having cesarean births. The comparison was based on two independent variables: primary or repeat cesarean and early or late in the postoperative hospitalization. No main effects or interaction effects of the independent variables were found. Further analysis indicated, however, that among women having primary cesarean births, more negative responses occurred in women who had attended childbirth education classes than in those who had not.

RELATIONAL/PREDICTIVE RESEARCH

Mercer et al. (1983) studied predictors of childbirth perceptions in a sample of 294 first-time mothers aged 15 to 42. Both obstetric and psychosocial variables were used to predict childbirth perceptions in multiple regression analysis. Thirty-nine percent of the variance in childbirth perception was explained by social support, infant separation, self-concept, maternal illness, and type of delivery. Among those predictors, mate emotional support explained 20 percent of the variance and type of delivery explained only 1 percent.

In a follow-up of this sample, Mercer (1985) examined the relationship of birth perceptions and mothering behaviors at 1, 4, 8, and 12 months postpartum. For teenagers, perceptions of birth were significantly related to mothering on all occasions. For mothers in the 20- to 29-year age group, perceptions and mothering were also related except at the 8-month observation. For mothers aged 30 to 42, however, there was no relation between perception of birth and mothering. Relatedly, older mothers demonstrated greater readiness for pregnancy than younger mothers.

In another study of first-time mothers, Kearney and Cronenwett (1989) examined the relation of perceived perinatal complications and satisfaction to the childbirth experience. Both variables were measured by responses to one-item questions. Perceived complications were associated with less satisfaction with the labor and delivery experience. Lower satisfaction was specifically associated with cesarean delivery, longer hospitalizations of mother and baby, and lower 1-minute Apgar scores.

INTERVENTION RESEARCH

Three interventive studies were related to preparation for cesarean birth. (*Note:* Studies of preparation for childbirth by vaginal delivery are contained in Chapter 4, on coping.) Hart (1980) reported on maternal attitudes after cesarean birth in a group who had attended a cesarean preparation class (n = 17) and a group who had not (n = 21). Details of group assignment and preexisting group differences were sketchy or not reported. Class content covered reason for cesarean birth, anesthesia, procedures, the father's role, newborn differences, and postoperative care. Mothers who attended the class had more positive attitudes on one of four attitudes: desire to actively participate in delivery.

Fawcett and Burritt (1985) conducted a field test of an informational pamphlet aimed at preparing parents for cesarean birth should it occur. Content of the pamphlet was arranged according to Roy's (1976) four adaptive modes: physical-physiological, self-concept, role function, and interdependence. Information within each mode described procedures, sensory experiences, and coping. Pamphlets were distributed to couples at childbirth classes, and the couples also received a home visit or telephone call to review pamphlet content. Of 81 couples, 18 subsequently experienced a cesarean birth. A follow-up questionnaire was mailed to cesarean birth couples. Those couples reported that the prenatal telephone call or home visit was helpful in clarifying pamphlet content. Suggestions for additional pamphlet content were provided by couples. Couples' responses to cesarean birth were analyzed by using Roy's four adaptive modes. In comparing adaptive and ineffective responses, the following significant differences occurred: Mothers had more adaptive than ineffective responses in the physical-physiological mode, and fathers had more ineffective than adaptive responses in the role function and interdependence modes. Fathers' ineffective role function responses occurred almost exclusively when cesarean birth was unplanned rather than planned.

In a second field test, Fawcett and Henklein (1987) extended the earlier test by incorporating cesarean birth content in Lamaze childbirth classes and gathering postpartal reactions to the cesarean content from both vaginal birth and cesarean birth parents. Cesarean birth content was provided by both pamphlet and focused discussion during the Lamaze classes. Seventy-five percent of the study participants returned a follow-up questionnaire. Participants reflected 13 of 15 cesarean births and 31 of 43 vaginal births occurring within the original sample. Responses to the follow-up questionnaire were content-analyzed. Regardless of type of birth, men and women had significantly more positive than negative responses to the informational pamphlet. In addition, most men and women were satisfied with the information provided by the combination of pamphlet and class discussion.

FUTURE RESEARCH DIRECTIONS

Childbirth has been studied from multiple perspectives. The fundamental experience of childbirth is elaborated in such concepts as body image, body boundaries, pain, and time, which are the focus of research by such investigators as Rich (1973), Beck (1983), and Richardson (1979). Others, such as Lowe (1987) and Gaston-Johansson, Fridh, and Turner-Norvell (1988), have initiated nursing research on the fundamental pain component of childbirth (Chapter 3). A second tier of studies addressed reactions to the birth experience (e.g., Hott, 1980; Cronenwett & Newmark, 1974; Tcheng, 1984) as well as their relation to other such variables as parenting (e.g., Mercer, 1985). Additional research related to childbirth emanates from a coping perspective, presented in Chapter 4, and is directed at dealing with pain in childbirth and maintaining control through active participation in the childbirth process. Finally, clinicians have given high priority to research that evaluates the effectiveness or impact of current childbirth practices (Thomas, 1984). As impressive as the scope of childbirth research may be, at least two weaknesses are evident. First, there is a paucity of research on the fundamental components of the childbirth experience: investigation of body image, body boundaries, pain, and time in childbirth. Second, linkages across related fields of childbirth research and fundamental components of childbirth are not well developed. In large measure, the second problem is tied to the limited amount of research now going on in the areas of fundamental components of childbirth.

Of the types of research reported in this chapter, the most complex and difficult is research related to study of the fundamental components of the childbirth experience. That is true because investigating fundamental components of childbirth requires well-developed methods to access phenomena that are complex and often are not easily measured. Further, study of fundamental components of childbirth necessarily places the investigator in a complex social situation in which the needs of women in labor may overshadow the researcher's need to know. Still further, since most births occur in institutional settings, gaining clinical access to undertake the research may be troublesome. Still, without more research of the fundamental components, research at the second tier as well as practice itself must be undertaken without core knowledge about childbirth.

Table 12–2 shows that although a number of measures for studying the experience of childbirth exist, there is no one commonly used instrument that cuts across studies. In this chapter the most frequently used scale is the Perception of Birth Scale (Marut & Mercer, 1979). With regard to the pain component of childbirth, the McGill Pain Questionnaire (Melzack, 1983) has also been used in several studies (Chapter 3). Future research would be aided by the use of several instruments or observational methods that recur in diverse studies; knowledge building would thereby be helped.

Ideally, such indices would include one or more of the fundamental components of childbirth such as body image, time perception, and pain.

REFERENCES

Affonso, D. D., & Stichler, J. F. (1978). Exploratory study of women's reactions to having a cesarean birth. *Birth and the Family Journal, 5*(2), 88–94

Bakeman, R., & Gottman, J. M. (1986). *Observing interaction: An introduction to sequential analysis.* Cambridge, England: Cambridge University Press.

Beck, C. T. (1983). Parturients' temporal experiences during the phases of labor. *Western Journal of Nursing Research, 5,* 283–295.

Berry, K. H. (1983). The body image of a primigravida following cesarean delivery. *Issues in Health Care of Women, 6,* 367–376.

Birch, E. R. (1986). The experience of touch received during labor: Postpartum perceptions of therapeutic value. *Journal of Nurse-Midwifery, 31,* 270–276.

Butani, P., & Hodnett, E. (1980). Mothers' perceptions of their labor experiences. *Maternal-Child Nursing Journal, 9,* 73–82.

Cox, B. E., & Smith, E. C. (1982). The mother's self-esteem after a cesarean delivery. *MCN, The American Journal of Maternal/Child Nursing, 7,* 309–314.

Cranley, M. S., Hedahl, K. J., & Pegg, S. H. (1983). Women's perceptions of vaginal and cesarean deliveries. *Nursing Research, 32,* 10–15.

Cronenwett, L. R., & Newmark, L. L. (1974). Fathers' responses to childbirth. *Nursing Research, 23,* 210–217.

Fawcett, J. (1981). Needs of cesarean birth parents. *Journal of Obstetric, Gynecologic, and Neonatal Nursing, 10,* 372–376.

Fawcett, J., & Burritt, J. (1985). An exploratory study of antenatal preparation for cesarean birth. *Journal of Obstetric, Gynecologic, and Neonatal Nursing, 14,* 224–230.

Fawcett, J., & Henklein, J. C. (1987). Antenatal education for cesarean birth: Extension of a field test. *Journal of Obstetric, Gynecologic and Neonatal Nursing, 16,* 61–65.

Gabel, H. (1982). Childbirth experiences of unprepared fathers. *Journal of Nurse-Midwifery, 27,* 5–8.

Gaston-Johansson, F., Fridh, G., & Turner-Norvell, K. (1988). Progression of labor pain in primiparas and multiparas. *Nursing Research, 37,* 86–90.

Hart, G. (1980). Maternal attitudes in prepared and unprepared cesarean deliveries. *Journal of Obstetric, Gynecologic, and Neonatal Nursing, 9,* 243–245.

Hott, J. R. (1980). Best laid plans: Pre- and postpartum comparison of self and spouse in primiparous Lamaze couples who share delivery and those who do not. *Nursing Research, 29,* 20–27.

Humenick, S. S., & Bugen, L. A. (1981). Correlates of parent-infant interaction: An exploratory study. In R. P. Lederman, B. S. Raff, & P. Carroll (Eds.), *Perinatal parental behavior: Nursing research and implications for newborn health.* New York: Liss. March of Dimes Birth Defects Foundation. *Birth Defects, Original Article Series, 17*(6), 181–199.

Kearney, M., & Cronenwett, L. R. (1989). Perceived perinatal complications and childbirth satisfaction. *Applied Nursing Research, 2,* 140–142.

Littlefield, V. M., & Adams, B. N. (1987). Patient participation in alternative perinatal care: Impact on satisfaction and health locus of control. *Research in Nursing & Health, 10,* 139–148.

Lowe, N. K. (1987). Parity and pain during parturition. *Journal of Obstetric, Gynecologic, and Neonatal Nursing, 16,* 340–346.

MacLaughlin, S. M., & Taubenheim, A. M. (1983). A comparison of prepared and unprepared first-time fathers' needs during the childbirth experience. *Journal of Nurse-Midwifery, 28,* 9–16

Marut, J. S., & Mercer, R. T. (1979). Comparison of primiparas' perceptions of vaginal and cesarean births. *Nursing Research, 28,* 260–266.

May, K. A., & Sollid, D. T. (1984). Unanticipated cesarean birth from the father's perspective. *Birth, 11*(2), 87–95.

Melzack, R. (1983). The McGill pain questionnaire. In R. Melzack (Ed.), *Pain measurement and assessment.* New York: Raven Press.

Mercer, R. T. (1985). Relationship of the birth experience to later mothering behaviors. *Journal of Nurse-Midwifery, 30,* 204–211.

Mercer, R. T., Hackley, K. C., & Bostrom, A. G. (1983). Relationship of psychosocial and perinatal variables to perception of childbirth. *Nursing Research, 32,* 202–207.

Norr, K. L., Block, C. R., Charles, A. G., & Meyering, S. (1980). The second time around: Parity and birth experience. *Journal of Obstetric, Gynecologic, and Neonatal Nursing, 9,* 30–36.

Palkovitz, R. (1987). Fathers' motives for birth attendance. *Maternal-Child Nursing Journal, 16,* 123–129.

Penny, K. S. (1979). Postpartum perceptions of touch received during labor. *Research in Nursing and Health, 2,* 9–16.

Rich, O. J. (1973). Temporal and spatial experience as reflected in the verbalizations of multiparous women during labor [Monograph]. *Maternal-Child Nursing Journal, 2,* 239–325.

Richardson, P. (1979). Approach and avoidance behaviors by women in labor toward others. *Maternal-Child Nursing Journal, 8,* 1–21.

Roy, C. (1976). *Introduction to nursing: An adaptation model.* Englewood Cliffs, NJ: Prentice-Hall.

Rubin, R. (1984). *Maternal identity and the maternal experience.* New York: Springer.

Tcheng, D. M. (1984). Emotional response of primary and repeat cesarean mothers to the cesarean method of childbirth. *Health Care for Women International, 5,* 323–333.

Thomas, B. S. (1984). Identifying priorities for prepared childbirth research. *Journal of Obstetric, Gynecologic, and Neonatal Nursing, 13,* 400–408.

Tilden, V. P., & Lipson, J. G. (1981). Caesarean childbirth: Variables affecting psychological impact. *Western Journal of Nursing Research, 3,* 127–149.

VanMuiswinkel, J. (1984). Hand behaviors of women during childbirth. *Maternal-Child Nursing Journal, 13,* 205–288.

CHAPTER 13

Parent-Infant Nursing Research on the Experience of Early Parenting

DEFINITIONS AND DESCRIPTIONS OF THE EXPERIENCE OF EARLY PARENTING

Research presented in this chapter is broadly defined as work that directly or indirectly reflects Rubin's framework of maternal role attainment and identity (Rubin, 1961a, 1961b, 1963, 1967a, 1967b, 1977, 1984). In some cases, that influence is easy to detect by citations to Rubin's work; in others, the relationship is more subtle and is revealed in a focus on cognitive or role-related dimensions of the early parenting experience. For example, studies of parental concerns and needs are placed in this chapter, although many were not initiated explicitly from a Rubinian perspective. Still, the emphasis of the studies on cognitive and affective dimensions of the parent-infant relationship and parenting role and on the postpartal physical and emotional experiences of the mother are congruent with phenomena described in Rubin's perspective.

Further, role attainment and identity are viewed here as entailing the processes and experiences of both mothers and fathers, but because little if any nursing research has focused on role attainment and identity processes inherent in fathering, mothers' experiences predominate in this chapter. (*Note:* Some studies of fathering from an attachment perspective have been undertaken. They are presented in Chapter 14.)

Finally, as noted in Chapter 10, on the transition to parenthood, there is not a hard, fast line between that theoretical perspective and the role attainment and identity perspective. Thus, some of the research presented in this chapter is relevant to the transition perspective, and research on the transition to parenthood bears some relevance to role attainment and identity.

DEFINING THE EXPERIENCE OF PARENTING

Table 13–1 presents nursing investigators' definitions and descriptions of phenomena related to experience of early parenting. Terms defined cover role-related needs and concerns as well as definitions related to role functions.

Table 13–1
DEFINITIONS AND DESCRIPTIONS RELATED TO THE EARLY PARENTING EXPERIENCE

Definitions of Concepts Used to Study the Early Parenting Experience

Concerns: "Areas of special interest or worry to mothers as indicated by questions pertaining to particular areas of care." (Adams, 1963, p. 72.)

Concern: "Questions, worries, or areas of marked preoccupation or interest related to the puerperium." (Bull, 1981, p. 391.)

Needs: "Practical, social, and emotional circumstances that require courses of action." (Young, Creighton, & Sauve 1988, p. 188.)

Role: Behavior expected of an individual because of the position that person holds in society." (Julian, 1983, p. 224.)

Definitions Related to the Maternal Role

"Maternal role attainment is defined as a process in which the mother achieves competence in the role and integrates the mothering behaviors into her established role set, so that she is comfortable with her identity as a mother. Mothering behaviors reflect social norms, which are common beliefs about what mothers should and should not do." (Mercer, 1985a, p. 198.)

"Maternal role behavior is defined as that set of behaviors a woman performs in providing nurturance and care for her child." (Walz & Rich, 1983, p. 186.)

Perceived maternal role competence: "The mother's view of her own ability to function with mothering behavior." (Julian, 1983, p. 227.)

Demonstrated maternal role competence: "Actions by the mother during infant feeding." (Julian, 1983, p. 227.)

Internal working model of feeding: "A mother's construction of the feeding reality, [it] includes a mother's sense of herself, her infant, and feeding events as well as the processes she uses to obtain and act on information." (Pridham et al., 1989a, pp. 31–32.)

THEORETICAL MODELS OF THE EXPERIENCE OF PARENTING

Few studies reported in this chapter fully explicate theoretical models of the experience of early parenting as a basis for investigation. That may be partially accounted for by the extensive amount of descriptive research in this area. Exceptions were found, however. Mercer's research (1985a) was heavily based on her theoretical model of factors affecting the maternal role (Mercer, 1981). Brown (1975) carefully derived assumptions for intervention from Rubin's theory of maternal role attainment as a basis for delineating when to provide infant-related information to a new mother. Other theoretical models used in research on the early parenting experience include Julian's (1983) and Flagler's (1988) maternal role competence frameworks and Pridham, Knight, and Stephenson's (1989a) internal working models of feeding.

One theoretical model was the outcome of a research study. Based on analysis of qualitative data, Hewat & Ellis (1984) constructed a theoretical framework for the breast-feeding relationship. In that framework, initiation, maintenance, and resolution of breast feeding are dependent on satisfactory negotiation and integration of maternal and infant needs. Maternal needs center around fulfillment of expectations and ability to cope; infant needs revolve around food and contentment. Each of these is in turn affected by such influencing variables as support and physical attributes.

MEASUREMENT

GENERAL STRATEGIES

The subjective (intrapersonal) nature of much of the early parenting experience (Table 13–1) heavily influences the types of measures that may be used in investigations of that experience. Probably more than in the study of any other phenomenon covered in this book, interviews have served as a basis for descriptive investigations. Checklists and other self-report instruments also provide a means of tapping the subjective dimensions of parenting. To a lesser extent, observation of parenting behaviors may be suitable indicators of the process of role attainment and identity or other related dimensions of parental role development.

Specific Tools

Table 13–2 presents tools used in parent-infant nursing investigations of the early parenting experience. The most frequently used tool reported in Table 13–2 is the Neonatal Perception Inventories (Broussard & Hartner,

Table 13–2
MEASURES/TOOLS FOR THE CONCEPT OF EXPERIENCE OF PARENTING

Tool	Source Described in	Studies Using Tool
	ATTITUDINAL & KNOWLEDGE MEASURES	
Postpartum Self-Evaluation Questionnaire: Nine-item subscale for adaptation to the motherhood role	Lederman, Weingarten, and Lederman (1981)	Jordan (1987) Cronenwett (1985) Shaw (1986) Lederman & Lederman (1987)
Gratification in the Maternal Role: Self-report scale of role enjoyment	Russell (1974)	Mercer et al. (1984b) Mercer (1985a) Mercer (1986a) Mercer (1985b) Mercer et al. (1984a)
Parental Sense of Competence: Seventeen-item scale of parenting competence	J. Gibaud-Wallston c/o Library Peabody College Nashville, TN 37023	Ferketich & Mercer (1989) Julian (1983)
Role Competence Index: Six-item index of perceived parenting ability	Roberts (1983)	Roberts (1983)
Pharis Self-Confidence Scale: Thirteen-item scale of maternal self-confidence in caregiving	Pharis (1978) as cited in Walker et al. (1986a)	Walker et al. (1986a) Walker et al. (1986b)
Self-Confidence Scale: Measure of self-confidence using paired comparisons	Seashore, Leifer, Barnett, & Leiderman (1973)	Poley-Strobel & Beckmann (1987)
Confidence Scale: Twelve-item scale about confidence in knowing baby's cues	Golas & Parks (1986)	Golas & Parks (1986)

Paternal Competence Index: Three-item scale of father's perceived parenting competence	Jones & Lenz (1986)	Jones & Lenz (1986)
Myself as Mother: Eleven-item semantic differential scale	Walker et al. (1986a)	Walker (1989a, 1989b) Walker et al. (1986a) Walker et al. (1986b)
My Baby: Six-item semantic differential scale	Walker et al. (1986a)	Walker et al. (1986a) Walker et al. (1986b)
Semantic differential scales: Fifteen adjective pairs related to four concepts	Flagler (1988)	Flagler (1988)
Maternal Attitude Scale: Five subscales of attitudes toward motherhood	Cohler, Grunebaum, & Weiss (1970)	Brouse (1985) Flagler (1988) Virden (1988) Mercer (1986a) Choi & Hamilton (1986)
Knowledge test: Twenty-item test of maternal and infant care for postpartum period	Petrowski (1981)	Petrowski (1981)
Content Quiz: Nine-item quiz on infant care	Leff (1988)	Leff (1988)
Knowledge Questionnaire: Twenty-item test about infant characteristics and capabilities	Golas & Parks (1986)	Golas & Parks (1986)
Infant Care Self-Efficacy: Scale of self-efficacy related to infant care	Froman & Owen (1989)	—
How Parents Problem-Solve Regarding Infant Care: Eleven-item tool of perceived competence in problem solving related to infant care	Pridham et al. (1987)	Pridham et al. (1987) Pridham (1989)

Table 13–2
MEASURES/TOOLS FOR THE CONCEPT OF EXPERIENCE OF PARENTING *(Continued)*

Tool	Source Described in	Studies Using Tool
	ATTITUDINAL & KNOWLEDGE MEASURES (Continued)	
Neonatal Perception Inventories: Ten-item perception scales for average and own baby	Broussard & Hartner (1970, 1971)	White & Dawson (1981) Mercer et al. (1984b) Wiles (1984) Roberts (1983) Lee (1982) Harrison & Twardosz (1986) Mercer (1980) Winkelstein & Carson (1987) Feller, Henson, Bell, Wong, & Bruner (1983) Cranley (1981) Croft (1982) Hall (1980) Jones (1981) Lotas & Willging (1979) Jones & Parks (1983) Koniak-Griffin & Rummell (1988) Koniak-Griffin & Ludington-Hoe (1987) Bee et al. (1982) Perry (1983) Mitchell, Bee, Hammond & Barnard (1985)
Degree of Bother Inventory: Ten-item scale of infant behaviors which are bothersome to parent	Broussard & Hartner (1971)	Mercer (1980) Winkelstein & Carson (1987) Harrison & Twardosz (1986)

Degree of Comfort Scale: Five-item scale for mother's comfort in caretaking	Winkelstein & Carson (1987)	Winkelstein & Carson (1987)
Feelings about Baby: Nine-item self-report scale; modified slightly by some researchers in later studies	Leifer (1977)	Mercer et al. (1984b) Cranley, Hedahl, & Pegg (1983) Mercer (1985a) Mercer (1986a) Mercer et al. (1984a)
Blank Infant Tenderness Scale: Thirty-six-item scale of perception of infant tenderness needs	Blank (1985)	Blank (1986)
ASSESSMENT OF PARENTING AND PARENTING BEHAVIOR		
Martell Questionnaire: Twenty-two item scale of taking-in and taking-hold	Martell & Mitchell (1984)	Martell & Mitchell (1984)
Maternal Behavior Scales: Scales for observer ratings of maternal behavior	Blank (1964)	Mercer et al. (1984b) Mercer (1985a) Mercer (1986a) Mercer (1986b) Mercer et al. (1984a)
Assessment of Early Mothering: Clinical guide for assessment of early mothering	Hayes (1983)	—
Assessing Adaptation to Motherhood: Clinical guide to assessment of early mothering	Sheehan (1981)	—
Pridham questionnaire: Sixty-eight items on perceptions of childbearing and competence in infant feeding, care, etc.	Rutledge & Pridham (1987)	Rutledge & Pridham (1987)

Table 13–2
MEASURES/TOOLS FOR THE CONCEPT OF EXPERIENCE OF PARENTING *(Continued)*

Tool	Source Described in	Studies Using Tool
	ASSESSMENT OF PARENTING AND PARENTING BEHAVIOR (Continued)	
Ways of Handling Irritating Child Behaviors: Self-report measure of parenting behaviors	Disbrow, Doerr, & Caulfield (1977)	Mercer et al. (1984b) Mercer (1985a) Mercer (1986a) Mercer (1984a) Brandt (1984)
How My Baby Feeds: Self-report tool for use in interviews about infant feeding	Pridham et al. (1989b)	Pridham et al. (1989a)
Postnatal Research Inventory: Ninety-one-item scale about behaviors and reactions of mothers	Schaefer & Manheimer (1960)	Meleis & Swendsen (1978)
Michigan Screening Profile of Parenting: Fifty-item scale for screening for parent-child problems	Helfer, Schneider, & Hoffmeister (1978) cited in Lee (1982)	Lee (1982)
Observation checklist: Eighteen-item scale for observing maternal behavior during feeding	Harrison & Twardosz (1986)	Harrison & Twardosz (1986)
Frequency of calls or visits to intensive care nursery	Harrison & Twardosz (1986)	Harrison & Twardosz (1986)
Evidence of milk-ejection reflex (e.g., leaking milk)	Princeton (1986)	Princeton (1986)
Duration of breastfeeding (in weeks)	Princeton (1986)	Princeton (1986)
Teaching priorities questionnaire: Forty-four items on teaching needs related to maternal & infant care	Davis, Brucker & MacMullen (1988)	Davis et al. (1988)

PARENTAL NEEDS AND CONCERNS		
Newborn Information Checklist: Thirteen-item checklist for expressing areas of needed information about newborns	Golas & Parks (1986)	Golas & Parks (1986)
Concerns questionnaire: Fifty-item tool of concerns about self, baby, etc.	Bull (1981)	Bull (1981)
In Hospital and at Home Questionnaires: Two questionnaires about knowledge acquired and its subsequent usefulness	Bull & Lawrence (1984)	Bull & Lawrence (1984) Bull & Lawrence (1985)
Card sort of 61 topics related to mother, infant, and family concerns	Moss (1981)	Moss (1981) Hiser (1987)
Written logs of maternal issues related to the infant and parenting	Pridham, Hansen, Bradley, & Heighway (1982)	Pridham et al. (1982) Pridham et al. (1987)
Health education needs questionnaire: Fifty-six health items	Howard & Sater (1985)	Howard & Sater (1985) Degenhart-Leskosky (1989)
Teaching priorities care sort: Twenty-four cards related to priorities in short-stay maternity program	Martell, Imle, Horwitz, & Wheeler (1989)	Martell et al. (1989)
Needs questionnaire: Scale of needs of adoptive parents	Walker (1978)	Walker (1978) Walker (1981)
Patient problem questionnaire: Thirty-four problems derived from nursing diagnoses	Tribotti, Lyons, Blackburn, Stein, & Withers (1988)	Triboti et al. (1988) Blackburn et al. (1988)

1970, 1971). Unfortunately, it has been the subject of some criticism (Palisin, 1980, 1981). A promising instrument for postpartal assessment developed by a nurse investigator is the Postpartum Self-Evaluation Questionnaire (Lederman, Weingarten, & Lederman, 1981). Other than the Martell and Mitchell (1984) questionnaire, few tools present an explicit effort to operationalize dimensions of early parenting from the vantage point of Rubin's theoretical work. For assessing parents' needs, concerns, and related dimensions of early parenting, the methods most frequently used include questionnaires, interviews, card sorts, and daily logs or diaries.

SUMMARY OF RESEARCH

SCOPE OF RESEARCH ON THE EXPERIENCE OF EARLY PARENTING

The study of the early parenting experience is dominated by descriptive research that elaborates the complex processes inherent in early parenthood (Table 13–3). Descriptive accounts of parental needs, concerns, and related aspects of early parenting in a variety of subpopulations are presented. Descriptive studies also elaborate postpartal cognitive operations and dynamics of maternal thinking relative to infant care. Changes in or trajectories of parenting phenomena across time also are investigated. Comparative studies highlight differences between subpopulations in regard to parenting. By contrast, substantially fewer studies have examined the network of relationships among early parenting variables or the means to intervene from a nursing perspective. (*Note:* Studies that span the prenatal to the postpartum period are reviewed in Chapter 11, on the experience of pregnancy. Studies about reactions to the cesarean birth experience are contained in Chapter 12, on the experience of childbirth. For additional studies of role attainment in relation to social support, see Chapter 5.)

DESCRIPTIVE RESEARCH

Descriptions of Parental Concerns and Needs

A number of studies have investigated needs, concerns, and related dimensions of the early parenting experience. These studies are presented in Table 13–4. Overall, the findings of the studies cited in Table 13–4 show that needs and concerns of parents are functions of time since birth and also functions of such special circumstances as parity, infant health status, adoption, and feeding method. Needs and concerns in the first few postpartum days emphasize the care and physical well-being of mother and infant and infant feeding. Later in the postpartum period, infant behavioral

Table 13–3
PARENT-INFANT NURSING RESEARCH ON THE EARLY PARENTING EXPERIENCE

DESCRIPTIVE
Concerns, Needs, and Related Dimensions of Early Parenting
Adams (1963), primiparous mothers
Brooten, Gennaro, Knapp, Brown, & York (1989), parents of very low birth weight infants
Bull & Lawrence (1985), primiparous and multiparous mothers
Chapman, Macey, Keegan, Borum, & Bennett (1985), breast-feeding mothers
Davis et al. (1988), primiparous and multiparous mothers
Graef et al. (1988), breast-feeding mothers
Gruis (1977), primiparous and multiparous mothers
Hiser (1987), multiparous mothers
Howard & Sater (1985), adolescent mothers
Martell et al. (1989), new mothers in a short-stay program
Moss (1981), multiparous mothers
Pridham (1987), primiparous and multiparous mothers
Pridham et al. (1982), primiparous and multiparous mothers
Sumner & Fritsch (1977), primiparous and multiparous mothers
Tribotti et al. (1988), new mothers
Walker (1978), adoptive mothers and fathers
Young et al. (1988), families of oxygen-dependent infants
Descriptions of Early Parenting
Bampton et al. (1981), low-income, black primiparas
Chao (1979), multiparas and primiparas
Grubb (1980), multiparas
Kikuchi (1980), mothers of infants with congenital defects
Mercer (1980), teenage mothers
Pickens (1982), career-oriented primiparas
Walz & Rich (1983), mothers giving birth to a second child
Descriptions of Maternal Thinking
Pridham (1988)
Pridham (1989)
Pridham et al. (1987)
Pridham et al. (1989a)
Patterns of the Early Parenting Experience
Hewat & Ellis (1984), breast-feeding relationship
Morse & Bottorff (1988), breast milk expression
Morse & Bottorff (1989), breast milk leakage
Zabielski (1984), balance of giving and receiving in postpartum
Changes during the Experience of Early Parenting
Bull (1981), during first week postpartum
Bull & Lawrence (1984), during first week postpartum
Lederman & Lederman (1987), during first 6 wk
Martell & Mitchell (1984), during first 3 d
Mercer (1985a), during the first 12 mo
Mercer (1986b), during the 8 months postpartum
Walker et al. (1986a), during the first 4 to 6 wk

Table 13–3 *(Continued)*
DESCRIPTIVE
Differences in the Early Parenting Experience
Degenhart-Leskosky (1989), adolescent vs. nonadolescent mothers
Jordan (1987), employed vs. unemployed mothers
Martell et al. (1989), primiparas vs. multiparas
Mercer (1986a), mothers in three age groups
Mercer (1986b), mothers in three age groups
Mercer et al. (1983), mothers in three age groups
Mercer et al. (1984a), mothers in three age groups
Virden (1988), breast-feeding vs. bottle-feeding mothers
RELATIONSHIPS AMONG VARIABLES/PREDICTIVE MODELS
Blackburn et al. (1988), congruence of mother-nurse dyads
Curry (1983), correlates of maternal adaptation
Julian (1983), perceived and demonstrated role competence
Mercer (1985b), correlates of role attainment
Mercer (1986a), predictors of role attainment
Mercer (1986b), correlates of role attainment
Rutledge & Pridham (1987), predictors of maternal competence
Walker (1981), adoptive parents' needs and characteristics
Walker et al. (1986b), subjective and behavioral role components
INTERVENTION RESEARCH
Brown (1975), information about infant
Flagler (1988), infant behavioral information
Golas & Parks (1986), infant behavioral information
Harrison & Twardosz (1986), information on preterm infants
Leff (1988), instructional videotape on infant care
Princeton (1986), deliberative nursing intervention
Winkelstein & Carson (1987), rooming-in

concerns and maternal concerns about self (time for self, regaining figure) emerge. Further, concerns of multiparas may extend to family relationships and adjustment, not just the mother-infant dyad.

Descriptions of Maternal Thinking

In an extension of research on parental needs and concerns, Pridham has undertaken a series of studies on maternal thinking about infant and parenting issues in the first 3 months of life. In the first study, Pridham, Chang, and Hansen (1987) use daily logs of 62 mothers (38 primiparas and 24 multiparas) to trace parenting issues from delivery to 90 days later.

Table 13–4
NEEDS, CONCERNS, AND RELATED DIMENSIONS OF THE EXPERIENCE OF EARLY PARENTING

Citation: Sample	Method*	Focus†	Major Findings
Adams (1963): Twenty primiparous mothers of preterm infants; 20 primiparous mothers of term infants	I	C	At 2 d postpartum, infant feeding, bathing, and navel and/or circumcision care predominated. At 1 wk and 1 mo after assuming care at home, infant feeding and other concerns (e.g., hiccoughs, sleeping) predominated.
Gruis (1977): Seventeen primiparas; 23 multiparas (both low-risk)	Q	C	At 1 mo postpartum both groups were concerned about return of normal figure, regulating family demands, and emotional tension. Also, primiparas were concerned about infant behavior and feeding and multiparas were concerned about fatigue and time for self.
Sumner & Fritsch (1977): Two hundred seventy phone calls to health facility (62% primiparas, 38% multiparas)	O	C	During the first 6 wk after birth, 80% of calls focused on (in descending order): feeding, gastrointestinal concerns, skin, other, postpartum, and sleep/cry. Calls were most frequent during the first 2 wk and decreased markedly by 6 wk. Primiparas called more often, but multiparas asked more questions per call.
Walker (1978): Eighty-nine mothers and 78 fathers adopting primarily infants	Q	N	At least 50% of parents expressed needs related to information and feelings. Predominant informational needs related to adoption and preparing for and adjusting to the arrival of the child. The predominant feeling needs related to the adoption process.
Moss (1981): Fifty-six multiparas	O	C	On the third postpartum day, mothers were more frequently concerned about family relationships, especially other children's reactions to the baby, than about themselves or their babies.
Pridham et al. (1982): Thirty-eight primiparas, 24 multiparas	O	O	From delivery to 91 days postpartum, the three most frequenct daily "issues" were baby care, illness, and development. The groups had similar issues, but multiparas had more parenting issues than primiparas.

Table 13–4
(Continued)

Citation: Sample	Method*	Focus†	Major Findings
Bull & Lawrence (1985): Seventy-eight new mothers of mixed parity	Q	O	After 1 wk at home with a new baby, at least 70% reported information on self-care and infant physical care and feeding was helpful. More information on infant behavior would have been useful.
Chapman et al. (1985): Fifty breast-feeding mothers	O	C	From birth to 4 mos, three types of concerns occurred: breast, infant, and postpartum. Breast concerns included milk supply, sore nipples, frequency of feeds, infant preferred one breast, milk expression/storage.
Howard & Sater (1985): Sixty-six adolescent mothers in teenaged parent programs	Q	N	During the first 6 wk, needs of adolescent mothers were rank-ordered as follows: baby medical needs, baby's daily physical needs, mother-baby psychosocial needs, and mothers' physical care.
Hiser (1987): Twenty low-risk multiparas	O	C	At 10 to 14 ds postpartum, concerns that mothers worried about most often were meeting needs of everyone at home, finding time for self, being a good mother, and mother's weight. Overall, mothers had proportionately more family concerns than mother or baby concerns.
Pridham (1987): Forty-eight primiparas, 35 multiparas	Q	O	Based on observations at 7 d and 1 and 3 mo postpartum, the leading changes at each time point were, respectively, perceptions of life, life-style, and life-style. The leading satisfaction associated with parenthood was perception of life at all three times. The most difficult aspects of parenthood were infant care tasks (7 d and 1 mo) and resources, especially not enough time (3 mo). Aids needed to ease difficulties were related to life-style, especially a predictable schedule (7 d), and resources, especially having help (1 and 3 mo).

Table 13–4
(Continued)

Citation: Sample	Method*	Focus†	Major Findings
Davis et al. (1988): One hundred seventeen low-risk mothers of various parity and age groups	Q	O	Mothers' teaching priorities in immediate postpartum (1–3 d) for own care were postpartum complications, episiotomy care. Teaching priorities for infant care were feeding baby, cord care, taking temperature, and infant medications.
Graef et al. (1988): Thirty-two first-time breast-feeding mothers	O	C	During the first 4 wk postpartal, predominant concerns focused on infant and mother, not family or friends. Infant concerns covered mainly feeding and infant behavior (sleeping, crying). Maternal concerns centered on physical and emotional matters.
Martell et al. (1989): Fourteen primiparas and 28 multiparas in a short-stay program	O	O	Informational priorities for the first three postpartal days in the home ranked as high included warning signs of infant and maternal illness, infant care, and infant feeding. Moderate priorities were breast care, uterine massage, comfort measures, involution, and rest. Low priorities were pericare, bowel function, family changes, and sexuality.
Tribotti et al. (1988): Two hundred thirty-one new mothers (mixed parity and delivery method)	Q	O	Nursing diagnoses pertinent to mothers during the first 72 h as identified by mothers were alteration in comfort, potential for growth, fluid volume excess or deficit, impaired mobility, sleep pattern disturbance, and alteration in bowel elimination.
Young et al. (1988): Forty-four families with oxygen-dependent child at home; 20 health professionals	I	N/C	Predominant parental concerns at discharge of infants included infant health, infant weight gain, and mobility of oxygen equipment. Later parental needs included qualified babysitters. Professionals viewed the following as parental needs: information about postdischarge services, infant nutrition, family and personal impact of infant care, and length of oxygen therapy.

Table 13–4
(Continued)

Citation: Sample	Method*	Focus†	Major Findings
Brooten et al. (1989): Nurses' family teaching logs for care of 36 very low birth weight infants (predischarge to 18 months after discharge)	O	N	Content analysis of logs showed predischarge teaching focused on infant caretaking, infant health, growth and development, managing the health care system, and resources needed. Postdischarge teaching focused mainly on infant caretaking (especially feeding), infant health (especially current health problems), and growth and development.

*I = interview; Q = questionnaire; O = other.
†N = needs; C = concerns; O = other.

In addition to issues, mothers rated the importance of issues, need for actions to be taken, and help used. Mothers also rated their overall perceived competence in problem-solving baby care issues. Issues were classified in seven categories such as development, temperament, baby care, illness, and behavior. Overall, importance of issues was rated as moderate and need for action was rated slightly lower, especially in the instances of development and temperament. Ratings of importance and need for action were moderately to highly correlated except with regard to temperament issues. Ratings for importance showed little change across time, but the need for action showed significant declines for two issues: baby care and illness. Parity was not related to either importance or need for action. Predictors of perceived competence and use of help were studied in regression analyses. Need for action in regard to behavior issues was negatively related to perceived competence. Importance of behavior issues was positively related to use of help, whereas importance of temperament issues was negatively related to use of help.

In a second study investigating the cognitive structures that mothers use in thinking about infant feeding, Pridham (1988) interviewed 52 mothers (29 primiparas and 23 multiparas) when infants were 3 and 11 weeks old. Interviews were conducted after feedings, and responses were coded for three content areas: goals, commitments, and criteria. Mothers also gave assessments of their feeding satisfaction and confidence about feeding decisions. At both times, the most frequent maternal feeding goals related to the baby's feeding experience and nutritional intake. Satisfaction with feeding most often related to length/amount of feeding, infant behavior, and infant alertness. Infant behaviors were most often used as the criteria for feeding initiation; at the older feeding, external criteria, such as breast fullness, were most often used. Infant behavior was the most often used criterion for feeding termination. Primiparas used nutritional intake as a feeding goal more than multiparas. Mothers' goals, commitments, and criteria remained fairly constant across the two feeding observations. Neither maternal feeding satisfaction nor maternal confidence was associated with parity or time of observation.

In a third study, Pridham (1989) identified mothers' decision rules for problem naming and taking action with regard to two simulated infant problems (a short feeding and unexplained crying). Data were collected via telephone interviews of 41 mothers conducted twice during the first 3 postpartal months. Mothers' perceived competence was also assessed. For problem naming, mothers most often used analysis of the situation. For taking action, mothers' decision rules varied. In the first interview, nonspecific actions were used, but in the second interview, problem-specific actions were used. Maternal parity was not associated with decision rules for naming problems or taking actions. Also, there was little relation between decision rules for naming and taking action. Further, most correlations between perceived competence and decision rules for naming and taking action were small and not significant except that the action rule of "self-evident/intuition" was positively related to maternal confidence in three of four simulated situations.

Finally, in a study of mothers' internal working models of feeding, Pridham et al. (1989a) further investigated maternal thinking by specifically investigating mothers' decision rules and concepts of feeding regulation. Telephone interviews of 122 mothers were conducted when infants were 2 months old. In interviews, mothers were presented with feeding situations to which they gave responses that were open-ended or selected from predetermined options. Mothers used types of decision rules (i.e., observation, principle, or generalization) that varied with feeding events (e.g., initiating or ending feeds). Observation was the most frequent type of decision rule for initiating a feed; principles were used most often for ending and patterning feeds; and generalizations were most often used in relation to maintaining feeds. Regulatory functions (maternal, infant or mutual) also varied with feeding events: Infant regulation predominated in initiating feeds; maternal regulation predominated in burping; and mutual regulation predominated in patterning feeds. Overall, types of decision rules and regulatory functions were not associated with each other except in the burping context. Decision rules and regulatory functions were not associated with parity or feeding method (breast or bottle). When feeding method was held constant, however, associations between regulatory functions and decision rules were identified. For example, among bottle-feeders, those reporting maternal or infant regulation more often used principles to end feeds, whereas those reporting mutual regulation used observations.

Descriptions of Early Parenting

In a study of adolescent motherhood, Mercer (1980) followed 12 teenaged mothers from shortly after birth until 1 year later. Interviews were conducted at 12 time points during that period. Over most of the first year, teenaged mothers perceived the costs of motherhood to exceed its rewards; only at hospitalization for delivery, 8 months, and 12 months were rewards judged to exceed costs. Two mothers never reported feelings of motherliness during the year of study. Teenagers' mates and mothers were the two most frequent sources of support, and friends were the least. Teenage mothers expressed marked increases in hostility from 2 to 4 weeks after delivery; this leveled out at about the fifth month. Half of the teenagers' infants experienced illnesses in the first month. Over the first year, the most frequent infant illnesses were upper respiratory infections and diarrhea. Two infants were identified as having failure to thrive at 4 months. Over the course of the study, teenagers made a total of 19 changes in residence. Four critical periods for infants of teenaged mothers were identified: first days after birth, 1 month, 3 to 4 months, and 6 to 9 months.

Bampton, Jones, and Mancini (1981) conducted a descriptive study of early mothering behaviors of black, low-income primiparas to validate earlier descriptions of maternal touch proposed by Rubin (1963). Twenty-four new mothers were observed at their first and last infant feedings in the hospital and at home 4 weeks later. At first contact with their babies, 75 percent of mothers touched infants with arms and hands. Across the three observations, 69 percent of mothers looked at their babies at least for 30 minutes during feeding; 67 percent made verbal comments to their babies; and 79 percent referred to their babies by gender ("he" or "she") versus by name; 52 percent held their babies throughout the entire feeding. Mothers held their babies progressively less from the hospital to the home setting.

A number of studies have been undertaken to describe particularly the subjective experience of early parenting. For the most part, these studies have focused on analysis of maternal behavior and maternal verbalizations as a means of delineating maternal experience during postpartum. The studies of Chao (1979), Grubb (1980), Kikuchi (1980), Walz and Rich (1983), and Pickens (1982) that follow are of this type.

Chao (1979) studied new mothers' cognitive operations related to concept formation about their infants and themselves in the maternal role. Data for the study came from spontaneous verbalizations of 11 new mothers (six primiparas and five multiparas). Each mother was observed on three successive days during the morning feeding of her infant. Written process recordings of maternal verbalizations were made within 2 hours of each feeding observation. Data were coded by using content analysis of process recordings. Codes covered (1) baby (appearance, physical state, body function, and social characteristics); (2) self as mother (caregiving, integrating baby within family); and (3) cognitive operations (orienting, evaluating, delineating). Of 2195 cognitive operations recorded, 54 percent were orienting, 38 percent evaluating, and 8 percent delineating. The referent of operations was the infant (67 percent) more than the mother herself (33 percent). Mothers' orienting operations that focused on their infants most often addressed body function, especially feeding, followed by appearance, physical state, and social characteristics. Caregiving dominated mothers' orienting operations related to the maternal role; among caregiving activities, feeding and burping were most frequently the focus. Evaluating operations that focused on the infant were most often concerned with function and were most often positive; nearly half of mothers' self-evaluating operations were concerned with their role performance, and they were mostly negative (89 percent). Delineating operations focused on baby more often than on mother and concentrated on the baby's appearance. Maternal age, parity, and feeding method affected maternal concept-forming operations about the infants, but they had little effect on concept-forming operations about roles as mothers.

In an exploratory study of the postpartum, Grubb (1980) studied new mothers' perceptions of time in regard to themselves and others. Using unstructured interviews, Grubb followed eight married multiparas weekly for 4 weeks after delivery. Written records of interviews were made within 6 hours of interview completion. The records were then content-analyzed for the occurrence of time themes. Time was coded as (1) a commodity (enough, not enough) or (2) as a criterion for (A) organization (orient, disorient); (B) motivation (activate, inhibit); or (C) evaluation (compare, predict). Data were also coded in terms of the person/area to which time themes referred, for example, the mother, her baby, or others. Across 4 weeks, mothers' statements coded as time as commodity increased from 32 to 40 percent, a significant increase. Breast feeding, but not number of children or baby's health, was associated with more frequent statements about time as a commodity. Further, statements about not having enough time greatly exceeded (90 percent) those about having enough time. The most frequently cited persons for whom mothers had insufficient time were themselves. About three eighths of mothers' statements dealt with time as a commodity; about five eighths dealt with time as a criterion. Among the three categories of time as a criterion, organization comprised the majority of statements; it was followed by evaluation and then motivation. Within the organization category, the bulk of statements concerned use of time to orient the mothers to their babies and other children.

To determine what maternal responses occur when infants are born with congenital defects, Kikuchi (1980) interviewed five mothers (two primiparas and three multiparas) during the first postpartum month. All mothers were separated from their infants after birth as a result of the transfer of the infants to a children's hospital. Infants were hospitalized from 11 to 42 days. Their diagnoses included spina bifida, duodenal atresia, choanal atresia, and respiratory distress. The investigator, as participant observer, conducted unstructured interviews during hospital and clinic visits made by mothers and telephone and home visits made by the investigator. Process recordings of interviews were made within 2 to 4 hours after the interviews occurred. Coding categories, inductively developed, covered two major dimensions: (1) maternal responses to the infant and (2) infant dimensions to which mothers responded. Maternal responses were coded as assimilative (identifying, comparing) or accommodative (preparing, optimizing, protesting, avoiding). Infant dimensions included body structure, body function, and medical treatments. The vast majority of maternal responses were assimilative, not accommodative; mothers responded primarily to infants' functional capacities and less to their body structure or medical treatment. Mothers' assimilative responses primarily focused on identifying, rather than comparing, dimensions of their infants. The majority of mothers' accommodative responses focused on preparing for the positive and negative aspects of the infants' capacities and care. The ratio of assimilative and accommodative maternal responses remained 4:1 across the 4 weeks of observation. Mothers' assimilative responses focused primarily on abnormal aspects of their babies; in their concerns about infant functioning, concern about feeding and retaining food predominated.

Walz and Rich (1983) examined maternal postpartum tasks related to the birth of a second child. Data were collected by interview and observation of 14 mothers during the 2 to 3 days of hospitalization after childbirth. Written recordings of observations and interviews were made within 24 hours after the observations or interviews occurred. Six behavioral codes were used to analyze the recordings. The codes, in descending order of frequency, were for (1) promoting acceptance of the second child by the first child, (2) grieving for the past relationship with the first child, (3) planning for the new family life, (4) reformulating the relationship with the first child, (5) identifying the second child, and (6) assessing self as capable of mothering two children. Mothers' extensive focusing on their relationships with their first children resulted in minimal attention to the husband-wife relationships during the first postpartal days.

In a study of identity reformulation among career-oriented primiparas, Pickens (1982) interviewed five women at 13 to 26 days and 16 to 17 weeks postpartum. All five women, aged 30 to 33, had active careers for at least 7 years. Based on brief notes made during interviews, written accounts of interviews were made within 24 hours after occurrence. Six behavioral clusters were used to code statements about self or the maternal role: reviewing, projecting, planning, cost accounting, weighing, and assessing. Reviewing the past aspects of self and career was the most frequent behavior at the first interview; assessing (appraising self as mother) and cost accounting (views on rewards and costs of motherhood) were the most frequent at the second interview. At the first interview, statements about costs (e.g., loss of rest and sleep, isolation, disorganization) greatly exceeded rewards; at the second interview, statements about costs and rewards were more balanced. Although mothers self-assessed with more negative than positive statements at the first interview, that pattern was reversed at the second interview. Thus, with more experience in the role of mother, women became more positive in self-assessments.

Patterns of Early Parenting

Using a case study design, Zabielski (1984) described the effects of perceived imbalance of giving and receiving on maternal responses during the neonatal period. The subject, a primipara who unexpectedly gave birth to twins, was followed from delivery to 10 weeks later. The smaller of the twins spent 13 days in the premature nursery; the other twin had a normal neonatal course. Based on analysis of 13 process recordings, themes were identified. The major theme was giving; the secondary theme was receiving. Subtypes of giving and receiving also were specified. During three consecutive time periods in which giving and receiving moved progressively from balance to imbalance, psychic depletion and resentment ensured.

Three studies investigated breast-feeding phenomena from a qualitative approach. Hewat & Ellis (1984) examined perceptions of breast feeding in a sample of 40 mothers who varied in duration of breast feeding. Mothers were interviewed on two occasions to record their perceptions of their breast-feeding experiences. Based on analysis of themes, five maternal and three infant factors were identified as influencing the breast-feeding relationship. Maternal factors included personal priorities, congruence of expectations and experience, physical recovery, interpretation of infant behavior, and support. Infant factors involved amount and frequency of feeds, infant behavior and temperament, and physical attributes.

In two additional qualitative studies of the breast-feeding experience, Morse and Bottorff examined the problem of milk leakage and milk expression. Morse and Bottorff (1989) conducted interviews of 61 women monthly via telephone and interviewed 9 other women in-depth about milk leakage. Among the 61 mothers, 95 percent at 2 months postpartum and 66 percent at 6 months reported milk leakage. Mothers perceived leaking to be involuntary and unpredictable and viewed it negatively. Mothers coped with leaking by (1) patterns of dress, including use of padding, (2) searching for cues that foretold leaking, (3) actions to stop leakage, and (4) acceptance of leaking as a part of breast feeding.

In addition, Morse and Bottorff (1988) examined women's emotional responses to expressing milk from their breasts. In interviews with 61 breast-feeding mothers, the investigators used grounded theory methods to analyze the data gathered by telephone interviews. Four categories of data related to milk expression were identified: (1) acquiring the skill to express milk, (2) justifying one's choice to express, (3) tolerating the objectionable aspects of expressing, and (4) expressing successfully. The four categories were used to build descriptive models of success and failure in milk expression among breast-feeding mothers.

Changes during the Experience of Early Parenting

Bull (1981) examined changes in maternal concerns from the third postpartal day to 1 week after discharge. Thirty first-time, low-risk mothers indicated concerns in the five areas of self, infant, spouse, family, and community. Contrary to prediction, there were no significant differences in the five major areas. Further analysis of the subcomponents of self and infant showed that while concern about physical discomforts decreased, concerns about emotional state increased. Although concerns about infant behavior remained unchanged, there was a decrease in concerns about infant physical care.

In a related study, Bull and Lawrence (1984) compared knowledge that mothers had acquired by the time of hospital discharge with usefulness of that knowledge 1 week later. Seventy-eight low-risk mothers completed both testing occasions. At least 70 percent of the mothers indicated knowledge of the areas of pericare, breast care, and infant physical care at discharge. One week later, at least 70 percent of the sample found information in the following areas helpful to them: pericare, breast care, elimination, food and fluids, activity and rest, social interaction, infant physical care, infant feeding, and infant behavior. No inferential significance tests were applied to data from the two occasions.

Lederman and Lederman (1987) compared maternal adaptation within multiparas at 3 days and 6 weeks postpartum. Adaptation was assessed by the Post-partum Self-Evaluation Questionnaire (PSQ), comprised of seven dimensions, and interviews whose content paralleled that of the questionnaire as well as tapped four other dimensions such as physical discomforts. Both questionnaires and interviews showed significant changes in maternal self-confidence over time and significant decreases in both husband's participation in infant care and satisfaction with life circumstances. However, changes in self-confidence on the PSQ became more favorable, whereas those assessed by interview became less favorable. Interviews detected significant changes in three other dimensions that were included but failed to reach significant levels in the PSQ. In addition, interviews showed significant increases in physical discomforts. Three clusters of phenomena (husband, infant, and maternal coping) were identified in correlations among scales.

In a related investigation, Walker, Crain, and Thompson (1986a) studied stability and change in attitudinal indicators of role attainment and identity in 64 primiparas and 58 multiparas. Measures of maternal evaluation, maternal self-confidence, and infant evaluation were administered at both 1 to 3 days and 4 to 6 weeks postpartum. Significant main effects for time of testing and parity were found in both maternal and infant evaluation, but whereas the former increased over time, the latter decreased. In addition, primiparas showed greater gains in self-confidence over time than multiparas. Greater interrelatedness was found among primiparas' attitudes than among multiparas' attitudes.

In the most extensive study of changes in self-concept and maternal role development during the first year of motherhood, Mercer (1986b) studied three groups of mothers: teenagers, mothers from 20 to 29 years, and mothers from 30 to 42 years. Contrary to expectations, mothers in the two older age groups experienced significant decreases in self-concept from 1 to 3 days to 8 months after childbirth. Decreases in teenaged mothers' self-concept were not significant. Also, there were no significant changes in personality integration scores over time for any of the three groups. Further, when the development of the maternal role at 1, 4, 8, and 12 months was assessed by using multiple indicators, a positive linear trend was not found (Mercer, 1985a). Instead, in all three groups, feelings toward the baby peeked at 4 months. Maternal behaviors also were at their highest at 4 months and then declined progressively. For gratification in the maternal role and ways of handling irritating child behaviors, each age group displayed somewhat distinct trajectories. For example, for gratification in the maternal role, 30- to 42-year-olds remained relatively unchanged after 4 months; in contrast, at 8 months, teenagers and 20- to 29-year-olds changed in opposite directions, with teens dropping in gratification.

In an effort to test Rubin's (1961b) concept of puerperal change in which initial taking-in (first 3 days) is later superseded by taking-hold (3 to 10 days), Martell and Mitchell (1984) studied 20 low-risk new mothers. A questionnaire containing items on taking-hold and taking-in was administered each of three mornings that mothers were in the hospital. Score ranges showed little evidence of taking-in, but taking-hold was evident. Statistical tests showed, however, that taking-in scores decreased significantly and taking-hold scores increased, particularly between the first and second days. The latter support in part the hypothesized pattern, but the time period for gains in taking-hold did not conform to Rubin's description.

Differences in the Experience of Early Parenting

In comparing teaching priorities of 14 primiparas and 28 multiparas participating in a short-stay postpartum program, Martell, Imle, Horwitz, and Wheeler (1989) used a Q-sort to assess mothers' views. Mothers and infants remained in the hospital for 6 to 8 hours after birth. Teaching priorities were assessed when mothers returned for clinic appointments at about 72 hours after birth. Of 12 areas assessed, primiparas' and multiparas' teaching priorities differed significantly in only two areas: Primiparas gave higher priority to pericare; multiparas gave higher priority to rest.

In an investigation of differences among three maternal-age groups

(15 to 19, 20 to 29, and 30 to 42), Mercer, Hackley, and Bostrom (1984a) compared 294 new mothers over a 12-month period. All three groups reported similar feelings of love for their babies. The three groups differed significantly on three measures of role attainment across the first year. Over most of the first year, teenaged mothers reported more gratification in the maternal role compared to older mothers. (See also Mercer, 1985b.) Over the 12 months, however, both groups of older mothers consistently were rated more positively than teenaged mothers by raters of mothering behaviors. At 12 months, when a composite measure of role attainment based on five indicators was used to test group differences, both groups of older mothers had higher maternal role scores than teenaged mothers (Mercer, 1986a). (See also Hackley, Mercer, and Bostrom [1982] and Mercer [1985a].)

In related analyses of Mercer's sample at 8 months after delivery (Mercer, 1986b; Mercer, Hackley, & Bostrom, 1983), both groups of older mothers demonstrated more competent maternal behaviors than teenagers. Mothers from 30 to 42 years also had higher self-concept and personality integration than teenaged mothers at both 1 to 3 days and 8 months postpartum.

In another study comparing effects of age, Degenhart-Leskosky (1989) compared the health education needs of 22 adolescent and 30 nonadolescent mothers in the immediate postpartum period. No differences in educational needs were found with regard to mother-baby psychosocial needs or the physical care needs of the babies. However, adolescent mothers had greater needs related to infant medical care, whereas nonadolescent mothers had greater needs related to mothers' physical care.

Jordan (1987) compared employed and unemployed mothers on postpartal adaptation. All the women were second-time mothers. On a multidimensional measure of adaptation at 6 weeks and 6 months postpartum, mothers differed in only one of nine dimensions: support for parental role from friends/family at 6 weeks. Unemployed mothers experienced greater support than employed mothers at that time.

To examine the association of feeding method with maternal adjustment, Virden (1988) compared three groups of mothers at 4 to 6 weeks postpartum: 33 breast-feeding primiparas, 13 bottle-feeding primiparas, and 14 using both methods. The three groups did not differ in age, education, prenatal classes, or ethnicity. Significant differences were found in two measures of maternal adjustment: maternal anxiety and mother-infant mutuality. In each case, breast-feeding mothers scored most favorably, followed by those using both methods. Bottle-feeders scored least favorably.

RELATIONAL/PREDICTIVE RESEARCH

To study congruence of nurse and patient perceptions of health-related concerns during postpartum, Blackburn, Lyons, Stein, Tribotti, & Withers

(1988) studied 236 new mother-nurse dyads. By use of questionnaires derived from nursing diagnostic labels and descriptors, the mothers indicated their problems, and the nurses who cared for the mothers independently assessed their patients' problems. Overall, the most frequently occurring problems selected by mothers were similar to those selected by nurses. When the congruence between dyads was assessed, however, significant incongruency in some diagnoses was found. For example, nurses were likely to identify knowledge deficit as a problem when mothers did not.

In a study of 167 parents adopting mostly infant children, Walker (1981) examined relations between parental needs and parental characteristics. Parental needs (informational, feeling, and judgment-development) were related to parental gender, age of parent, number of other children, amount of previous child care experience, and preparedness for parenthood. Overall, mothers adopting a first or second child reported higher needs than other adoptive parents reported.

Relations between perceived and behavioral aspects of the maternal role have been studied by several investigators. Julian (1983) examined relations between perceived and demonstrated (behavioral) maternal role competence in 32 adolescent primiparas. Data were collected between 12 and 24 hours after delivery. Perceived role competence was measured by questionnaire, and demonstrated role competence was assessed by behavioral observations recorded during infant feeding. Perceived and demonstrated role competence were unrelated to each other.

In a related study, Walker, Crain, and Thompson (1986b) examined the relations of subjective and behavioral components of the maternal role. Sixty-four primiparas and 60 multiparas completed three attitudinal indicators related to the maternal role at 1 to 3 days and 4 to 6 weeks postpartum. At the second testing, mothers also were videotaped during a feeding interaction that was later coded for maternal sensitivity and responsiveness. Among primiparas, two of six correlations of subjective and behavioral components of the maternal role were significant. In particular, maternal self-confidence at the second testing was related to maternal behavior. For multiparas, only maternal self-evaluation at the first testing was related to maternal behavior.

Correlates and predictors of the maternal role have been the focus of several studies. Rutledge and Pridham (1987) examined predictors of maternal perceived competence in infant feeding and care during the early postpartum period (less than 1 week postpartum). One hundred forty mothers of varying parity completed survey items. Results showed that perceived competence was related to amount of in-hospital preparation for bottle-feeding mothers; for breast-feeding mothers, the amount of rest was related to higher perceived competence. Competence was also associated with parity, but not with type of delivery.

Curry (1983) explored variables related to maternal adaptation among 20 medically low-risk primiparas. Mothers were classified into easy and difficult adapters primarily on the basis of their postpartal self-reports. Data collection (self-concept, observations of attachment, and interviews) commenced prenatally and continued until 3 months after delivery. Easy adapters (n = 15) and difficult adapters (n = 5) did not differ significantly in attachment behaviors, self-concept, age, income, education, length of labor, perception of birth, or whether the pregnancy was planned. Comments of easy adapters indicated they had previous child care experience and that their husband were involved with the infants. Difficult adapters had either limited or no previous child care experience and commented on their loneliness and the long hours their husbands were working.

In the most extensive study of correlates and predictors of maternal role attainment during the first year of motherhood, Mercer (1985b, 1986a, 1986b) investigated three subsamples: teenaged mothers, mothers 20 to 29 years old, and mothers 30 to 42 years old. In personality correlates of maternal behavior at 8 months postpartum, each age group showed a different set of relations: Teenager maternal behavior was related most highly to personality integration, empathy, and intensity of temperament; among older mothers, maternal behavior was more related to self-concept, flexibility, adaptability, and mood (Mercer, 1986b). In examining correlates of gratification in the maternal role at 8 months postpartum in these subsamples, Mercer (1985b) found no significant correlates in teenaged mothers' gratification; for mothers aged 20 to 29, there were four significant correlates of gratification, for example, role strain and mate relationship; for mothers aged 30 to 42, there were five significant correlates, for example, education and age. When the subsamples were combined in regression analysis, five significant predictors of gratification were identified, and they accounted for 23.7 percent of the variance: role strain, physical support, mate relationship, size of support network, and empathy. Finally, Mercer (1986a) tested predictors of maternal role attainment at 12 months by using a composite index of role attainment based on five separate scales, including infant growth. After controlling four demographic variables, the variable contributing the most (16.9 percent) to the prediction of maternal role attainment was self-concept.

INTERVENTION RESEARCH

To test an intervention aimed at increasing maternal competence, Flagler (1988) randomly assigned low-risk primiparas to control and experimental groups. Mothers in the latter group received a 15- to 20-minute teaching and demonstration session in their hospital rooms during which their infants' behavioral responses were explained. At 4 to 6 weeks postpartum both groups completed measures of maternal competence and infant behavioral style, an intervening variable. No significant group differences were found by any of three measures of maternal competence. However, two maternal competence measures were significantly related to infant behavioral style.

In a related study, Golas and Parks (1986) tested an intervention aimed at teaching mothers about infant capabilities and characteristics by film, demonstration, and instruction. Forty-six mothers, randomly assigned, received the experimental intervention, served as a contrast group (filled out an information checklist), or acted as a control group. The intervention was provided when infants were 2 weeks old. At 1 month, mothers in the intervention group showed significantly greater knowledge of infant behavior, but not greater self-confidence, than those in the other two groups.

Princeton (1986) tested the efficacy of a deliberative nursing intervention on reducing maternal distress in breast-feeding mothers. Mothers were assigned to a control group receiving routine care (n = 12), a control group receiving routine care plus extra attention (n = 12), or an experimental group (n = 12). The experimental group received a deliberative nursing intervention that focused on assessing and meeting mothers' needs and providing breast-feeding instruction. Experimental group mothers had significantly more signs of activation of the milk-ejection reflex (e.g., uterine cramping during feeding) than either control group. Also, significant differences were found in the number of mothers still breast-feeding at 8 weeks postpartum, but the direction of this was not clearly specified.

To determine if infant care taught by televised videotape was as effective as live group instruction, Leff (1988) used an experimental design to test the merits of each instructional method. Mothers of normal newborns were randomly assigned to the televised (n = 106) or live (n = 115) instructional groups. Mothers completed an infant care quiz and attitude scale immediately after instruction. The groups did not differ significantly in posttest quiz scores on infant care or in their attitudes about what they learned. However, mothers in both groups preferred live to videotaped instruction because, for example, they could receive immediate answers to questions.

Winkelstein and Carson (1987) used a quasiexperimental design to compare effects of rooming-in on an adolescent sample. Mothers delivered at two inner-city, urban teaching hospitals, one with rooming-in and the other without, were compared on questionnaires at 2 days and 4 weeks postpartum. Rooming-in mothers had infants in their rooms about 16 hours per day; they reported receiving more teaching about cord care and were more satisfied with nursing care than mothers without rooming-in. No significant differences between groups were found in mothers' perceptions of their infants or in their degree of bother and comfort with their infants and their care.

To test the impact of instructing mothers of preterm infants about the physical and behavioral characteristics of their babies, Harrison and Twardosz (1986) randomly assigned mothers to control, attention, and experimental groups. The experimental group received instruction about preterm infants' special characteristics, such as reflexes' appearances, and parental reactions; instructional approaches included discussion, videotape, and written format. In addition to routine care, the attention group discussed nonmedical concerns about their infants with the investigators. On average, both the experimental instruction and attention occurred when infants were 15 days old. Dependent measures of mothers' perceptions of their infants and maternal behaviors were made on home visits after discharge. No group differences were found in mothers' perceptions of their infants, numbers of visits or calls to the nursery during the infants' hospitalization, or subsequent maternal behaviors during feeding.

Finally, Brown (1975) used Rubin's (1967a, 1967b) theory of maternal role attainment as a framework for assessment and intervention in a case study of a 21-year-old multipara with a normal infant. Rubin's theory, specifically, the type of maternal cognitive operation, was used to determine maternal readiness for nursing intervention. Intervention consisted of informative and interpretive comments the investigator made with regard to infant behaviors. The investigator interviews with the mother began at 5 hours postdelivery and covered 4 days. The investigator identified predominance of grief work as a barrier to readiness to learn about the infant; mimicry and introjection-projection-rejection were seen respectively as early and late role-taking operations. The investigator adjusted her intervention based on the patterning of operations over time. At the conclusion, the investigator judged Rubin's theory to be helpful in assessing the mother's readiness for nursing intervention in the form of information about and interpretation of infant behaviors.

FUTURE RESEARCH DIRECTIONS

Rubin's influence is broadly evident in nurses' research of early parenting by virtue of the amount of attention given to the mother's subjective experience and role taking. Still, the field contains few studies that originate in a thorough analysis of Rubin's work. The studies of Martell and Mitchell (1984) and Brown (1975) are indeed noteworthy in their efforts to advance understanding of the strengths and weaknesses of Rubin's ideas about postpartal maternal experience.

Clearly, nurse investigators have generated a wealth of descriptive information about mothers' postpartal experiences. Now the need is to move the research to well thought out, hypothesis-based studies. To complete the next step, however, measures that have a solid conceptual base and adequate psychometric properties must be developed or refined. If we assume that Rubin's theoretical work has provided a distinctly nursing perspective on maternal experience and identity, then effort is needed to link that perspective to reproducible methods of measurement.

Although qualitative studies may continue to be important in exploring and perhaps testing some dimensions of Rubin's work, certain methodological features of past research need improvement. For example, writing down mothers' statements from memory several hours after interviews have been completed is no longer defensible. Particularly when such methods as content analysis are used, tape recording and transcription are essential to credibility. Even when frequency counts of thematic material are not formally done, an audit trail is necessary to show on what basis an investigator arrived at generalizations about mothers' experiences.

No topic in this book has omitted men as research subjects to the extent evidenced in this chapter. Based on the literature surveyed here, paternal role attainment and identity have not been nursing research concerns. Although this may in part stem from Rubin's focus on mothers, not fathers, it leaves nurses without knowledge and understanding of male parental development. Attention to fathers' role attainment and identity is overdue.

REFERENCES

Adams, M. (1963). Early concerns of primigravida mothers regarding infant care activities. *Nursing Research, 12* 72–77.

Bampton, B., Jones, J., & Mancini, J. (1981). Initial mothering patterns of low-income black primiparas. *Journal of Obstetric, Gynecologic, and Neonatal Nursing, 10,* 174–178.

Bee, H. L., Barnard, K. E., Eyres, S. J., Gray, C. A., Hammond, M. A., Spietz, A. L., Snyder, C., & Clark, B. (1982). Prediction of IQ and language skill from perinatal status, child performance, family characteristics, and mother-infant interaction. *Child Development, 53,* 1134–1156.

Blackburn, S., Lyons, N., Stein, M., Tribotti, S., & Withers, J. (1988). Patients' and nurses' perceptions of patient problems during the immediate postpartum period. *Applied Nursing Research, 3,* 141–142.

Blank, D. M. (1985). Development of the infant tenderness scale. *Nursing Research, 34,* 211–216.

Blank, D. M. (1986). Relating mothers' anxiety and perception to infant satiety, anxiety, and feeding behavior. *Nursing Research, 35,* 347-351.

Blank, M. (1964). Some maternal influences on infants' rates of sensorimotor development. *Journal of American Academy of Child Psychiatry, 3,* 668-687.

Brandt, P. A. (1984). Stress-buffering effects of social support on maternal discipline. *Nursing Research, 33,* 229-234.

Brooten, D., Gennaro, S., Knapp, H., Brown, L., & York, R. (1989). Clinical specialist pre- and postdischarge teaching of parents of very low birth weight infants. *Journal of Obstetric, Gynecologic and Neonatal Nursing, 18,* 316–322.

Brouse, S. H. (1985). Effect of gender role identity on patterns of feminine and self-concept scores from late pregnancy to early postpartum. *Advances in Nursing Science, 7*(3), 32–48.

Broussard, E. R., & Hartner, M. S. S. (1970). Maternal perception of the neonate as related to development. *Child Psychiatry and Human Development, 1*(1), 16–25.

Broussard, E. R., & Hartner, M. S. S. (1971). Further considerations regarding maternal perception of the first born. In J. Hellmuth (Ed.), *Exceptional infant: Vol. 2. Studies in abnormalities* (pp. 432–449). New York: Brunner/Mazel.

Brown, P. W. (1975). The use of a descriptive theory in planning nursing intervention. *Maternal-Child Nursing Journal, 4,* 171–182.

Bull, M. J., & Lawrence, D. (1984). A pilot study: Postpartum mothers' perception of the information received in the hospital and its usefulness during the first weeks at home. *Journal of Community Health Nursing, 1*(2), 111-124.

Bull, M. J., & Lawrence, D. (1985). Mothers' use of knowledge during the first postpartum weeks. *Journal of Obstetric, Gynecologic, and Neonatal Nursing, 14,* 315-320.

Bull, M. J. (1981). Change in concerns of first-time mothers after one week at home. *Journal of Obstetric, Gynecologic, and Neonatal Nursing, 10,* 391-394.

Chapman, J. J., Macey, M. J., Keegan, M., Borum, P., & Bennett, S. (1985). Concerns of breast-feeding mothers from birth to 4 months. *Nursing Research, 34,* 374-377.

Chao, Y. Y. (1979). Cognitive operations during maternal role enactment [Monograph]. *Maternal-Child Nursing Journal, 8,* 211-275.

Choi, E. S. C., & Hamilton, R. K. (1986). The effects of culture on mother-infant interaction. *Journal of Obstetric, Gynecologic and Neonatal Nursing, 15,* 256-261.

Cohler, B., Grunebaum, H. U., & Weiss, J. (1970). Child care attitudes and emotional disturbances among mothers of young children. *Genetic Psychology Monographs, 82,* 3-47.

Cranley, M. S. (1981). Roots of attachment: The relationship of parents with their unborn. In R. P. Lederman, B. S. Raff & P. Carroll (Eds.), *Perinatal parental behavior: Nursing research and implications for newborn health.* New York: Liss. March of Dimes Birth Defects Foundation. *Birth Defects, Original Article Series, 17*(6) 59-83.

Cranley, M. S., Hedahl, K. J., & Pegg, S. H. (1983). Women's perceptions of vaginal and cesarean deliveries. *Nursing Research, 32,* 10-15.

Croft, C. A. (1982). Lamaze childbirth education: Implications for maternal-infant attachment. *Journal of Obstetric, Gynecologic, and Neonatal Nursing, 11,* 333-336.

Cronenwett, L. R. (1985). Network structure, social support, and psychological outcomes of pregnancy. *Nursing Research, 34,* 93-99.

Curry, M. A. (1983). Variables related to adaptation to motherhood in "normal" primiparous women. *Journal of Obstetric, Gynecologic, and Neonatal Nursing, 12,* 115-121.

Davis, J. H., Brucker, M. C., & MacMullen, N. (1988). A study of mothers' postpartum teaching priorities. *Maternal-Child Nursing Journal, 17,* 41-50.

Degenhart-Leskosky, S. M. (1989). Health education needs of adolescent and nonadolescent mothers. *Journal of Obstetric, Gynecologic, and Neonatal Nursing, 18,* 238-244.

Disbrow, M. A., Doerr, H., & Caulfield, C. (1977). Measuring the components of potential for child abuse and neglect. *Journal of Child Abuse and Neglect, 1,* 279-296.

Feller, C. M., Henson, D., Bell, L., Wong, S., & Bruner, M. (1983). Assessment of adolescent mother-infant attachment. *Issues in Health Care of Women, 4,* 237-250.

Ferketich, S. L., & Mercer, R. T. (1989). Men's health status during pregnancy and early fatherhood. *Research in Nursing & Health, 12,* 137-148.

Flagler, S. (1988). Maternal role competence. *Western Journal of Nursing Research, 10,* 274-290.

Froman, R. D., & Owen, S. V. (1989). Infant care self-efficacy. *Scholarly Inquiry for Nursing Practice, 3,* 199-211.

Golas, G. A., & Parks, P. (1989). Effect of early postpartum teaching on primiparas' knowledge of infant behavior and degree of confidence. *Research in Nursing & Health, 9,* 209-214.

Graef, P., McGhee, K., Rozycki, J., Fescina-Jones, D., Clark, J. A., Thompson, J., & Brooten, D. (1988). Postpartum concerns of breastfeeding mothers. *Journal of Nurse-Midwifery, 33,* 62-66.

Grubb, C. A. (1980). Perceptions of time by multiparous women in relation to themselves and others during the first postpartal month [Monograph]. *Maternal-Child Nursing Journal, 9,* 225-331.

Gruis, M. (1977). Beyond maternity: Postpartum concerns of mothers. *MCN, The American Journal of Maternal/Child Nursing, 2,* 182-188.

Hackley, K. C., Mercer, R. T., Bostrom, A. (1982). Motherhood in the 30's: A preview of their experience. *Communicating Nursing Research, 15,* 61.

Hall, L. A. (1980). Effect of teaching on primiparas' perceptions of their newborn. *Nursing Research, 29,* 317–322.

Harrison, L. L., & Twardosz, S. (1986). Teaching mothers about their preterm infants. *Journal of Obstetric, Gynecologic, and Neonatal Nursing, 15,* 165–172.

Hayes, E. E. (1983). Assessment of early mothering: A tool. *Issues in Health Care of Women, 6,* 361–366.

Hewat, R. J., & Ellis, D. J. (1984). Breastfeeding as a maternal-child team effort: Women's perceptions. *Health Care for Women International, 5,* 437–452.

Hiser, P. L. (1987). Concerns of multiparas during the second postpartum week. *Journal of Obstetric, Gynecologic, and Neonatal Nursing, 16,* 195–203.

Howard, J. S., & Sater, J. (1985). Adolescent mothers self-perceived health education needs. *Journal of Obstetric, Gynecologic, and Neonatal Nursing, 14,* 399–404.

Jones, C. (1981). Father to infant attachment: Effects of early contact and characteristics of the infant. *Research in Nursing and Health, 4,* 193–200.

Jones, L. C., & Lenz, E. R. (1986). Father-newborn interaction: Effects of social competence and infant state. *Nursing Research, 35,* 149–153.

Jones, C., & Parks, P. (1983). Mother-, father-, and examiner-reported temperament across the first year of life. *Research in Nursing and Health, 6,* 183–189.

Jordan, P. L. (1987). Differences in network structure, social support, and parental adaptation associated with maternal employment status. *Health Care for Women International, 8,* 133–150.

Julian, K. C. (1983). A comparison of perceived and demonstrated maternal role competence of adolescent mothers. *Issues in Health Care of Women, 4,* 223–236.

Kikuchi, J. F. (1980). Assimilative and accommodative responses of mothers to their newborn infants with congenital defects [Monograph]. *Maternal-Child Nursing Journal, 9,* 141–221.

Koniak-Griffin, D., & Ludington-Hoe, S. M. (1987). Paradoxical effects of stimulation on normal neonates. *Infant Behavior and Development, 10,* 261–277.

Koniak-Griffin, D., & Rummell, M. (1988). Temperament in infancy: Stability, change, and correlates. *Maternal-Child Nursing Journal, 17,* 25–40.

Lederman, R. P., & Lederman, E. (1987). Dimensions of post-partum adaptation: Comparisons of multiparas 3 days and 6 weeks after delivery. *Journal of Psychosomatic Obstetrics and Gynaecology, 7,* 193–203.

Lederman, R. P., Weingarten, C. T., & Lederman, E. (1981). Postpartum self-evaluation questionnaire: Measures of maternal adaptation. In R. P. Lederman, B. S. Raff, & P. Carroll (Eds.), *Perinatal parental behavior: Nursing research and implications for newborn health,* New York: Liss. March of Dimes Birth Defects Foundation. *Birth defects. Original Article Series, 17*(16), 201–231.

Lee, G. (1982). Relationship of self-concept during late pregnancy to neonatal perception and parenting profile. *Journal of Obstetric, Gynecologic, and Neonatal Nursing, 11,* 186–190.

Leff, E. W. (1988). Comparison of the effectiveness of videotape versus live group infant care classes. *Journal of Obstetric, Gynecologic, and Neonatal Nursing, 17,* 338–344.

Leifer, M. (1977). Psychological changes accompanying pregnancy and motherhood. *Genetic Psychology Monographs, 95,* 55–96.

Lotus, M. B., & Willging, J. M. (1979). Mothers, babies, perception. *Image, 11,* 45–51.

Martell, L. K., Imle, M., Horwitz, S., & Wheeler, L. (1989). Information priorities of new mothers in a short-stay program. *Western Journal of Nursing Research, 11,* 320–327.

Martell, L. K., & Mitchell, S. K. (1984). Rubin's "puerperal change" reconsidered. *Journal of Obstetric, Gynecologic and Neonatal Nursing, 13,* 145–149.

Meleis, A. I., & Swendsen, L. A. (1978). Role supplementation: An empirical test of a nursing intervention. *Nursing Research, 27,* 11–18.

Mercer, R. T. (1980). Teenage motherhood:

The first year. *Journal of Obstetric, Gynecologic, and Neonatal Nursing, 9,* 16–27.

Mercer, R. T. (1981). A theoretical framework for studying factors that impact on the maternal role. *Nursing Research, 30,* 73–77.

Mercer, R. T. (1985a). The process of maternal role attainment over the first year. *Nursing Research, 34,* 198–204.

Mercer, R. T. (1985b). The relationship of age and other variables to gratification in mothering. *Health Care for Women International, 6,* 295–308.

Mercer, R. T. (1986a). Predictors of maternal role attainment at one year postbirth. *Western Journal of Nursing Research, 8,* 9–25.

Mercer, R. T. (1986b). The relationship of developmental variables to maternal behavior. *Research in Nursing & Health, 9,* 25–33.

Mercer, R. T., Hackley, K. C., & Bostrom, A. (1983). Impact of motherhood after thirty. *Communicating Nursing Research, 16,* 51–52.

Mercer, R. T., Hackley, K. C., & Bostrom, A. (1984a). Adolescent motherhood. *Journal of Adolescent Health Care, 5*(1), 7–13.

Mercer, R. T., Hackley, K. C., & Bostrom, A. (1984b). Social support of teenage mothers. In K. E. Barnard, P. A. Brandt, B. S. Raff, & P. Carroll (Eds.), *Social support and families of vulnerable infants.* White Plains, NY: March of Dimes Birth Defects Foundation. *Birth Defects, Original Article Series, 20*(5), 245–272.

Mitchell, S. K., Bee, H. L., Hammond, M. A., & Barnard, K. E. (1985). Prediction of school and behavior problems in children followed from birth to age eight., In W. K. Frankenburg, R. N. Emde, & J. W. Sullivan (Eds.), *Early identification of children at risk* (pp. 117–132). New York: Plenum.

Morse, J. M., & Bottorff, J. L. (1988). The emotional experience of breast expression. *Journal of Nurse-Midwifery, 33,* 165–170.

Morse, J. M., & Bottorff, J. L. (1989). Leaking: A problem of lactation. *Journal of Nurse-Midwifery, 34,* 15–20.

Moss, J. R. (1981). Concerns of multiparas on the third postpartum day. *Journal of Obstetric, Gynecologic, and Neonatal Nursing, 10,* 421–424.

Palisin, H. (1980). The neonatal perception inventory: Failure to replicate. *Child Development, 51,* 737–742.

Palisin, H. (1981). The neonatal perception inventory: A review. *Nursing Research, 30* 285–289.

Perry, S. E. (1983). Parents perceptions of their newborn following structured interactions. *Nursing Research, 32,* 208–212.

Petrowski, D. D. (1981). Effectiveness of prenatal and postnatal instruction in postpartum care. *Journal of Obstetric, Gynecologic, and Neonatal Nursing, 10,* 386–389.

Pickens, D. S. (1982). The cognitive processes of career-oriented primiparas in identity reformulation. *Maternal-Child Nursing Journal 11,* 135–164.

Poley-Strobel, B. A., & Beckmann, C. A. (1987). The effects of a teaching-modeling intervention on early mother-infant reciprocity. *Infant Behavior and Development, 10,* 467–476.

Pridham, K. F. (1987). The meaning for mothers of a new infant: Relationship to maternal experience. *Maternal-Child Nursing Journal 16,* 103–122.

Pridham, K. F. (1988). Structures of maternal information processing for infant feeding. *Western Journal of Nursing Research, 10,* 566–575.

Pridham, K. F. (1989). Mothers' decision rules for problem solving. *Western Journal of Nursing Research, 11,* 60–74.

Pridham, K. F., Chang, A. S., & Hansen, M. F. (1987). Mothers' problem-solving skill and use of help with infant-related issues: The role of importance and need for action. *Research in Nursing & Health, 10,* 263–275.

Pridham, K. F., Hansen, M. F., Bradley, M. E., & Heighway, S. M. (1982). Issues of concern to mothers of new babies. *The Journal of Family Practice, 14*(6), 1079–1085.

Pridham, K. F., Knight, C. B., & Stephenson, G. (1989a). Decision rules for infant feeding: The influence of maternal expertise, regulating functions, and feeding method. *Maternal-Child Nursing Journal, 18,* 31–48

Pridham, K. F., Knight, C. B., & Stephenson, G. (1989b). Mothers' working models of infant feeding: Description and influencing factors. *Journal of Advanced Nursing, 14,* 1051-1061.

Princeton, J. C. (1986). Incorporating a deliberative nursing care approach with breast feeding mothers. *Health Care for Women International, 7,* 277-293.

Roberts, F. B. (1983). Infant behavior and the transition to parenthood. *Nursing Research, 32,* 213-217.

Rubin, R. (1961a). Basic maternal behavior. *Nursing Outlook, 9,* 683-686.

Rubin, R. (1961b). Puerperal change. *Nursing Outlook, 9,* 753-755.

Rubin, R. (1963). Maternal touch. *Nursing Outlook, 11,* 828-831.

Rubin, R. (1967a). Attainment of the maternal role: 1. Processes. *Nursing Research, 16,* 237-245.

Rubin, R. (1967b). Attainment of the maternal role: 2. Models and referrants. *Nursing Research, 16,* 342-346.

Rubin, R. (1977). Binding-in in the postpartum period. *Maternal-Child Nursing Journal, 6,* 67-75.

Rubin, R. (1984). *Maternal identity and the maternal experience.* New York: Springer.

Russell, C. S. (1974). Transition to parenthood: Problems and gratifications. *Journal of Marriage and the Family, 36,* 294-301.

Rutledge, D. L., & Pridham, K. F. (1987). Postpartum mothers' perceptions of competence for infant care. *Journal of Obstetric, Gynecologic, and Neonatal Nursing, 16,* 185-194.

Schaefer, E. S., & Manheimer, H. (1960, April). Dimensions of Prenatal Adjustment. Paper presented at the Eastern Psychological Association, New York, NY.

Seashore, M. J., Leifer, A. D., Barnett, C. R., & Leiderman, P. H. (1973). The effects of denial of early mother-infant interaction on maternal self-confidence. *Journal of Personality and Social Psychology, 26,* 369-378.

Shaw, H. S. W. (1986). Telephone audiotapes for parenting education: Do they really help? *MCN, The American Journal of Maternal/Child Nursing, 11,* 108-111.

Sheehan, F. (1981). Assessing postpartum adjustment: A pilot study. *Journal of Obstetric, Gynecologic, and Neonatal Nursing, 10,* 19-23.

Sumner, G., & Fritsch, J. (1977). Postnatal parental concerns: The first six weeks of life. *Journal of Obstetric, Gynecologic, and Neonatal Nursing, 6,* 27-32.

Tribotti, S., Lyons, N., Blackburn, S., Stein, M., & Withers, J. (1988). Nursing diagnoses for the postpartum woman. *Journal of Obstetric, Gynecologic, and Neonatal Nursing, 17,* 410-416.

Virden, S. F. (1988). The relationship between infant feeding method and maternal role adjustment. *Journal of Nurse-Midwifery, 33,* 31-35.

Walker, L. O. (1978). A survey of the needs of adoptive parents. *Pediatric Nursing, 4*(2), 28-31.

Walker, L. O. (1981). Identifying parents in need: An approach to adoptive parenting. *MCN, The American Journal of Maternal/Child Nursing, 6,* 118-123.

Walker, L. O. (1989a). A longitudinal analysis of stress process among mothers of infants. *Nursing Research, 38,* 339-343.

Walker, L. O. (1989b). Stress process among mothers of infants: Preliminary model testing. *Nursing Research, 38,* 10-16.

Walker, L. O., Crain, H., & Thompson, E. (1986a). Maternal role attainment and identity in the postpartum period: Stability and change. *Nursing Research, 35,* 68-71.

Walker, L. O., Crain, H., & Thompson, E. (1986b). Mothering behavior and maternal role attainment during the postpartum period. *Nursing Research, 35,* 352-355.

Walz, B. L., & Rich, O. J. (1983). Maternal tasks of taking-on a second child in the postpartum period. *Maternal-Child Nursing Journal, 12,* 185-216.

White, M., & Dawson, C. (1981). The impact of the at-risk infant on family solidarity. In R. Lederman & B. Raff (Eds.), *Perinatal parental behavior: Nursing research and implications for newborn health.* New York. Liss. March of Dimes Birth Defects Foundation. *Birth Defects. Original Article Series, 17*(6), 253-284.

Wiles, L. S. (1984). The effect of prenatal breastfeeding education on breastfeeding success and maternal perception of the infant. *Journal of Obstetric, Gynecologic, and Neonatal Nursing, 13,* 253–257.

Winkelstein, M. L., & Carson, V. J. (1987). Adolescents and rooming-in. *Maternal-Child Nursing Journal, 16,* 75–88.

Young, L. Y., Creighton, D. E., & Sauve, R. S. (1988). The needs of families of infants discharged home with continuous oxygen therapy. *Journal of Obstetric, Gynecologic, and Neonatal Nursing, 17,* 187–193.

Zabielski, M. T. (1984). Giving and receiving in the neomaternal period. A case of distributive inequity. *Maternal-Child Nursing Journal, 13,* 19–46.

CHAPTER 14

Parent-Infant Nursing Research on Attachment

DEFINITIONS AND DESCRIPTIONS OF ATTACHMENT

DEFINING ATTACHMENT

Definitions of attachment formulated in parent-infant nursing research are presented in Table 14–1. Definitions from other fields, such as those of Ainsworth (1973, p. 1) and Klaus and Kennell (1976, p. 2), have also been used in parent-infant nursing research (e.g., Fortier, 1988; Taubenheim, 1981). Across definitions, key components of attachment—particularly parental attachment—are an affective tie to another and the specificity and enduring nature of the tie. Although a few investigators distinguish between attachment and bonding (e.g., Tony, 1983), the terms are used interchangeably for the most part. *Acquaintance* is an additional term used by a few (e.g., Furr & Kirgis, 1982) to refer to the formative period of the parent-infant relationship.

THEORETICAL MODELS OF ATTACHMENT

Although many parent-infant studies contain definitions of attachment, few manifest theoretical models of attachment that guide the research. The following illustrates the incorporation of theoretical models in nursing research. Gottlieb (1978), as a result of her qualitative research,

Table 14–1
DEFINITIONS AND DESCRIPTIONS OF ATTACHMENT

Maternal attachment was conceptualized in terms of maternal statements that "reflected a developing growth of positive feelings on the part of the mother toward her infant, and included such dimensions as wanting to possess, to prolong, or to seek contact, and to be proud of and to love her infant." (Gottlieb, 1978, p. 40.)

Maternal-fetal attachment: "The extent to which women engage in behaviors which represent an affiliation and interaction with their unborn child." (Cranley, 1981b, p. 65.)

"Maternal attachment may be thought of as the extent to which a mother feels that her infant occupies an essential position in her life." (Schroeder, 1977, p. 37.)

"Maternal attachment—an affectional tie formed between a mother and her child which endures through time and is manifested by specific maternal behaviors." (Avant, 1981, p. 416.)

"Attachment is the emotional and affectional tie that a mother feels toward her child that develops through their interactions." (Carson & Virden, 1984, p. 356.)

proposed a conceptual framework for maternal bonding based on disbelief and discovery and complementary and antagonistic behavioral systems.

More recently, Mercer, Ferketich, May, DeJoseph, and Sollid (1988) proposed a theoretical model of predictors of prenatal attachment to the fetus. In that model, negative life events and pregnancy risk status influence a second set of variables: self-esteem, health perception, family functioning, mate relationship, and social support. The second set of variables influences mastery, which in turn affects anxiety and depression. The latter two variables are proposed to directly affect parents' prenatal attachment. Unfortunately, initial tests of this model have been disappointing. (See findings of model testing presented below.)

Other frameworks used to guide the exploration of attachment include Rogers' (1970) model of life processes (Schodt, 1989) and Bowlby's (1969) attachment framework in conjunction with the Johnson (1980) Behavioral System Model. (Holaday, 1981). In addition, a number of studies have derived hypotheses from the idea of a sensitive period (Klaus & Kennell, 1976) in which early or extended parent-infant contact is thought to be essential to the developing parent-infant relationship (Table 14–4).

MEASUREMENT

GENERAL STRATEGIES

Most definitions of attachment characterize it as an emotional tie to another. Thus, with regard to parental attachment, operationalizing it takes two forms: (1) measuring the tie by a self-report method such as a questionnaire or interview or (2) measuring the behavioral correlates of the tie. Often, unfortunately, no empirical substantiation is given for the validity of behavioral measures of attachment; that is, the correlation of a measure to the emotional tie is not empirically demonstrated before the use of the measure in research.

The study of infant attachment has a long history (Ainsworth, 1973), and perhaps for that reason it has not been a focus of most nursing research on attachment. Approaches to measurement of infant attachment have relied heavily on longitudinal observations of mothers and infants in naturalistic settings (Ainsworth, Blehar, Waters, & Wall, 1978).

SPECIFIC TOOLS

Table 14–2 presents measures of attachment that have been used in parent-infant nursing research. (*Note:* If tools were specifically designed for studies of attachment, they were included in this chapter regardless of their overlap with other topics covered in this book.)

The most widely used self-report tool for measuring attachment is the Maternal-Fetal Attachment Scale (MFAS) and its paternal adaptation (Cranley, 1981a). Grace (1989), however, has noted that "although the instrument's title invokes the attachment paradigm, the items and subscales conceptually represent antepartal task of maternal role attainment" (p. 228).

Among behavioral measures of attachment, a vast number have been used in parent-infant nursing research. In many cases these measures have been used in single studies and have had no further research application. Thus, cumulative information about their reliability and validity is unavailable.

With regard to measurement of infant attachment, the "strange situation procedure," which involves episodes of caregiver-infant separation and reunion and introduction of a stranger, is the definitive measure of that phenomenon at this time (Ainsworth et al., 1978). Training in the setup and scoring of this procedure is essential before using the procedure in research.

SUMMARY OF RESEARCH

SCOPE OF ATTACHMENT RESEARCH

Nurses have made attachment a major area of parent-infant nursing research by virtue of the number of studies of the phenomenon. Unlike such areas as role attainment, attachment intervention studies have been almost as frequent as descriptive studies. Indeed, the areas given least attention

Table 14–2
MEASURES/TOOLS FOR THE CONCEPT OF ATTACHMENT

Tool	Source Described in	Studies Using Tool
	ATTITUDINAL OR SELF-REPORT MEASURES:	
Maternal-Fetal Attachment Scales: Twenty-four-item prenatal scale; modified for fathers as the Paternal-Fetal Attachment Scale	Cranley (1981a) Weaver & Cranley (1983)	Koniak-Griffin (1988) Cranley (1984) Curry (1987) Cranley (1981b) Mercer et al. (1988) Weaver & Cranley (1983) Schodt (1989) Kemp & Page (1987a) Gaffney (1986) Heidrich & Cranley (1989) Grace (1989) Davis & Akridge (1987)
Questionnaire on father attitude to newborn: Thirty-four-item scale	Leonard (1976) as cited in Taubenheim (1981)	Taubenheim (1981)
Postnatal interview: Items related to thoughts and feelings about baby and rooming-in	Schroeder (1977)	Schroeder (1977)
Affectional Bond Questionnaire: Twenty-five-item scale for quality of bond with infant	Bills (1980)	Bills (1980)
Task Sequence Questionnaire: Eight-item scale related to caregiving	Bills (1980)	Bills (1980)

BEHAVIORAL MEASURES		
Maternal Attachment Scale: Observational tool of maternal attachment behaviors	Avant (1982)	Norr, Nacion, & Abramson (1989) Martone & Nash (1988) Avant (1981) Avant (1979) Davis & Akridge (1987) Norr, Roberts, & Freese (1989)
Observation tool: Rating scale and coding guide for fathers' attachment behaviors	Taubenheim (1981)	Taubenheim (1981)
Paternal attachment behaviors: Time sampling of six behaviors related to attachment	Bowen & Miller (1980)	Bowen & Miller (1980)
Mother-infant interaction: Time-sampling tool for maternal affectionate bonding	Grace (1984)	Grace (1984)
Care-Giving & Play Checklist: Self-report tool for frequency of activities with infant	Jones (1981)	Jones (1981)
Maternal Attachment Tool: Clinical assessment tool for maternal behavior	Cropley, Lester, & Pennington (1976)	Boudreaux (1981)
Postnatal Attachment Test: Specific maternal attachment behaviors	Crater-Jessop (1981)	Carter-Jessop (1981) Carson & Virden (1984)
Observation of Maternal Infant Behavior: Observational measure of maternal affectionate behavior	deChateau & Wiberg (1977)	Hepworth et al. (1987) Curry (1983) Feller et al. (1983) Curry (1982)

Table 14–2
MEASURES/TOOLS FOR THE CONCEPT OF ATTACHMENT *(Continued)*

Tool	Source Described in	Studies Using Tool
	BEHAVIORAL MEASURES (Continued)	
Observation checklist: Time sampling of caregiver behaviors in initial handling of infant	Tulman (1985)	Tulman (1985) Tulman (1986)
Father-infant observation protocol: Time sampling of fathers' behaviors during play interaction	Jones (1981)	Fortier (1988) Jones (1981)
Interaction assessment tool: Observational tool of bonding behaviors of new fathers	Toney (1983)	Toney (1983)
Codes for sibling behavior: Coding scheme for sibling attachment behaviors	Marecki et al. (1985)	Marecki et al. (1985)
Thirty-six behavioral codes for father and infant behavior during well-baby visit	Pannabecker & Emde (1977)	Pannabecker & Emde (1977)
Narrative coding of attachment related behaviors	Holaday (1981)	Holaday (1981)
Strange Situation Procedure: Laboratory test of infant attachment	Ainsworth et al. (1978)	Barnard et al. (1988)

have been relational or predictive studies linking attachment to antecedent or consequent events for parents or infants (Table 14–3). The scope of attachment research reviewed in this chapter begins with the prenatal period and includes attachment among mothers, fathers, and siblings of infants. (*Note:* For additional studies of attachment in relation to social support, see Chapter 5.)

DESCRIPTIVE RESEARCH

Description of Prenatal Attachment

Cranley (1981b) explored mothers' and fathers' prenatal attachment to the fetus. In the first study, 30 mothers were assessed during the last 6 weeks of pregnancy and on the third postpartum day. Prenatal attachment was measured by questionnaire. Of five dimensions of attachment, mothers engaged most often in giving of self and least often in interacting with the fetus. Ninety-three percent of mothers reported at least sometimes engaging in giving of self, but only 55.5 percent reported at least sometimes interacting with the fetus.

In the second study, Cranley (1981b) measured 100 fathers' prenatal attachment by questionnaire. Fathers reported most often engaging in attachment behaviors related to differentiating of self and least often in behaviors related to interacting with the fetus. The percent of fathers engaging in specific dimensions of prenatal attachment was as follows: differentiating of self (89 percent), role taking (86 percent), giving of self (66 percent), attributing qualities to the fetus (49 percent), and interacting with the fetus (40 percent).

Descriptions of Postnatal Attachment

In two studies about the development of attachment, Cogan and Edmunds (1980) studied pronoun use in parents' retrospective descriptions of their infants at birth. In the first study, 107 couples provided survey data with regard to childbirth and subsequent events. Based on responses to an open-ended question, parents were classified according to whether they referred to their child with a neuter pronoun or a gender-specific one. Fathers (57 percent) more often than mothers (36 percent) used the neuter pronoun. In the second study, Cogan and Edmunds (1980) again classified new parents regarding use of the neuter pronoun based on survey responses gathered about one month after birth. Mothers using the neuter pronoun were more likely to be multiparas and older and to have attended childbirth classes than were mothers who used gender-specific pronouns. Among fathers, those using neuter pronouns tended to attend childbirth classes, to feel confident about their knowledge of birth, and to have

Table 14–3
PARENT-INFANT NURSING RESEARCH ON ATTACHMENT

DESCRIPTIVE
Descriptions of Attachment
Anderberg (1988), siblings of newborn infants
Avant (1979), new mothers
Brown et al. (1989), parents of very low birth weight infants
Cogan & Edmunds (1980), new parents
Cranley (1981b), expectant mothers
Cranley (1981b), expectant fathers
Marecki et al. (1985), siblings of newborn infants
Mercer (1974), mothers of handicapped infants
Palkovitz (1986), laypersons
Palkovitz (1988), laypersons
Taubenheim (1981), new fathers
Patterns of Attachment
Gottlieb (1978), attachment processes
Changes in Attachment
Cranley (1984), early vs. late pregnancy
Feller et al. (1983), from birth to 1 mo postpartum
Grace (1989), from first prenatal visit to end of pregnancy
Differences in Attachment
Fortier (1988), fathers of infants with vaginal vs. cesarean birth
Heidrich & Cranley (1989), expectant mothers who varied with regard to fetal movement, ultrasound, and amniocentesis
Holaday (1981), mothers of normal vs. chronically ill infants
Kemp & Page (1987a), women with high- vs. low-risk pregnancies
Kemp & Page (1987b), women with high- vs. low-risk pregnancies
Martone & Nash (1988), bottle- vs. breast-feeding mothers
Mercer et al. (1988), expectant fathers vs. mothers and low- vs. high-risk men and women
Tulman (1985), new mothers vs. student nurses
Tulman (1986), vaginal vs. cesarean birth mothers
RELATIONSHIPS AMONG VARIABLES/PREDICTIVE MODELS
Avant (1981), correlate of postnatal attachment
Cranley (1981b), correlates of prenatal attachment
Fortier (1988), correlates of postnatal attachment
Gaffney (1986), correlates of prenatal attachment
Mercer et al. (1988), predictive model of prenatal attachment
Schodt (1989), attachment correlates of couvade
Weaver & Cranley (1983), correlates of prenatal attachment
INTERVENTION RESEARCH
Bills (1980), infant caregiving
Boudreaux (1981), three nursing interventions (e.g., review of pregnancy, labor, and delivery)

Table 14–3 *(Continued)*
INTERVENTION RESEARCH (Continued)
Bowen & Miller (1980), presence at birth, preparenthood classes
Brodish (1982), early contact
Carson & Virden (1984), prenatal fetal awareness and massage
Carter-Jessop (1981), prenatal fetal awareness and massage
Croft (1982), Lamaze classes
Curry (1982), skin-to-skin contact after birth
Davis & Akridge (1987), prenatal fetal awareness and massage
Furr & Kirgis (1982), teaching about infant
Grace (1984), amniocentesis, ultrasound, knowledge of fetal gender
Hall (1980), teaching about infant
Jones (1981), early contact
Lotas & Willging (1979), rooming-in
Marecki et al. (1985), sibling preparation classes
Norr et al. (1989), rooming-in
Pannabecker & Emde (1977), early contact
Schroeder (1977), rooming-in
Toney (1983), holding infant at birth

attended the births of their infants. No association between pronoun use and later parenting was found.

Avant (1979) described attachment behaviors of 15 new mothers during a feeding to assess proposed behaviors as part of a validation study of the process of diagnosis development. The most frequently occurring maternal behaviors were looks at infant, en face gaze, finger/palm touching of infant, close contact, cradling, bottle out of mouth of infant, encompassing infant, and talking. These favorably paralleled the theoretical criteria of attachment: visual contact, touch, positive affect, reciprocal interaction, and vocalization.

Paternal attachment was the focus of Taubenheim's study (1981) of 10 first-time fathers during the first three postpartum days. Fathers' attachment behaviors were coded during three 30-minute observations of fathers during infant feedings in mothers' hospital rooms. The most frequently occurring behavior was talking to another about the baby. Fathers who were ranked highest on bonding behaviors fed their infants during observations, and those with the greatest number of bonding behaviors also engaged more often in en face positioning, holding infants, and talking to infants.

Mercer (1974) described attachment within the context of handicapping conditions. She examined five new mothers' attachment and aversion responses to their handicapped infants, each of whom had a visible defect. Observations and interviews were conducted across four time periods: the first 8 days, 2 weeks to 1 month, 2 months, and 3 months. Maternal attachment and aversion responses were assessed within three broad categories of maternal behavior: maternal assessments (stated perceptions of an infant's appearance and function), maternal contact (communicative responses to the baby), and maternal care activities (mothering acts). Among assessment responses, attachment predominated over aversion at all times; attachment responses increased proportionately at both 2 and 3 months compared to preceding periods. Mothers' assessment responses focused proportionately more on function than appearance, particularly after the first 8 days. With regard to maternal contact behaviors, although attachment behaviors predominated in all periods, the proportion of aversion increased progressively from birth to 3 months. Among care activities, again attachment predominated but aversion increased progressively with time. Despite those changes, over all categories of behavior, attachment and aversion responses remained relatively constant from birth to 3 months.

In a study of two behaviors related to attachment, parental visiting and telephoning, Brown, York, Jacobsen, Gennaro, and Brooten (1989) followed families of 65 low birth weight infants. Using chart review, family visits and telephone calls regarding the infant were tabulated during the first 6 weeks of the infants' hospitalization. Mothers were the most frequent visitors averaging 2 to 3 visits per week. Fathers averaged 1.5 visits during the first week and 0.03 visit thereafter. Joint visits by parents occurred about once per week. Mothers averaged three telephone calls per week; fathers' average calls were about zero. On average, more frequent visits occurred if parents were married, had higher incomes, had private insurance, and owned a car.

In a study of sibling attachment to the newborn, Marecki, Wooldridge, Dow, Thompson, and Lechner-Hyman (1985) videotaped 30 siblings aged 3 to 5 years during visits with the newborns on the day of hospital discharge. Videotapes were coded by using a time-sampling technique. Most siblings spent most of the time in close proximity to the newborns. Sibling behaviors involved mainly looking at the infant's head/face (96.7 percent) rather than touching (86.7 percent) or talking about the infant (60 percent). Over half of the siblings kissed and/or hugged the infants.

Anderberg (1988) investigated acquaintance and attachment behaviors of newborns' siblings at their first meeting. Thirty siblings aged 17 months to 11 years were observed for 15 to 20 minutes. Also, parent interviews were conducted to assess the children's preparation and background. During their visits, siblings interacted more with mothers than with newborns. The most frequent response of siblings to the newborns was to look at them. Less often, siblings touched or talked about the newborns. Siblings with previous loss experiences displayed less acquaintance and attachment behaviors than siblings without loss experiences. Several mothers reported that siblings displayed prenatal attachments to fetuses. Some younger siblings displayed troubled behaviors such as demanding the newborn be moved from the parent or ignoring the mother.

Finally, Palkovitz (1988) investigated sources of laypersons' beliefs about father-infant bonding. Seventeen laypersons (eight females and nine males) who participated in a larger survey of beliefs about bonding were interviewed for detailed information about their beliefs about bonding. Eighty-three percent of the subjects agreed that scientific evidence conclusively showed that, at birth, fathers bond to babies, and 41 percent indicated the source of that information was general knowledge. Other sources cited included television (35 percent), classes (18 percent), and popular written material (18 percent). However, only 12 percent agreed that there was firm evidence that the father-infant relationship was impaired by not attending the birth, and 47 percent agreed that evidence was strong that early contact increased fathers' involvement. Again the bases for those beliefs were general knowledge, television, classes, and popular literature.

In a related report, Palkovitz (1986) examined characteristics of subjects (N = 224) who viewed birth attendance as essential for the father-infant relationship. The sample included high school and college students, expectant parents, and people surveyed at a shopping mall. Based on agreement with specific statements in a survey instrument, persons who viewed birth attendance as essential were identified. The demographic characteristics of those with the strongest beliefs about the critical nature of birth attendance were high school graduates with no further educational plans who had one child or three or more children and had a low income and were attending childbirth classes.

Attachment Patterns

Gottlieb (1978) began her qualitative study of maternal attachment by questioning the equivalence of mothering and attachment behaviors. Eleven primiparas with healthy newborns were interviewed and observed during infant feeding on three occasions: during the first day, fifth day, and fourth week postpartum. Maternal attachment was operationally defined in terms of feelings represented in maternal verbalizations. A core concept of Gottlieb's analysis of data was the discovery process whereby a newly born, but unfamiliar, infant is transformed into one's familiar and personal child. Gottlieb proposed that a feeling of disbelief following birth provides motivation for the discovery process. The mother's senses are used in discovery and sensory input leads to three forms of discovery about the infant: identifying, relating, and interpreting. In particular, Gottlieb noted that mothers made a greater proportion of interpreting statements on the fifth day than earlier. Mothers especially made interpreting statements that were likely to enhance the maternal bond to the infant. For example, mothers made statements that elicited positive feelings toward the infant or construe infant behaviors as recognizing or acknowledging the mother.

Changes in Attachment

Cranley (1984) studied fetal-attachment levels in two groups of expectant couples: those in the first half of gestation (n = 145) and those in the second half (n = 181). As expected, couples in the latter group evidenced levels of fetal attachment higher than those in the former group.

To further study the development of maternal-fetal attachment, Grace (1989) administered the MFAS at 4-week intervals during pregnancy to 69 women. (*Note*: Grace's [1989] comment concerning the conceptual inconsistencies of the MFAS that was cited earlier in this chapter). The MFAS, comprising five subscales, had internal consistency values exceeding 0.80 for the total scale, but values for two subscales were below 0.60 on at least one occasion. Only total scale findings are reported here. Correlations between MFAS scores on different occasions ranged from 0.55 to 0.95. With regard to MFAS changes over time, statistically significant effects for time and subject were found. A significant interaction between time and subject also occurred. Overall, expectant mothers' MFAS scores increased over the course of pregnancy. Further, as the number of children women had increased, less positive change in MFAS scores occurred during pregnancy. Of note, some significant relationships between MFAS subscale scores and postpartal adaptation were found.

To assess maternal attachment in adolescent mothers, Feller, Henson, Bell, Wong, and Bruner (1983) followed 15 adolescents from 12 hours after birth until 1 month later. Adolescents were observed interacting with their infants at 12 hours, 24 to 48 hours, 10 days, and 30 days. Also, maternal perceptions were measured at 1 to 2 days and 30 days. Forty-seven percent of the mothers viewed their babies positively at the first assessment, and that increased to 86 percent at the second assessment. The one mother who viewed her baby negatively at the second assessment reported her pregnancy was unplanned and unwanted. Mothers' attachment behaviors were not specifically different from birth to day 10 and day 30.

Differences in Prenatal Attachment

Mercer et al. (1988) compared attachment to the fetus in four subsamples: medically high-risk pregnant women (n = 153), partners of high-risk women (n = 75), medically low-risk pregnant women (n = 218), and partners of low-risk women (n = 147). Both high- and low-risk women had significantly higher prenatal attachment to their fetuses than their partners had (see also Schodt, 1989). Risk groups did not differ significantly in regard to prenatal attachment.

In a related study, Kemp and Page (1987b) assessed the effects of high-risk status on maternal attachment. They compared 54 women having normal pregnancies with 32 women having high-risk pregnancies. All the latter were receiving prenatal care at a high-risk clinic. The two groups differed in several characteristics: race, parity, and whether pregnancies were planned. The two groups did not differ on a measure of prenatal attachment, but mothers with high-risk pregnancies had significantly lower self-esteem than mothers with normal pregnancies. In addition, both maternal age and education were inversely related to prenatal attachment. In a second report, Kemp and Page (1987a) again compared prenatal attachment in women with normal and high-risk pregnancies. In that study, a different measure of prenatal attachment was used. Again, the investigators found no significant differences in attachment between the two groups of mothers. Further, demographic and other variables were unrelated to prenatal attachment.

Heidrich and Cranley (1989) examined differences in prenatal attachment in women who had felt fetal movement, had experienced ultrasound scans, or had undergone amniocentesis. Prenatal attachment and perception of the fetus was assessed at 16 and 20 weeks of gestation in 91 women. There was a significant main effect for fetal movement; women who had experienced fetal movement had higher attachment. The procedures of amniocentesis and ultrasound were not associated with overall differences in attachment. However, a specific contrast of mothers prior to amniocentesis compared to mothers not having amniocentesis showed the former did have lower scores at that point. With regard to perception of the fetus, there were no significant main effects of fetal movement or the two obstetric procedures. There was a significant interaction between fetal movement and time; mothers who had not felt movement at the first testing had greater gains in perception of the fetus than those who had already felt movement.

Differences in Postnatal Attachment

To assess the specificity of mothers' initial handling of their infants (Klaus, Kennell, Plumb, & Zuehlke, 1970) as an attachment index, Tulman (1985) compared 36 new mothers' behavior with the behavior of 36 student nurses having first contact with particular infants. New mothers' behavior following vaginal delivery was observed during infants' first postpartum visit; infants ranged in age from 3 to 12 hours. Student nurses were observed during contact with infants on the first day of their newborn nursery rotation; infants ranged in age from 4 to 144 hours. Mothers and students did not differ in demographic variables. Observations focused on handling behaviors used by mothers and students; eye contact and vocalizations were not recorded. Except for two behaviors, mothers exceeded students in the amount of handling behaviors during 15-minute observations. Although students and mothers did not differ in how soon they initiated finger exploration of the infants, mothers initiated palm, arm, and trunk contact sooner than students, and students initiated exploration of infants' extremities sooner than mothers. Statistical analyses indicated that students, but not mothers, followed a significant behavioral sequence in the use of their own body parts during initial handling. Students' sequence of use of their own body parts more closely resembled the theoretically proposed attachment sequence (finger tips to palms to arms and upper torso) than did the mothers' sequence. With regard to infant body parts touched, both mothers and students followed statistically significant sequences of contact with infants' bodies. Mothers' sequence of contact with infants' bodies, however, was the reverse of the theoretically proposed sequence.

Tulman (1986) further assessed maternal handling differences between 36 new mothers having vaginal births and 36 mothers having cesarean births. Both groups of mothers were similar in background variables except that cesarean birth mothers were older, initially handled infants later after delivery, received more pain medication, and were less likely to handle their infants in the delivery or recovery rooms than mothers with vaginal births. Observations of maternal handling behaviors were made during infants' first visits to their mothers' postpartal rooms. The two groups differed in the frequency of a number of maternal handling behaviors, with vaginal birth mothers exceeding in number the cesarean birth mothers. For most behaviors, the two groups did not differ in how soon they initiated specific behaviors during their initial postpartum handling of infants. In regard to their own body parts, neither group of mothers followed a statistically significant sequence of initial handling behaviors. Both groups demonstrated a similar and statistically significant sequence of touching infant body parts. Presence of fathers during maternal handling of the infants was associated with less frequent maternal behaviors among cesarean birth mothers, but the association did not hold true for vaginal birth mothers.

Two studies respectively examined the effects of intrapartal factors and feeding method on attachment. Fortier (1988) considered intrapartal influences on attachment by comparing fathers whose wives had had vaginal (n = 30) and planned (n = 15) and unplanned (n = 15) cesarean births. Observational and questionnaire data were collected during a home visit at 1 month postpartum. Because infant state was correlated with attachment behaviors, it was used as a covariate in statistical analysis. When state was controlled, there were no significant differences between groups of fathers in regard to attachment. Further, to determine if attachment differences occurred in breast-feeding (n = 15) versus bottle-feeding mothers (n = 15), Martone and Nash (1988) observed feedings on the second postpartal day. Observations were coded by using an attachment protocol. No significant differences in overall attachment were found.

In a study of differences between mothers with chronically ill infants and mothers with normal infants, Holaday (1981) made home observations at 3-week intervals when infants were 4 to 6 months of age. Six mothers with chronically ill infants were observed, and data on 26 mothers with normal infants were obtained from an extant database. The attachment behavior of infant crying—duration and frequency—and maternal interventions for crying were the focuses of the study. Chronically ill infants cried more often than normal infants. In both groups, mothers' most frequent intervention was picking up the infants. Chronically ill infants in some cases demonstrated alterations in cry patterns such as waxing and waning of cry intensity. Compared to mothers of normal infants, mothers of chronically ill infants ignored their cries less often, responded more quickly to crying, maintained greater proximity to the infants, and used a series of interventions rather than just one. Further, duration of the cry was a key variable influencing maternal response.

RELATIONAL/PREDICTIVE RESEARCH

In a series of two studies, Cranley (1981b) identified correlates of prenatal attachment in both mothers and fathers. Among expectant mothers, self-esteem, trait anxiety, and perception of the infant were unrelated to fetal attachment. In contrast, social support and stress were significantly related to fetal attachment. Among expectant fathers, prenatal attachment was moderately related to the marital relationship but only modestly related to couvade symptoms.

In a further examination of relations to fathers' prenatal attachment, Weaver and Cranley (1983) assessed physical symptoms, the marital relationship, and attachment in 100 expectant fathers. Attachment was measured by a questionnaire composed of five subscales, an example of which was differentiating self from fetus. As predicted, prenatal attachment was significantly related to physical symptoms and the marital relationship. Of the five attachment subscales, all but one—interaction with the fetus—were related to the marital relationship. Only two subscales were related to physical symptoms: attributing characteristics/intentions to the fetus and role taking.

Using Rogers' (1970) principle of integrality, Schodt (1989) examined prenatal attachment and couvade symptoms in 110 low-risk expectant couples. Variables were measured during the third trimester of pregnancy. Predicted relations between parental attachment and men's couvade symptoms were not found. Further, men's and women's fetal attachment scores were *inversely* related to each other. Finally, the level of maternal-fetal attachment did not influence the relations between paternal-fetal attachment and couvade symptoms.

Gaffney (1986) examined self-concept and anxiety as correlates of maternal-fetal attachment among 100 expectant mothers during the third trimester. Contrary to expectations, self-concept was unrelated to attachment. Both state and trait anxiety were inversely correlated with attachment, but only the correlation between state anxiety and attachment was significant.

In a study of postpartal maternal attachment, Avant (1981) examined the relation between anxiety and attachment in 30 healthy new mothers.

Maternal attachment was measured by observation of maternal feeding behaviors on the first and third postpartal days. As expected, overall attachment and anxiety were inversely related on both the first and third days. Further, on the first day, maternal age was related to both variables with younger mothers showing higher anxiety and lower attachment than older mothers.

In a study of 60 fathers' postnatal attachment, Fortier (1988) identified predictors of two attachment measures. For an observation measure of attachment, no significant amount of variance was explained by predictors. For a caretaking questionnaire related to attachment, significant predictors included previous children, infant gender, and early contact.

Mercer et al. (1988) tested a hypothesized model predicting prenatal attachment in four subsamples: medically high-risk pregnant women, mates of high-risk women, medically low-risk pregnant women, and mates of low-risk women. Of 10 predictors in the hypothesized model, only two variables were predicted to directly affect prenatal attachment: anxiety and depression. Tests of the hypothesized model conducted separately for each subsample accounted for from 0 to 3.8 percent of the variance in prenatal attachment. Respecified models as of predictors of attachment produced only modest increases in the amount of explained variance, except for mates of high-risk women. Four variables accounted for 31 percent of the variance in the latter's prenatal attachment: depending on parents for help, family functioning, mate relationship, and received support.

INTERVENTION RESEARCH

Because a number of studies have tested interventions related to fostering attachment, they are presented in Table 14–4 for easier inspection. Although the attachment rubric—or its related terms, bonding or acquaintances—was invoked in all the studies listed in Table 14–4, there was great diversity among studies with regard to the independent and dependent variables. Further, some studies were broadly related to the attachment process, but they involved neither directly manipulating early contact (the mechanism most often thought to influence attachment) nor measuring conceptually related manifestations of attachment.

Of note, over half of the studies reviewed did not randomly assign subjects of the interventions. Thus, preexisting differences may have influenced outcomes. Several studies did not employ statistical analysis of data. Many studies are composed of small samples. Keeping in mind limitations of studies, nine studies that tested effects of early or extended contact, including rooming-in, resulted in about equal support for and against hypothesized effects of contact. The outcomes of nursing studies are not inconsistent with other reviews of research dealing with early and extended contact interventions (Lamb & Hwang, 1982; Palkovitz, 1985).

Table 14–4
INTERVENTIONS RELATED TO ATTACHMENT

Citation: Group/Population	Independent Variable(s)	Dependent Variable(s) and Study Outcomes*
Schroeder (1977): Twenty primiparas (10 in the experimental and 10 in control groups)	Nonrandomized rooming-in during postpartum hospital stay	Thoughts and feelings about baby on second postpartum day (+) Competence in infant care on second postpartum day (+) *Note:* No test statistics were used.
Pannabecker & Emde (1977): Forty-eight fathers of normal newborns: 16 each in experimental and two control groups	Randomized to (1) early contact with teaching at 12 and 36 h after birth or (2) (first control) teaching & videotape at 12 and 36 h; second control group not randomized and had only routine care	Fathers' attachment behaviors during infant well-baby appointment at one month postnatally; in 85 analyses only two significant differences were found (0)
Lotas & Willging (1979): Eighty-one healthy new mothers of mixed parity: 46 in experimental and 35 in control groups	Nonrandomized rooming-in during postpartum hospital stay	Maternal perception of infant at 1 to 2 d after birth (0) Maternal perception of infant at 4 wk after birth (0)
Bills (1980): New fathers (N = 30?); 15 in control and 15 in experimental groups	Nonrandomized, supervised infant caregiving in hospital by 48 h after birth	Fathers' affectional bond with infant by 48 h after birth (0) Fathers' nurturant personality traits (0) Fathers' evaluation of intervention (experimental group only) was positive
Bowen & Miller (1980): Forty-six new fathers: 21 had classes and were present at birth, 8 were present at birth, and 17 neither had classes or were present at birth	Nonrandomized to (1) present at birth and/or (2) preparenthood classes	If present at birth, total and distal, but not proximal, paternal attachment behaviors were greater during postpartum hospital stay (+) No significant effect of classes on attachment behaviors (0)

Table 14–4
INTERVENTIONS RELATED TO ATTACHMENT *(Continued)*

Citation: Group/Population	Independent Variable(s)	Dependent Variable(s) and Study Outcomes*
Hall (1980): Thirty primiparas: 15 in experimental and 15 in control groups	Randomized in-home teaching about infant behavior at 2 to 4 d after discharge	Maternal perception at 1 mo postpartum (+)? *Note:* The experimental group showed significant gains and the control group did not, but direct comparison of groups on outcomes was not given.
Boudreaux (1981): Ten ill new mothers; all received the interventions	Three nursing interventions (catharsis, infant examination, infant caretaking); no control condition	Maternal attachment behaviors increased during postpartum hospitalization *Note:* No test statistics used
Carter-Jessop (1981): Ten primiparas: 5 in the experimental and 5 in control groups	Randomized prenatal intervention of transabdominal tactile contact with fetus and awareness of fetal activity	Maternal attachment behaviors at 2 to 4 d postpartum (+)
Jones (1981): Fifty-one new fathers of first-born infants: 34 in experimental and 17 in control groups	Nonrandomized early contact in first hour after birth	Fathers' perceptions of infants at 14 to 72 h after birth (0) Fathers' perceptions of infants at 1 mo after birth (0) Fathers' verbal interaction at 1 mo after birth (0) Fathers' nonverbal interaction at 1 mo after birth (+) Fathers' self-reported play behavior at 1 mo after birth (0) Fathers' self-reported caretaking behavior at 1 mo after birth (0)

Brodish (1982): Eighty-five mothers and their full-term, bottle-fed infants: 57 with and 28 without early contact	Nonrandomized early contact in postpartum recovery room	Infant weight change during first three postnatal days (+) Amount of formula consumed during first three postnatal days (+)
Croft (1982): Sixty-one primiparas: 45 in experimental and 16 in control groups	Nonrandomized Lamaze childbirth preparation	Maternal perception of infant on first postpartum day (0) Maternal perception of infant at 1 mo postpartum (−)
Curry (1982): Twenty primiparas: 11 in control and 9 in experimental groups	Modified randomization to skin-to-skin contact with infant in first hour after birth (*Note:* Control mothers also had contact, but with blanketed infants.)	Maternal attachment behaviors 36 h after birth (0) Maternal attachment behaviors 3 mo after birth (0) Maternal self-concept 3 mo after birth (0)
Furr & Kirgis (1982): Forty primiparas: 10 in each group of a Solomon four-group design	Randomized to groups: Intervention comprised teaching about infant behaviors on third postpartum day	Maternal adaptive behavior during infant feeding at 2 wk after birth (+)
Toney (1983): Thirty-seven first-time fathers; *n*'s = ?	Randomized holding of infant at delivery for 10 min	Fathers' bonding behaviors at 12 to 36 h after birth (0)
Carson & Virden (1984): Sixty-nine pregnant women of mixed parity in public health dept. caseload: 25 in control, 21 in relaxation, and 23 in palpation groups	Randomized to (1) fetal palpation and massage in third trimester, (2) prenatal relaxation training for labor, or (3) control	Maternal attachment behaviors during first two postpartal weeks: main effect for groups (0) and interaction of parity and groups (+) with multiparas in both experimental groups benefiting more than the control group Advanced maternal attachment behaviors during first 2 wk postpartum: main effect for groups (0) and parity by group interaction (0)

Table 14–4
INTERVENTIONS RELATED TO ATTACHMENT *(Continued)*

Citation: Group/Population	Independent Variable(s)	Dependent Variable(s) and Study Outcomes*
Grace (1984): Sixty-seven pregnant women: 33 had amniocenteses, 28 knew gender of fetus, and 54 had ultrasound scans of fetuses	Nonrandomized to amniocentesis, knowledge of fetal gender, and ultrasound scan of fetus	Maternal attachment behaviors at 24 to 121 h after birth: effect of amniocentesis (0), effect for knowledge of gender (0), and effect for ultrasound (0)
Marecki et al. (1985): Thirty siblings (aged 3 to 5 years): of newborns: 10 in experimental and 20 in control groups	Nonrandomized sibling preparation classes	Sibling attachment behaviors on day mother and baby discharged from hospital (0)
Davis & Akridge (1987): Twenty-two pregnant women: 10 in experimental and 12 in control groups	Randomized prenatal intervention of transabdominal tactile contact with fetus and awareness of fetal activity	Maternal attachment behaviors at 2 to 4 d postpartum (0)
Norr et al. (1989): One hundred eighty-seven indigent primiparas: 80 in experimental, 72 in historical control, and 35 in current control groups	Nonrandomized to (1) rooming-in, (2) historical control (before rooming-in available), or (3) current control (wanted but did not have rooming-in)	Maternal attachment behaviors at 2 and 3 d after birth (+)

**Note:* A (+) indicates outcomes favored group(s) that received treatments hypothesized to enhance attachment over comparison/control groups; a (0) indicates no differences between treated and comparison/control groups: a (−) indicates outcomes favored comparison/control group(s) that did not receive treatment over groups that received treatments hypothesized to enhance attachment.

Equally mixed results occurred in the remainder of studies. For example, Davis and Akridge (1987) were unable to replicate Carter-Jessop's (1981) findings about prenatal intervention, and Carson and Virden (1984) found only one of four analyses supportive of prenatal intervention.

FUTURE RESEARCH DIRECTIONS

Parental bonding has received extensive attention in nursing and has considerable importance in the eyes of the lay public (Palkovitz, 1986, 1988). Still, critical reviews stress that there is no clear scientific support for a "sensitive period" during which parent-infant contact has long-term and important effects on the subsequent parent-child relationship (Tulman, 1981; Lamb & Hwang, 1982; Lamb, 1982; Goldberg, 1983; Palkovitz, 1985). Those reviews do not claim that a deep and committed emotional tie to the infant is not important. Rather, the critical nature of singular early events in forging that tie is at issue. In retrospect, Lamb and Hwang (1982, p. 33) have pointed out that ungulates—species initially cited by Klaus et al (1972)—are a poor analogy to humans. Ungulates exist in herds and bear precocious young who are mobile shortly after birth, a marked contrast to human infants.

Nurse investigators could profitably redirect their attention to a number of unsolved research problems related to attachment. Included among those problems is the need for careful scientific work to build and refine measures of prenatal and postnatal parental attachment (Gaffney, 1988). Scientific work is also needed to determine the extent of continuity between the prenatal and postnatal periods of attachment development. Research on interventions to enhance the parent-infant relationship should continue. As the programmatic research of Barnard et al. (Chapter 5) on supportive inventions has shown, however, it is unlikely that brief interventions will have major impacts. Rather, researchers should attempt to design interventions that reflect the complex processes involved in the parent-infant relationship and the influence of parents' social context.

REFERENCES

Ainsworth, M. D. S. (1973). The development of infant-mother attachment. In B. M. Caldwell & H. N. Ricciuti (Eds.), *Review of child development research* (Vol. 3, pp. 1-94). Chicago: University of Chicago Press.

Ainsworth, M. D. S., Blehar, M. D., Waters, E., & Wall, S. (1978). *Patterns of attachment: A psychological study of the strange situation.* Hillsdale, NJ: Erlbaum.

Anderberg, G. J. (1988). Initial acquaintance and attachment behavior of siblings with the newborn. *Journal of Obstetric, Gynecologic, and Neonatal Nursing, 17,* 49–54.

Avant, K. (1979). Nursing diagnosis: Maternal attachment. *Advances in Nursing Science, 2*(1), 45–55.

Avant, K. C. (1981). Anxiety as a potential factor affecting maternal attachment. *Journal of Obstetric, Gynecologic, and Neonatal Nursing, 10,* 416–419.

Avant, K. C. (1982). A maternal attachment

assessment strategy. In S. S. Humenick (Ed.), *Analysis of current assessment strategies in the health care of young children and childbearing families* (pp. 171–178). East Norwalk, CN: Appleton-Century-Crofts.

Barnard, K. E., Magyary, D., Sumner, G., Booth, C. L., Mitchell, S. K., & Spieker, S. (1988). Prevention of parenting alterations for women with low social support. *Psychiatry, 51*(3), 248–253.

Bills, B. J. (1980). Enhancement of paternal-newborn affectional bonds. *Journal of Nurse-Midwifery, 25,* 21–26.

Boudreaux, M. (1981). Maternal attachment of high-risk mothers with well newborns: A pilot study. *Journal of Obstetric, Gynecologic, and Neonatal Nursing, 10,* 366–369.

Bowen, S. M., & Miller, B. C. (1980). Paternal attachment behavior as related to presence at delivery and preparenthood classes: A pilot study. *Nursing Research, 29,* 307–311.

Bowlby, J. (1969). *Attachment and loss. Vol. 1. Attachment.* New York: Basic Books.

Brodish, M. S. (1982). Relationship of early bonding to initial infant feeding patterns in bottle-fed newborns. *Journal of Obstetric, Gynecologic, and Neonatal Nursing, 11,* 248–252.

Brown, L. P., York, R., Jacobsen, B., Gennaro, S., & Brooten, D. (1989). Very low birthweight infants: Parental visiting and telephoning during initial infant hospitalization. *Nursing Research, 38,* 233–236.

Carson, K., & Virden, S. (1984). Can prenatal teaching promote maternal attachment? Practicing nurses test Carter-Jessop's prenatal attachment intervention. *Health Care for Women International, 5,* 355–369.

Carter-Jessop, L. (1981). Promoting maternal attachment through prenatal intervention. *MCN, The American Journal of Maternal/Child Nursing, 6,* 107–112.

Cogan, R., & Edmunds, E. P. (1980). Pronominalization: A linguistic facet of the maternal-paternal sensitive period. *Nursing Research, 29,* 225–227.

Cranley, M. S. (1981a). Development of a tool for the measurement of maternal attachment during pregnancy. *Nursing Research, 30,* 281–284.

Cranley, M. S. (1981b). Roots of attachment: The relationship of parents with their unborn. In R. P. Lederman, B. S. Raff, & P. Carroll (Eds.), *Perinatal parental behavior: Nursing research and implications for newborn health.* New York: Liss. March of Dimes Birth Defects Foundation. *Birth Defects, Original Article Series, 17*(6), 59–83.

Cranley, M. S. (1984). Social support as a factor in the development of parents' attachment to their unborn. In K. E. Barnard, P. A. Brandt, B. S. Raff, & P. Carroll (Eds.), *Social support and families of vulnerable infants.* White Plains, NY: March of Dimes Birth Defects Foundation. *Birth Defects, Original Article Series, 20*(5), 100–109.

Croft, C. A. (1982). Lamaze childbirth education: Implications for maternal-infant attachment. *Journal of Obstetric, Gynecologic, and Neonatal Nursing, 11,* 333–336.

Cropley, C., Lester, P., & Pennington, S. (1976). Assessment tool for measuring maternal attachment behaviors. In L. K. McNall & J. T. Galeener (Eds.), *Current practice in obstetric and gynecologic nursing* (pp. 16–28). St. Louis: Mosby.

Curry, M. A. (1982). Maternal attachment behavior and the mother's self-concept: The effect of early skin-to-skin contact. *Nursing Research, 31,* 73–78.

Curry, M. A. (1983). Variables related to adaptation to motherhood in "normal" primiparous women. *Journal of Obstetric, Gynecologic, and Neonatal Nursing, 12,* 115–121.

Curry, M. A. (1987). Maternal behavior of hospitalized pregnant women. *Journal of Psychosomatic Obstetrics and Gynaecology, 7,* 165–182.

Davis, M. S., & Akridge, K. M. (1987). The effect of promoting intrauterine attachment in primiparas on postdelivery attachment. *Journal of Obstetric, Gynecologic, and Neonatal Nursing, 16,* 430–437.

deChateau, P., & Wiberg, B. (1977). *Long-term effect on mother-infant behavior of extra contact during the first hour postpartum.* Umea, Sweden: Departments of Pediatrics and Child Psychiatry, University of Umea.

Feller, C. M., Henson, D., Bell, L., Wong, S., &

Bruner, M. (1983). Assessment of adolescent mother-infant attachment. *Issues in Health Care of Women, 4,* 237–250.

Fortier, J. C. (1988). The relationship of vaginal and cesarean birth to father-infant attachment. *Journal of Obstetric, Gynecologic, and Neonatal Nursing, 17,* 128–134.

Furr, P. A., & Kirgis, C. A. (1982). A nurse-midwifery approach to early mother-infant acquaintance. *Journal of Nurse-Midwifery, 27,* 10–14.

Gaffney, K. F. (1986). Maternal-fetal attachment in relation to self-concept and anxiety. *Maternal-Child Nursing Journal, 15,* 91–101.

Gaffney, K. F. (1988). Prenatal maternal attachment. *Image, 20,* 106–109.

Goldberg, S. (1983). Parent-infant bonding: Another look. *Child Development, 54,* 1355–1382.

Gottlieb, L. (1978). Maternal attachment in primiparas. *Journal of Obstetric, Gynecologic, and Neonatal Nursing, 7,* 39–44.

Grace, J. T. (1984). Does a mother's knowledge of fetal gender affect attachment? *MCN, The American Journal of Maternal/Child Nursing, 9,* 42–45.

Grace, J. T. (1989). Development of maternal-fetal attachment during pregnancy. *Nursing Research, 38,* 228–232.

Hall, L. A. (1980). Effect of teaching on primiparas' perceptions of their newborn. *Nursing Research, 29,* 317–322.

Heidrich, S. M., & Cranley, M. S. (1989). Effect of fetal movement, ultrasound scans and amniocentesis on maternal-fetal attachment. *Nursing Research, 38,* 81–84.

Hepworth, J. T., Bell, L., Feller, C., Hanson, D., Sands, D., & Muhlenkamp, A. (1987). Gynecologic age: Prediction in adolescent female research. *Nursing Research, 36,* 392–394.

Holaday, B. (1981). Maternal response to their chronically ill infants attachment behavior of crying. *Nursing Research, 30,* 343–348.

Johnson, D.E. (1980). The Johnson behavioral system model. In J.P. Riehl & C. Roy, Sr (Eds.), *Conceptual Models for nursing practice,* (2nd ed.) (pp. 207–216). New York: Appleton-Century-Crofts.

Jones, C. (1981). Father to infant attachment: Effects of early contact and characteristics of the infant. *Research in Nursing and Health, 4,* 193–200.

Kemp, V. H., & Page, C. K. (1987a). Maternal prenatal attachment in normal and high-risk pregnancies. *Journal of Obstetric, Gynecologic, and Neonatal Nursing, 16,* 179–184.

Kemp, V. H., & Page, C. (1987b). Maternal self-esteem and prenatal attachment in high-risk pregnancy. *Maternal-Child Nursing Journal, 16,* 195–206.

Klaus, M.H., Jerauld, R., Kreger, M.C., McAlpine, W., Steffa, M., & Kennell, J.H. (1972). Maternal attachment: Importance of the first post-partum days. *New England Journal of Medicine, 286,* 460–463.

Klaus, M. H., & Kennell, J. H. (1976). *Maternal-infant bonding.* St. Louis: Mosby.

Klaus, M.H., Kennell, J.H., Plumb, N., & Zuehlke, S. (1970). Haman maternal behavior at the first contact with her young. *Pediatrics, 46,* 187–192.

Koniak-Griffin, D. (1988). The relationship between social support, self-esteem, and maternal-fetal attachment in adolescents. *Research in Nursing and Health, 11,* 269–278.

Lamb, M. E. (1982). The bonding phenomenon: Misinterpretations and their implications. *Journal of Pediatrics, 101,* 555–557.

Lamb, M. E., & Hwang, C. (1982). Maternal attachment and mother-neonate bonding: A critical review. In M. E. Lamb & A. L. Brown (Eds.), *Advances in developmental psychology* (Vol. 2, pp 1–39). Hillsdale, NJ: Erlbaum.

Lotas, M. B., & Willging, J. M. (1979). Mothers, babies, perception. *Image, 11,* 45–51.

Marecki, M., Wooldridge, P., Dow, A., Thompson, J., & Lechner-Hyman, C. (1985). Early sibling attachment. *Journal of Obstetric, Gynecologic, and Neonatal Nursing, 14,* 418–423.

Martone, D. J., & Nash, B. R. (1988). Initial differences in postpartum attachment behavior in breastfeeding and bottle-feeding mothers. *Journal of Obstetric, Gynecologic, and Neonatal Nursing, 17,* 212–213.

Mercer, R. T. (1974). Mothers' responses to

their infants with defects. *Nursing Research, 23,* 133–137.

Mercer, R. T., Ferketich, S., May, K., DeJoseph, J., & Sollid, D. (1988). Further exploration of maternal and paternal fetal attachment. *Research in Nursing & Health, 11,* 83–95.

Norr, K. F., Nacion, K. W., & Abramson, R. (1989). Early discharge with home follow-up: Impacts on low-income mothers and infants. *Journal of Obstetric, Gynecologic, and Neonatal Nursing, 18,* 133–141.

Norr, K. F., Roberts, J. E., & Freese, U. (1989). Early postpartum rooming-in and maternal attachment behaviors in a group of medically indigent primiparas. *Journal of Nurse-Midwifery, 34,* 85–91.

Palkovitz, R. (1985). Fathers' birth attendance, early contact, and extended contact with their newborns: A critical review. *Child Development, 56,* 392–406.

Palkovitz, R. (1986). Laypersons' beliefs about the "critical" nature of father-infant bonding: Implications for childbirth educators. *Maternal-Child Nursing Journal, 15,* 39–46.

Palkovitz, R. (1988). Sources of father-infant bonding beliefs: Implications for childbirth educators. *Maternal-Child Nursing Journal, 17,* 101–113.

Pannabecker, B. J., & Emde, R. N. (1977). Effect of extended contact on father-newborn interaction. *Communicating Nursing Research, 10,* 97–114.

Rogers, M. E. (1970). *An introduction to the theoretical basis of nursing.* Philadelphia: Davis.

Schodt, C. M. (1989). Parental-fetal attachment and couvade: A study of patterns of human-environment integrality. *Nursing Science Quarterly, 2*(2), 88–97.

Schroeder, M. A. (1977). Is the immediate postpartum period crucial to the mother-child relationship? *Journal of Obstetric, Gynecologic, and Neonatal Nursing, 6,* 37–40.

Taubenheim, A. M. (1981). Paternal-infant bonding in the first-time father. *Journal of Obstetric, Gynecologic, and Neonatal Nursing, 10,* 261–264.

Toney, L. (1983). The effects of holding the newborn at delivery on paternal bonding. *Nursing Research, 32,* 16–19.

Tulman, L. J. (1981). Theories of maternal attachment. *Advances in Nursing Science, 3*(4), 7–14.

Tulman, L. J. (1985). Mothers' and unrelated persons' initial handling of newborn infants. *Nursing Research, 34,* 205–210.

Tulman, L. J. (1986). Initial handling of newborn infants by vaginally and cesarean-delivered mothers. *Nursing Research, 35,* 296–300.

Weaver, R. H., & Cranley, M. S. (1983). An exploration of paternal-fetal attachment behavior. *Nursing Research, 32,* 68–72.

CHAPTER 15

Parent-Infant Nursing Research on Loss and Separation

DEFINITIONS AND DESCRIPTIONS OF LOSS AND SEPARATION

DEFINING LOSS AND SEPARATION

In this chapter, loss and separation are defined to cover such perinatal events as miscarriage, stillbirth, and infant death as well as separation of parents and infants related to health, employment, and other events. The concepts of loss and separation apply to both parents and infants. Separation and loss are of particular significance for infants who are older than 6 months (Ainsworth, 1962/1969).

THEORETICAL MODELS OF LOSS AND SEPARATION

When frameworks were used to study loss and separation in the articles reviewed for this chapter, they varied from study to study. Williams and Nikolaisen (1982) applied a crisis framework in their study of parents' responses to sudden infant death syndrome (SIDS). In a study of the miscarriage experience, Hutti (1986) used a cognitive representation model that emphasized perception. Constructs of nursing practice served as the framework for Harris' (1984) study of perinatal loss.

MEASUREMENT

GENERAL STRATEGIES

Strategies for capturing parental responses to loss and separation include both questionnaires and interviews. Interviews are usually more suitable if there is any doubt about the appropriateness of applying existing tools to a new population or phenomenon. Questionnaires are more efficient and may be quite adequate if it is known that the tool is able to capture dimensions of a particular loss or separation experience. Studies of infant responses to loss and separation would be best chronicled through observational methods that note behavioral patterns as well as affective responses.

SPECIFIC TOOLS

Table 15–1 presents methods for measuring loss and separation experiences of parents. Dimensions of loss include tools for symptoms after loss as well as for the circumstances and experiences preceding and following the loss. Two tools are presented; for assessing maternal views and feelings about mother-infant separation as a result of maternal employment: the Maternal Separation Anxiety Scale and an interview-based rating scale (Pitzer & Hock, 1989).

SCOPE OF RESEARCH ON LOSS AND SEPARATION

Research about loss and separation during pregnancy, postpartum, and infancy (Table 15–2) is not extensively carried out by nurse investigators. However, the existing studies cover a variety of descriptive approaches. No studies that investigated variable relations or intervention effects are reported. (*Note:* For additional studies of loss in relation to social support, see Chapter 5.)

DESCRIPTIVE RESEARCH

Descriptions of Loss Experiences

To explore women's responses to a first-trimester spontaneous abortion, Wall-Haas (1985) had nine women complete survey questionnaires postabortion. Most women did not report eating or sleeping problems, but they did report the following: sadness, thinking and dreaming about the baby, irritability, thinking they had caused the abortion, anger, crying, praying, depression, and disbelief. Seven of nine women reported feeling closer to their mates after the abortion. Women also commented on the

Table 15–1
MEASURES/TOOLS FOR THE CONCEPTS OF LOSS AND SEPARATION

Tool	Source Described in	Studies Using Tool
	TOOLS RELATED TO LOSS	
Bereavement Health Assessment: Self-report tool of changes in physical health after a significant loss	Miles (1985)	Miles (1985)*
Benfield Questionnaire: Twenty-one-item questionnaire about miscarriage	Wall-Haas (1985)	Wall-Haas (1985)
Questionnaire of parents' perceptions of their crisis state following SIDS	Williams & Nikolaisen (1982)	Williams & Nikolaisen (1982)
	TOOLS RELATED TO SEPARATION	
Maternal Separation Anxiety Scale: Thirty-five-item scale about perceptions of maternal-infant separation	Pitzer & Hock (1989) Schroeder-Zwelling & Hock (1986)	Pitzer & Hock (1989) Schroeder-Zwelling and Hock (1986)
Interview-Based Rating Scale: Tool for assessing maternal separation anxiety	Pitzer & Hock (1989)	Pitzer & Hock (1989)

*Not a perinatal sample.

Table 15–2
PARENT-INFANT NURSING RESEARCH ON LOSS AND SEPARATION

DESCRIPTIVE
Descriptions of the Experience of Loss and Separation
Childs (1985), birth of a profoundly retarded infant
Wall-Haas (1985), first trimester spontaneous miscarriage
Williams & Nikolaisen (1982), sudden infant death syndrome
Patterns of the Experience of Loss and Separation
Harris (1984), dysfunctional perinatal grieving
Hutti (1986), miscarriage
Swanson-Kauffman (1988), miscarriage
Changes in the Experience of Loss and Separation
Pitzer & Hock (1989), from first- to second-born infant
Differences in the Experience of Loss and Separation
Schroeder-Zwelling & Hock (1986), diabetic vs. nondiabetic mothers
Williams & Nikolaisen (1982), fathers vs. mothers
Williams & Nikolaisen (1982), single vs. married parents
RELATIONSHIPS AMONG VARIABLES/PREDICTIVE MODELS
None
INTERVENTION RESEARCH
None

insensitive remarks made to them by some people and the insensitivity of some care providers.

Based on a survey of parents whose infants had died of SIDS, Williams and Nikolaisen (1982) reported findings about 54 parents' experiences. Only 29 percent of parents thought initially that SIDS was the cause of their babies' deaths. Even after counseling, some parents continued to believe the death was from other causes, such as punishment for the parents. Five mothers reported severe reactions requiring hospitalization after the SIDS event.

In studying mothers' responses to the birth of a retarded child, Childs (1985) interviewed 50 mothers of profoundly retarded infants. Interviews, conducted within 1 year of the infants' births, focused on the first 3 weeks after birth. Interview data were categorized according to maternal responses reported. Ninety-five percent of the mothers reported feeling guilt. Ninety percent reported experiencing denial, shame, confusion, and feelings of inferiority and questioning religious beliefs. Other reactions included wanting to die (80 percent), anger (80 percent), blaming others (80 percent), loneliness (70 percent), feeling unloved (60 percent), thinking about infanticide (40 percent), and helplessness (40 percent).

Patterns of Loss

In an exploratory study of the miscarriage experience, Hutti (1986) used qualitative methods to investigate two married women's experiences of miscarriage. One woman was a primigravida who miscarried at 7 weeks gestation. The other woman was a multigravida who miscarried at 12 weeks gestation: She had three living children and also had had a miscarriage with her first pregnancy. The women were interviewed twice about their miscarriages; both viewed their miscarriages as stressful, but the miscarriage was more of a threat to the primigravida's perceptions of her childbearing capacity. They reported experiencing numbness, depression, denial, and guilt after their first miscarriages. Both reported five common stages to their experience: recognition and assessment of the pregnancy, recognition of a possible miscarriage, recognition of the actual miscarriage, hospitalization and medical treatment, and returning home/aftermath. Both women reported marital conflict related to their first miscarriages because their husbands completed grieving more quickly than they did. During her second miscarriage, the multigravida's husband engaged in greater involvement with her and marital conflict did not occur subsequently.

In another qualitative study of the experience of miscarriage, Swanson-Kauffman (1988) explored its human-experience dimensions and the caring needs it evoked in women. The investigator interviewed a convenience sample of 20 women who lost pregnancies before the 16th week of gestation. All women were initially interviewed in their homes; a follow-up interview was conducted by telephone. Using a constant comparative method, six categories pertinent to the unfolding of the miscarriage experience were identified: coming to know, losing and gaining, sharing the loss, going public, getting through it, and trying again. Further, five caring needs of women who miscarry were identified: knowing, being with, enabling, doing for, and maintaining belief.

In a qualitative study of perinatal dysfunctional grieving, Harris (1984) analyzed cases from a private nursing counseling practice. Data were based on four couples and five individual mothers who had experienced spontaneous abortion, premature birth, stillbirth, infant death, or birth of a handicapped infant. Based on analysis of client records, characteristics of childbearing loss were generated, strategies for assessment and intervention were identified, and comparisons between study findings and existing literature were made. Characteristics of dysfunctional grieving the investigator reported were normalcy facade, role distress, repressing joy and humor, attributional guilt, and phantom baby experiences. Assessment strategies identified included the grief behavior paradox, and those for intervention included such methods as communication mapping and role playing. In comparing study findings to the literature, the investigator noted clients needed counseling support after the hospital experience, but the literature emphasized the nurses' in-hospital supportive role.

Changes in the Experience of Separation

To explore changes in mothers' concerns about infant separation, Pitzer and Hock (1989) used a longitudinal design to compare employed women when their first- and second-born infants were 7 months old. By using parallel questionnaires and interviews, changes in three dimensions of maternal separation anxiety were assessed: views about exclusive maternal care, views of effects of separation on the child, and specific work-related separation concerns. When comparisons of questionnaire responses for both occasions were made, mothers demonstrated less separation anxiety in two areas with their second-born infants (exclusive maternal care and effects of separation) and remained unchanged in the third (work-related concerns). Mothers' questionnaire and interview responses were correlated significantly across two of three parallel areas. Work preference was also associated with separation anxiety; mothers who preferred to stay at home had higher maternal separation anxiety than mothers who preferred to work.

Differences in Loss and Separation

Focusing on SIDS as a crisis for parents, Williams and Nikolaisen (1982) surveyed parents whose infants had died of SIDS over a 6-year period. Thirty-seven mothers and 17 fathers responded to the survey questionnaire, which was a combination of structured and open-ended items. Fathers and mothers differed significantly on four of five assessment areas. Fathers had a greater reality orientation about the SIDS event, experienced less intense feelings, dealt with the event by action-oriented problem solving, and viewed support received more positively than mothers. Also, married and single parents differed in four of five areas assessed. Married parents had a greater reality orientation about the SIDS event, had a greater expression of feelings after the event, dealt with the event with more action-oriented problem solving, and viewed support received more positively than single parents.

In a study of the effects of high-risk pregnancy, Schroeder-Zwelling and Hock (1986) compared 20 diabetic women (14 with chronic diabetes and 6 with gestational diabetes) to 20 nondiabetic, low-risk women with regard to separation anxiety. Maternal separation anxiety was assessed at 6 weeks postpartum. There were no significant differences in separation anxiety between diabetic and nondiabetic mothers or between the subsets of women with chronic and gestational diabetes.

FUTURE RESEARCH DIRECTIONS

Although the study of grief has a long history in the health professions (e.g., Lindemann, 1944), studies of loss and separation are not a frequent area of investigation for parent-infant nurses. The studies reported here indicate that perinatal loss in its many possible forms—for example, miscarriage, stillbirth, infant death—is perceived as relevant to the field of parent-infant nursing. With the increasing movement of women into the labor force, studies of the impact of separation on parents and infants are needed. Further, studies of the impact of maternal illness and circumstances that may render parents emotionally or physically unavailable to infants are needed. Although we no longer think of maternal deprivation (insufficient contact with a primary caregiver) as occurring in the manner described by Ainsworth (1962/1969), family ill fate can still expose infants to the effects of social and emotional neglect. As better descriptive understanding of perinatal loss and separation accumulates, predictive studies and nursing intervention studies will be needed.

REFERENCES

Ainsworth, M. (1962/1969). The effects of maternal deprivation: A review of findings and controversy in the context of research strategy. In *Deprivation of maternal care* (pp. 287-357). New York: Schocken.

Childs, R. E. (1985). Maternal psychological conflicts associated with the birth of a retarded child. *Maternal-Child Nursing Journal, 14,* 175-182.

Harris, C. C. (1984). Dysfunctional grieving related to childbearing loss: A descriptive study. *Health care for Women International, 5,* 401-425.

Hutti, M. H. (1986). An exploratory study of the miscarriage experience. *Health Care for Women International, 7,* 371-389.

Lindemann, E. (1944). Symptomatology and management of acute grief. *American Journal of Psychiatry, 101,* 141-148.

Miles, M. S. (1985). Emotional symptoms and physical health in bereaved parents. *Nursing Research, 34,* 76-81.

Pitzer, M. S., & Hock, E. (1989). Employed mothers' concerns about separation from the first- and second-born child. *Research in Nursing & Health, 12,* 123-128.

Schroeder-Zwelling, E., & Hock, E. (1986). Maternal anxiety and sensitive mothering behavior in diabetic and nondiabetic women. *Research in Nursing and Health, 9,* 249-255.

Swanon-Kauffman, K. (1988). Caring needs of women who miscarried. In M.M. Leininger (Ed.), Care: *Discovery and uses in clinical and community nursing* (pp. 55-70). Detroit: Wayne State University Press.

Wall-Haas, C. L. (1985). Women's perceptions of first trimester spontaneous abortion. *Journal of Obstetric, Gynecologic, and Neonatal Nursing, 14,* 50-53.

Williams, R. A., & Nikolaisen, S. M. (1982). Sudden infant death syndrome: Parents' perceptions and responses to the loss of their infant. *Research in Nursing & Health, 5,* 55-61.

PART FIVE

Behavioral Organization and Behavioral Interaction

CHAPTER 16

The Paradigm of Behavioral Organization and Behavioral Interaction

OVERVIEW OF THE PARADIGM

According to older ideas, infants existed in a blooming, buzzing confusion or came into the world as blank slates. In contrast, contemporary views of human infants stress the capabilities with which infants are born and their individual differences (Stone, Smith, & Murphy, 1973; Osofsky, 1979, 1987). One of the infant's capabilities is to organize its behavior relative to internal needs and external stimuli. For example, infants can orient to visual and auditory stimuli—especially the human face and voice—and can engage in some self-comforting behaviors such as hand-to-mouth maneuvers and hand sucking. Researchers do not impute intent or volition to newborns, but infants have behavioral capabilities beyond simple reflexes. Delineating those capabilities has led to a rash of research on infants in the areas of child development, behavioral pediatrics, and nursing, among others.

Two broad perspectives have guided much of nursing research on infants: behavioral organization and behavioral interaction. Unlike other paradigms presented in this book, those two are less substantive theories and more broad frameworks for studying behavior. Behavioral organization focuses on the infant's endogenous capacity to integrate biological or behavioral parameters, and behavioral interaction focuses on mutual influence of infant and parent or caregiver behaviors. Further, neither behavioral organization nor behavioral interaction reflects developmentally static perspectives; instead, each embodies conceptual and methodological approaches to study the developing infant in the context of the immediate environment.

The phenomenon of infant state is a key concept pertinent to both infant behavioral organization and behavioral interaction. Infant state refers to the infant's level of consciousness; it was described by Wolff (1959). One widely used typology of infant state is incorporated in the Neonatal Behavioral Assessment Scale (Brazelton, 1984). It includes six levels of consciousness: state 1—deep sleep (also called quiet sleep); state 2—light sleep (also called active sleep); state 3—drowsy; state 4—alert (also called quiet alert); state 5—active (also called active alert); and state 6—crying. Patterns of state represent one aspect of behavioral organization and influence behavioral interaction as well. Maturational changes in sleep and state-related behaviors, however, decrease the usefulness of the concept of state as one moves beyond early infancy (Emde, Gaensbauer, & Harmon, 1976, pp. 29–30).

KEY CONCEPTS AND RELATIONSHIPS

BEHAVIORAL ORGANIZATION

The perspective of behavioral organization views not only biological systems but also behavior in the human infant as reflecting endogenous—albeit immature—patterning. Exogenous influences will, of course, shape infant behavior, but infants possess inherent patterning in some domains of behavior. Coordination of sucking and swallowing is one primal example of early behavioral organization. Two areas of infant behavioral organization that have been of particular interest to nurses have been sucking and sleep.

Healthy infants are capable, however, of responding at higher than the reflex level. As items on the Neonatal Behavioral Assessment scale have shown, newborn infants are capable of a wide range of responses that take on social meaning, particularly to parents. From birth, for example, the healthy newborn is capable of orienting to some social stimuli when in alert states.

Organization of behavior versus its contrary, disorganization, is indicative of healthy development. Lack of organized responses or disorganized behavioral patterns may be a transitional state between pattern and repatterning, or it may indicate immaturity, deficits in current capabilities, or pathology. One cannot easily separate neurological and behavioral phenomena in the newborn. As a consequence, the integration of neurological and behavioral dimensions forms the core of behavioral organization. For these and related reasons, Medoff-Cooper (1988b) has called for adoption of behavioral organization as the framework for nursing care of very immature infants. In a related vein, Barnard and Blackburn (1985) stated:

> *It is in the organizational processes of neonatal self-regulation that nursing research will find a productive knowledge base for nursing practice. It is the newborn's capacity for self-regulation, response to the environment, and caregiving that comprise the phenomena for nursing science and nursing practice (p. 72).*

One of the most articulate expressions of the behavioral organization perspective has been provided by Als (1979; Als, Lester, & Brazelton, 1979). In her model of expanding infant organization within the infant-caregiver system (Fig. 16–1), Als presents a hierarchical model of four subsystems. Organization of one subsystem permits the system to begin differentiating another subsystem. Progressive differentiation and modulation of four subsystems is proposed: (1) physiological (autonomic) control of respiration and related biological parameters; (2) motoric regulation; (3) state regulation; and (4) control of the alert state in social interaction. Medoff-Cooper (1988a) has restated those subsystems from a nursing perspective as stages in the development of behavioral organization:

> *(a) stabilization and integration of respiration, heart rate, temperature control, digestive function and elimination competence; (b) restabilization and integration of all physiologic functions with increasing motor activity; (c) gradual emergence of the full range of states from sleep to awake and crying, with the states becoming clearly identifiable; and (d) the attainment of the alert state, which becomes robust and well differentiated. (pp. 132–133)*

Because behavioral organization is an abstraction, it may be applied to a broad or narrow dimension of infant behavior. In this book the rubric of behavioral organization is applied broadly to include the notion of temperament. As a dimension of individual differences, temperament refers generally to different behavioral styles of individuals (Chess, 1967). Behavioral style in children has been divided into nine categories such as activity, rhythmicity, and intensity (Chess, 1967).

A more restricted application of behavioral organization is evident in the construct of state organization delineated by Colombo and Horowitz (1987, p. 428). Colombo and Horowitz have proposed three parameters of

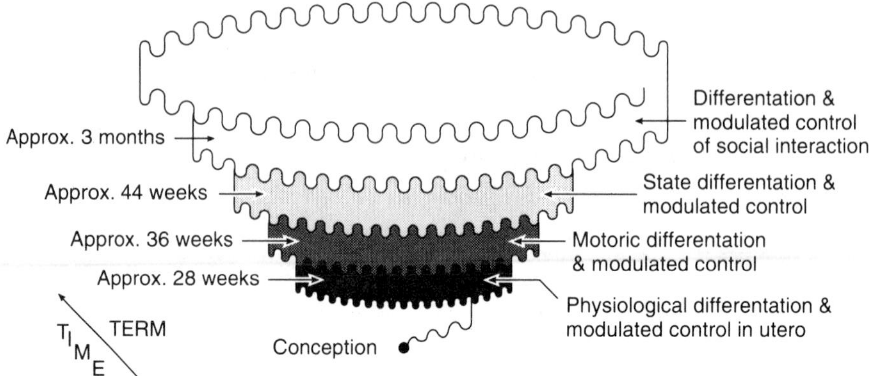

Figure 16–1.
Model for expanding infant organization within infant-caregiver system. (From Als, H. "Social interaction: Dynamic matrix for developing behavioral organization." In I.C. Uzgiris [Ed.], *Social Interaction and Communication During Infancy.* New Directions for Child Development, No. 4. San Francisco: Jossey-Bass, 1979, p. 26 [Fig. 1]. Used with permission of publisher.)

the construct of state organization in infants: (1) distinctiveness or quality of states, (2) state distribution both within and between several observations, and (3) state change patterns in response to stimulation from the environment.

In sum, behavioral organization represents a conceptual and research approach in which the integration of behavioral capacities of the newborn and maturing infant are described, interrelated, and facilitated within the context of the caregiving environment.

BEHAVIORAL INTERACTION

Behavioral interaction as a concept refers to patterns of mutual influence, usually at a microlevel rather than macrolevel, between partners in face-to-face or other forms of proximal contact with each other. For example, in Anderson's (1977) concept of mother and infant as mutual caregivers, neither parent nor infant is seen in isolation; each is seen in the context of the other. Interestingly, only in the last two decades has the infant been considered by researchers as having influence on the actions of parents (Bell, 1974). Behavioral interaction provides a rubric for studying mutual influence of parent and infant. Behavioral interaction also provides a viewpoint for describing early patterns of interaction as these relate to children's later development.

In parent-infant interaction, the behavior of both is orchestrated in varying ways and degrees for the purposes of such instrumental and communicative acts as feeding and social exchange. The part that each partner plays in interactions is, of course, influenced by the immaturity of the infant, attributes of the parent, and the bringing together of the two. Interactions may vary in the extent to which they are reciprocal (Brazelton, Koslowski, & Main, 1974) and in the degree to which they are adaptive (Sander, 1962, 1964, 1969). However, the concept of behavioral interaction is not identical with the idea of person-environment interaction. The latter typically refers to the mutual influences that occur at a macrolevel between persons, their environments, and their development (Chapter 19). Of course, patterns of behavioral interaction over time may comprise one of the major portions of a person's environment.

As with behavioral organization, behavioral interaction provides a broad rubric for the study of mutual influence. Investigators may inductively or deductively develop behavioral taxonomies for the observation of interactive behaviors. Thus, there is no one accepted conceptual scheme for the analysis of interaction. Instead, it is the purposes of an investigation that determine the most suitable conceptual scheme for studying behavioral interaction between parent and infant. For example, Keefe's (1988) theoretical model of irritable infant syndrome (Fig. 16–2) illustrates a mutual-influence model involving parent and infant. However, there are common threads in research undertaken from the viewpoint of behavioral interaction. Schaffer (1977) identified characteristics of studies of behavioral interaction in infancy as (1) focusing on dyads versus individuals, (2) viewing the infant as having some social capacity at birth, (3) focusing on temporal relationships, (4) using microanalytic methods, and (5) emphasizing process versus product.

INTERRELATIONSHIP OF BEHAVIORAL ORGANIZATION AND INTERACTION

Behavioral organization and behavioral interaction are highly interrelated. In a sense, behavioral organization sets the upper limit of the infant's ability to interact with parents or caregivers. In turn, the nature of the interaction between parents and infants—the patterning and sensitivity to the infants' needs—may enhance or disrupt behavioral organization in the infant.

METHODOLOGY

The core research method for conducting behavioral organization and behavioral interaction research is to observe behavior directly. Researchers whose methods focus on observing behavior face several issues outlined by Yarrow and Anderson (1979): selecting context or setting for observing behavior, choosing categories for coding behavior, and procedures for sampling and recording data. For example, differences in infant

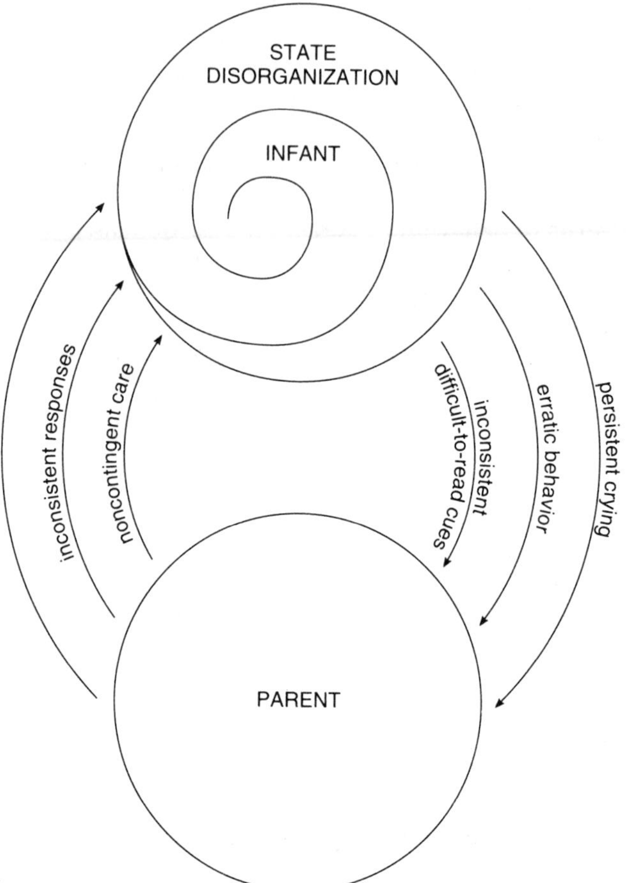

Figure 16–2.
Theoretical model of irritable infant syndrome. (From "Irritable infant syndrome: Theoretical perspectives and practice implications" by M.R. Keefe, 1988, *Advances in Nursing Science, 10,* p. 75. Copyright by Maureen Keefe. Reprinted with permission.)

state or setting, coding schemes for classifying behavior, and protocols for data recording may alter results of investigations. Thus, careful attention should be given to each of the dimensions. Sackett, Ruppenthal, and Gluck (1978) have written a readable guide for the investigator facing such methodological decisions.

Investigators who study parent-infant behavior by microanalysis of the flow of behavioral events face a number of choices about technology that may facilitate the research. Among the choices are advances in videotape technology and electronic data recording systems that interface with computers for data storage.

With regard to behavioral interaction, there are special issues that involve statistical methods. First, issues inherent in alternative ways of computing interrater reliability have been raised by several authors (Topf, 1986; Bakeman & Gottman, 1986, 1987). Second, behavioral interactive data also pose special data analytic issues. These have been examined in some detail by Lewis and Lee-Painter (1974), Bakeman and Gottman (1986), and Sackett (1987). One of the most fundamental issues is whether statistical methods selected indeed represent the interactive, that is, mutually influential, dimension of parent-infant behavior. For example, correlational procedures only examine relations between frequencies or other properties of behavior; they do not reflect the sequential interchange between interactants. Other statistical methods are needed to further unravel the dynamics of interaction. The issues are made even more complex if parent-infant interaction is considered within the context of the family and community. According to Parke and Tinsley (1987):

> *In order to understand the nature of parent-infant relationships within families, a multilevel and dynamic approach is required. Multiple levels of analysis are necessary in order to capture the individual, dyadic, and family unit aspects of operation within the family itself as well as to reflect the embeddedness of families within a variety of extra-familial social systems. The dynamic quality reflects the multiple developmental trajectories that warrant consideration in understanding the nature of families in infancy. (p. 581).*

In summary, to effectively study family interaction in infancy, Parke and Tinsley (1987) propose that multiple designs, data-gathering and data-analytic approaches are required.

For investigators who desire more global indicators of interaction, observation methods that result in summary ratings may be of value. Behavioral rating scales may be used for this purpose, and they have had some scientific utility (Parke & Tinsley, 1987). In addition, Waters and Deane (1985) have reported the use of Q-methodology for generating summary scores of infant behaviors following intensive observation. Parent report of characteristic infant patterns is another method that has been used to measure infant temperament. Parental reports have been shown, however, to be influenced by parental characteristics (Vaughn, Taraldson, Crichton, & Egeland, 1981). To minimize bias, Rothbart (Rothbart & Goldsmith, 1985) has avoided questionnaire items that request global, retrospective, or comparative judgments by parents about a child. Instead, parents are asked about relative frequency with which concrete infant behaviors have occurred in specifically delineated situations over the span of the most recent week or two.

REFERENCES

Als, H. (1979). Social interaction: Dynamic matrix for developing behavioral organization. In I. C. Uzgiris (Ed.), *New directions for child development: No. 4. Social interaction and communication during infancy* (pp. 21-39). San Francisco: Jossey-Bass.

Als, H., Lester, B. M., & Brazelton, T. B. (1979). Dynamics of the behavioral organization of the premature infant: A theoretical perspective. In T. M. Field, A. M. Sostek, S. Goldberg, & H. H. Shuman (Eds.), *Infants born at risk* (pp. 121–144). New York: SP Medical & Scientific Books.

Anderson, G. C. (1977). The mother and her newborn: Mutual caregivers. *Journal of Obstetric, Gynecologic and Neonatal Nursing, 6,* 50–57.

Bakeman, R., & Gottman, J. M. (1986). *Observing interaction: An introduction to sequential analysis.* Cambridge, England: Cambridge University Press.

Bakeman, R., & Gottman, J. M. (1987). Applying observational methods: A systematic view. In J. Osofsky (Ed.), *Handbook of infant development* (2nd ed., pp. 818–854). New York: Wiley.

Barnard, K. E., & Blackburn, S. (1985). Making a case for studying the ecologic niche of the newborn. In B. S. Raff, N. W. Paul, & F. Dickman (Eds.), *NAACOG invitational research conference.* White Plains, NY: March of Dimes Birth Defects Foundation. *Birth Defects, Original Articles Series, 21*(3), 71–88.

Bell, R. Q. (1974). Contributions of human infants to caregiving and social interaction. In M. Lewis & L. A. Rosenblum (Eds.), *The effect of the infant on its caregiver* (pp. 1–19). New York: Wiley.

Brazelton, T. B. (1984). *Neonatal behavioral assessment scale* (2nd ed.). Philadelphia: Lippincott.

Brazelton, T. B., Koslowski, B., & Main, M. (1974). The origins of reciprocity: The early mother-infant interaction. In M. Lewis & L. Rosenblum (Eds.), *The effect of the infant on its caregiver* (pp. 49–76). New York: Wiley.

Chess, S. (1967). Temperament in the normal infant. In J. Hellmuth (Ed.), *Exceptional infant: Vol. 1. The normal infant* (pp. 145–158). New York: Brunner/Mazel.

Colombo, J., & Horowitz, F. D. (1987). Behavioral state as a lead variable in neonatal research. *Merrill-Palmer Quarterly, 33,* 423-436.

Emde, R. N., Gaensbauer, T. J., & Harmon, R. J. (1976). Emotional expression in infancy: A biobehavioral study [Monograph 37]. *Psychological Issues, 10*(1), 3–198. New York: International Universities Press.

Keefe, M. R. (1988). Irritable infant syndrome: Theoretical perspectives and practice implications. *Advances in Nursing Science, 10*(3), 70–78.

Lewis, M., & Lee-Painter, S. (1974). An interactional approach to the mother-infant dyad. In M. Lewis & L. A. Rosenblum (Eds.), *The effect of the infant on its caregiver* (pp. 21–48). New York: Wiley.

Medoff-Cooper, B. (1988a). The effects of handling on preterm infants with bronchopulmonary dysplasia. *Image, 20,* 132–134.

Medoff-Cooper, B. (1988b, April). *NAACOG Research Task Force Proceedings,* Nurses' Association of the American College of Obstetrics and Gynecology, Washington, DC, p. 11.

Osofsky, J. D. (Ed.). (1979). *Handbook of infant development.* New York: Wiley.

Osofsky, J. D. (Ed.). (1987). *Handbook of infant development* (2nd ed.). New York: Wiley.

Parke, R. D., & Tinsley, B. J. (1987). Family interaction in infancy. In J. Osofsky (Ed.), *Handbook of infant development* (2nd ed., pp. 579-641). New York: Wiley.

Rothbart, M. K., & Goldsmith, H. H. (1985). Three approaches to the study of infant temperament. *Development Review, 5,* 237-260.

Sackett, G. P. (1987). Analysis of sequential social interaction data: Some issues, recent developments, and a causal inference model. In J. Osofsky (Ed.), *Handbook of infant development* (2nd ed., pp. 855–878). New York: Wiley.

Sackett, G. P., Ruppenthal, G. C., & Gluck, J. (1978). Introduction. In G. P. Sackett

(Ed.), *Observing behavior: Vol. 2. Data collection and analysis methods.* Baltimore: University Park Press.

Sander, L. W. (1962). Issues in early mother-child interaction. *Journal of the American Academy of Child Psychiatry, 1,* 141–166.

Sander, L. W. (1964). Adaptive relationships in early mother-child interaction. *Journal of the American Academy of Child Psychiatry, 3,* 231–264.

Sander, L. W. (1969). The longitudinal course of early mother-child interaction—cross-case comparison in a sample of mother-child pairs. In B. M. Foss (Ed.), *Determinants of infant behavior* (Vol. 4, pp. 189–225). London: Methuen.

Schaffer, H. R. (1977). Early interactive development. In H. R. Schaffer (Ed.), *Studies in mother-infant interaction* (pp. 3–16). London: Academic Press.

Stone, L. J., Smith, H. T., & Murphy, L. B. (Eds.). (1973). *The competent infant: Research and commentary.* New York: Basic Books.

Topf, M. (1986). Three estimates of interrater reliability for nominal data. *Nursing Research, 35,* 253–255.

Vaughn, B. E., Taraldson, B. J., Crichton, L., & Egeland, B. (1981). The assessment of infant temperament: A critique of the Carey infant temperament questionnaire. *Infant Behavior and Development, 4,* 1–17.

Waters, E., & Deane, K. E. (1985). Defining and assessing individual differences in attachment relationships: Q-methodology and the organization of behavior in infancy and early childhood. In I. Bretherton & E. Waters (Eds.), *Growing points of attachment theory and research* (pp. 41–65). *Monographs of the Society for Research in Child Development,* Serial No. 209, Vol. 50, Nos. 1–2.

Yarrow, L. J., & Anderson, B. J. (1979). Procedures for studying parent-infant interaction: A critique. In E. B. Thoman (Ed.), *Origins of the infant's social responsiveness* (pp. 209–223). Hillsdale, NJ: Erlbaum.

Wolff, P. H. (1959). Observations on newborn infants. *Psychosomatic Medicine, 21*(2), 110–118.

CHAPTER 17

Parent-Infant Nursing Research on Behavioral Organization in Infancy

DEFINITIONS AND DESCRIPTIONS OF BEHAVIORAL ORGANIZATION

DEFINING BEHAVIORAL ORGANIZATION

The study of behavioral organization in the human infant incorporates a strong neurobehavioral perspective (Medoff-Cooper, 1988). Thus, the study of behavioral organization includes such diverse phenomena as temperature and respiratory functions, reflex responses and sucking, sleep-wake states, and infant temperament. One of the most frequently defined aspects of infant behavioral organization is infant state (Keefe, Kotzer, Reuss, & Sander, 1989; Duxbury, Henly, Broz, Armstrong, & Wachdorf, 1984; Grauer, 1989). For example, according to Keefe et al. (1989), "The concept of infant state refers to patterns of behavior that comprise the sleep-wake cycle" (p. 344). Other terms related to behavioral organization that investigators have explicitly defined include nutritive sucking (Medoff-Cooper, Weininger, & Zukowsky, (1989) and nonnutritive sucking (Medoff-Cooper et al. 1989) and temperament (e.g., Houldin, 1987; Koniak-Griffin & Rummell, 1988).

THEORETICAL MODELS OF BEHAVIORAL ORGANIZATION

Many studies reviewed for this chapter focused on discrete phenomena such as sucking, temperature, and sleep. Thus, conceptualizing behavioral organization broadly was not an aim. Threaded implicitly throughout many studies, however, was concern with regulatory processes in the infant. That concern is explicitly described by Medoff-Cooper (1988) in her description of stages of behavioral organization in young infants. In her conceptualization, physiological and behavioral spheres are closely interrelated and hierarchically organized. (See Chapter 16 for a fuller description of Medoff-Cooper's description of stages of behavioral organization.)

One nursing conceptual model was used to study behavioral organization. Newport (1984) applied Levine's (1967) conservation principles in designing an intervention for infants immediately after birth.

MEASUREMENT

GENERAL STRATEGIES

Observational methods and biological assessment form the key methods for studying behavioral organization. As in all observation methods, it is vital that observers coding events receive adequate training and that their reliability be determined by using suitable methods (Bakeman & Gottman, 1986). With regard to biological and related forms of measurement, it is also vital that proper attention be given to calibration of equipment.

For one form of behavioral organization, temperament, use of parent-report questionnaires has emerged as a measurement method. One reason for use of parent-report is that temperament may be more accurately assessed if one has extensive contact with an infant. (*Note:* For a review of different temperament tools, see Rothbart & Goldsmith [1985].)

SPECIFIC TOOLS

Table 17–1 presents a variety of measures of behavioral organization. In addition to the widely used Neonatal Behavioral Assessment Scale (NBAS) (Brazelton, 1973, 1984), a number of tools have been employed to measure infant state, activity, sleep-wake patterns, and feeding. Among parent-report questionnaires, the most commonly used one in nursing has been the Revised Infant Temperament Questionnaire (Carey & McDevitt, 1978). In addition, a host of biological measures are pertinent to assessment of behavioral organization. Of note are several technologies pertinent to the early caregiving environment and young infant, such as a state-monitoring system (Keefe et al., 1989) and the suckometer (Anderson, McBride, Dahm, Ellis, & Vidyasagar 1982).

Table 17–1
MEASURES/TOOLS FOR THE CONCEPT OF BEHAVIORAL ORGANIZATION

Tool	Source Described in	Studies Using Tool
	OBSERVER-BASED TOOLS:	
Neonatal Behavioral Assessment Scale: Observational measure of behavioral organization	Brazelton (1973, 1984)	Anderson (1981) Barnard & Bee (1983) Zahr, Khoury, & Nugent (1988) Jones (1981) Kang & Barnard (1979) Becker et al. (1989) Jones & Parks (1983) Koniak-Griffin & Rummell (1988) Maloni, Stegman, Taylor, & Brownell (1986) Bee et al. (1982) Mitchell, Bee, Hammond, & Barnard (1985) Choi & Hamilton (1986) Jones & Lenz (1986) Riesch (1979) Riesch (1984) Koniak-Griffin & Ludington-Hoe (1987) Perry (1983) Poley-Strobel & Beckmann (1987) Snyder, Eyres, & Barnard (1979)
Medoff-Cooper Neurobehavioral Assessment Scale: Forty-one-item scale covering six areas of neurobehavioral assessment	Medoff-Cooper & Brooten (1987)	Medoff-Cooper & Brooten (1987)
Neurobehavioral assessment: Forty-nine items pertinent to very low birth weight infants	Medoff-Cooper (1988)	Medoff-Cooper (1988)

	—	Barnard & Bee (1983)
Neurological examination: Gestational age (total and neurological components)	L. Dubowitz, V. Dubowitz, & Goldberg (1970)	Barnard (1973)
Sleep-wake record: Seven-day record of sleep-wake states completed by parent	Barnard & Eyres (1979)	Barnard & Bee (1983) Bee et al. (1982) Mitchell et al. (1985) Barnard et al. (1987) Koniak-Griffin & Ludington-Hoe (1987)
Infant state: Classification of infant state of consciousness	Wolff (1966)	Bowen & Miller (1980) Salter (1978)
Infant state: Criteria for state in preterm infants	Dreyfus-Brisac (1974)	Duxbury et al. (1984)
Behavioral state: Six categories of infant state	Brazelton (1973)	Blank (1986)
Infant Behavioral State Scoring Criteria: System of five state categories	Keefe et al. (1989)	—
Infant state: Characteristics for assigning infant state	Lawson & Turkewitz (1985)	Grauer (1989)
Behavioral Inventory for Assessing States: Nine categories for coding infant state	Chappell (1970) as cited in Neeley (1979)	Neeley (1979)
Anderson Behavioral State Scale: Twelve categories for coding infant state	Gill et al. (1988)	Gill et al. (1988)
Activity Scale for Sleep Observation: Behavioral rating scale for activity and criteria for sleep-awake	Barnard (1973)	Barnard (1973)

Table 17–1
MEASURES/TOOLS FOR THE CONCEPT OF BEHAVIORAL ORGANIZATION *(Continued)*

Tool	Source Described in	Studies Using Tool
	OBSERVER-BASED TOOLS: (Continued)	
Activity Scale: Twelve categories for coding activity	Burroughs, Asonye, Anderson-Shanklin, & Vidyasagar (1978)	Burroughs et al. (1978)
Codes for infant behaviors: Coding system for infant behaviors in transitional nursery for use with keyboard entry on data	Gill et al. (1984)	Gill et al. (1984)
Time-lapse video recording coding system: Coding for infant activity and other events	Blackburn & Barnard (1985) Barnard & Bee (1983)	Blackburn & Barnard (1985) Barnard & Bee (1983)
Cry Scale: Scale for rating level of infant crying	Gill et al. (1984)	Gill et al. (1984)
Total crying duration	—	Lambesis, Vidyasagar, & Anderson (1979)
Feeding Evaluation Scale: Ten-item tool for rating first feeding of preterm infants	Measel & Anderson (1979)	Measel & Anderson (1979)
Feeding Scale: Six-category scale for rating first feeding of term infants	Anderson et al. (1982)	Anderson et al. (1982)
Clinical Feeding Scale: Six-category scale for rating first feeding of preterm infants	Weaver & Anderson (1988)	Weaver & Anderson (1988)
Complex Feeding Scale: Eight-category scale for rating first feeding of preterm infants	Weaver & Anderson (1988)	Weaver & Anderson (1988)
Feeding behaviors: Codes for aspects of sucking	Meier & Anderson (1987)	Meier & Anderson (1987)

Sucking scale: Three-category scale for rating preterm nonnutritive sucking	Anderson & Vidyasagar (1979)	Anderson & Vidyasagar (1979)
Hillard Interaction Tool: Codes for caretaker actions and infant behaviors in delivery room	Hillard (1973) as cited in Oliver & Oliver (1978)	Oliver & Oliver (1978)
PARENT REPORT TOOLS		
Survey of Infant Behavior: Twenty-two-item scale on infant behavioral style	Flagler (1988)	Flagler (1988)
Obligatory Infant Behavior Index: Fourteen-item index of infant behavior	Roberts (1983)	Roberts (1983)
Mother's Assessment of the Behavior of Her Baby: Maternal ratings of items adapted from the Neonatal Behavioral Assessment Scale	Field, Dempsey, Hallock, & Shuman (1978)	Becker (1987) Perry (1983) Poley-Strobel & Beckmann (1987)
Infant Behavior Questionnaire: Multidimensional scale of infant temperament	Rothbart (1978)	Ventura (1986, 1982) Tomlinson (1987)
Revised Infant Temperament Questionnaire: Ninety-five-item scale for nine areas of infant temperament	Carey & McDevitt (1978)	Medoff-Cooper & Schraeder (1982) Medoff-Cooper (1986) Houldin (1987) Koniak-Griffin & Rummell (1988) Koniak-Griffin & Ludington-Hoe (1988)
Toddler Temperament Questionnaire: Ninety-seven-item scale to assess nine dimensions of toddler temperament	Fullard, McDevitt, & Carey (1984)	Schraeder & Medoff-Cooper (1983) Medoff-Cooper (1986)

Table 17–1
MEASURES/TOOLS FOR THE CONCEPT OF BEHAVIORAL ORGANIZATION *(Continued)*

Tool	Source Described in	Studies Using Tool
	PARENT REPORT TOOLS (Continued)	
Perception of Baby Temperament: Card sort instrument of five dimensions of infant temperament	Pederson et al. as cited in Jones & Parks (1983)	Jones & Parks (1983)
	OTHER INSTRUMENTS AND MEASURES	
Computerized infant state monitoring system	Keefe et al. (1989)	—
Infant state monitoring system	Sander (1969)	Keefe (1987)
Accelerometer: Device for recording limb movements	Chapman (1978)	Chapman (1978) Chapman (1979)
Brain stem–evoked response	Barnard & Bee (1983)	Barnard & Bee (1983)
Sonagrams of infant cries: Spectrographic analysis	—	Krueger (1970)
Kron Nutritive Sucking Apparatus: Technology for measuring dimensions of nutritive sucking	Kron & Litt (1971)	Medoff-Cooper et al. (1989)
Suckometer and research nipple: Technology for measuring nonnutritive sucking	Anderson & Vidyasagar (1979) Anderson et al. (1982)	Ellison et al. (1979) Anderson et al. (1982) Weaver & Anderson (1988) Lambesis et al. (1979)
Transcutaneous oxygen tension	—	Updike et al. (1985) Burroughs et al. (1978) Meier & Anderson (1987) Meier (1988)
Apnea monitoring/apnea episodes	—	Updike et al. (1985) Jay (1982)

Infant temperature	—	Updike et al. (1985) Neal & Nauen (1968) Whitner & Thompson (1970) Gardner (1979) Lambesis et al. (1979) Britton (1980) Newport (1984) Oliver & Oliver (1978) Meier & Anderson (1987) Meier (1988) Jay (1982)
Respiratory rate	—	Lambesis et al. (1979) Newport (1984)
Pulse/heart rate or heart rate change	—	Updike et al. (1985) Neal (1979) Lambesis et al. (1979) Newport (1984) Segall (1972)
Incidence of bradycardia	—	Jay (1982)
Oxygen requirements	—	Jay (1982)
Physiologic Stability Index: Thirty-four variable index	Pollack, Yeh, Ruttiman, Holbrook, & Fields (1984)	Pohlman & Beardslee (1987)
Passage of urine and/or meconium	—	Lambesis et al. (1979) Boyer & Vidyasagar (1987)
Stooling frequency	—	Rausch (1981)
Visible jaundice	—	Boyer & Vidyasagar (1987)

Table 17–1
MEASURES/TOOLS FOR THE CONCEPT OF BEHAVIORAL ORGANIZATION *(Continued)*

Tool	Source Described in	Studies Using Tool
	OTHER INSTRUMENTS AND MEASURES (Continued)	
Serum indirect bilirubin	—	Boyer & Vidyasagar (1987)
Laboratory blood studies/values	—	Jay (1982)
Salivary cortisol	Bacon, Mucklow, Saunders, Rawlins, & Webb (1978) Walker, Riad-Fahmy, & Read (1978)	Grauer (1989)
Serum cortisol	Corning Medical & Scientific (1981) as cited in Blank (1986)	Blank (1986)
Serum glucose	Beckman Instruments (1981) as cited in Blank (1986)	Blank (1986)
Food preference	—	Brown & Grunfeld (1980)
Amount of food/fluid consumed	—	Brown & Grunfeld (1980) Lambesis et al. (1979) Collinge, Bradley, Perks, Rezny, & Topping (1982) Blank (1986) Rausch (1981)
Duration of feed	—	Meier & Anderson (1987)
Tolerance of oral nutrients	—	Jay (1982)
Weight gain or weight change	—	Barnard (1973) Boyer & Vidyasagar (1987) Koniak-Griffin & Ludington-Hoe (1987) Rausch (1981) Jay (1982)
Length of hospitalization	—	Jay (1982)

METHODOLOGICAL STUDIES

Three methodological studies pertinent to measurement of behavioral organization in infants have been reported. First, Medoff-Cooper and Brooten (1987) systematically examined the effect of time since last feeding on responses of preterm infants on neurobehavioral assessments. Nine healthy preterm infants, aged 30 to 38 weeks postconceptual age at the time of the study, received neurobehavioral assessments at each of three points in their 3-hour feeding cycle: 1 hour after, 10 minutes before, and 1 hour before a feeding. A 41-item assessment scale was used to examine infants in six areas: general assessment, cranial nerves, movement/tone, mental status, and both reflex and behavioral responses. Many items showed no variability across the three assessments. Fifteen items that showed some variability and that reflected the six areas of assessment were analyzed further. Only two items differed significantly across the three assessments: irritability and consolability. Infants were easier to console and less irritable 2 hours after feeding, that is, 1 hour before the next feeding. Thus, time within the feeding cycle did not have a major influence on outcomes of neurobehavioral assessments.

Second, Keefe et al. (1989) conducted a two-phase study to develop a computerized infant-state monitoring system. The system involved sensors built into a mattress to record movement, respiration, and heart rate. In the first phase, recordings of 22 infants' responses were made by using the computerized system 1 to 2 hours after feedings for periods of 60 to 120 minutes. From the monitoring system, investigators printed out continuous analog records of infants' responses, which were manually scored for infant state. Concurrent behavioral observations of infant state were made by observers at 1 minute intervals. Results showed mean agreement of 91.7 percent for state designations between observers and manual scorings of computer-generated recordings of infant responses.

In the second phase, Keefe et al. (1989) used data from the first phase to develop a computer program, Sleep State Evaluation Program, to translate computerized data into infant state categories. To test the software, 12 infants were again observed by raters, and concurrent recordings were made and classified by the computerized system. Overall agreement of the two methods was 79 percent. For individual infants, agreement varied from 63 to 93 percent.

Third, Becker, Lederman, and Lederman (1989) assessed the measurement properties and criterion-related validity of several measures of infant visual attention. Items or test components related to visual attention were extracted from the NBAS and the Bayley Scales for Infant Development (BSID) (Bayley, 1969). Analysis of the alternative measures was completed by using an existing dataset based on 56 term, normal infants. NBAS data were collected at 2 to 3 days after birth and were aggregated by using both a priori dimensions and cluster scores. Thus, two visual attention indices were extracted from the NBAS, Dimension I—Interactive Processes and Cluster 2—Orientation. The BSID was administered at 2 months and from it a seven-item visual attention index was constructed by using conceptually and empirically congruent items from the BSID Infant Behavior Record (IBR-ATT). The coefficient alpha for the Orientation Cluster was 0.78, and for the IBR-ATT it was 0.79. (*Note:* The NBAS Dimension scores do not lend themselves to this analysis.) For criterion-related validity, the three visual awareness measures were correlated with mental and psychomotor development as assessed by the BSID. The IBR-ATT was significantly related to both mental and psychomotor development, but the two NBAS visual attention indices were not.

SUMMARY OF RESEARCH

SCOPE OF RESEARCH ON BEHAVIORAL ORGANIZATION

Table 17-2 presents nursing studies pertinent to behavioral organization in infants. These studies have provided descriptions of a wide variety of behavioral and biological variables in infants, differences associated with subpopulations, and variables correlated with aspects of infant behavioral organization. (*Note:* See Chapter 3 for studies of infants from the perspective of stress.)

In addition, intervention studies have focused on early caregiving practices that may alter or enhance infant behavioral organization. Thus, studies have examined alternative approaches to such matters as feeding preterm infants, maintaining temperature in the newly born infant, and providing stimulation to infants. (For a summary of effects of stimulation programs on premature infants, see the Appendix).

DESCRIPTIVE RESEARCH

Descriptions of Crying and Sleep

Krueger (1970) examined the spectrographic properties of various cries of a 2-month-old infant girl. The mother's labeling of cries was the primary basis for differentiating six cry types: hungry, wet, playful, tired, plosive, and angry. Cries were tape-recorded, and then sonagrams were made of each type of cry. Each cry type had a visually distinct sonagram pattern and distinct relations of formants.

In a second study of infant crying, Gill, White, and Anderson (1984) described newborn infant behaviors that preceded crying after admission to the transitional nursery. Behaviors of 15 normal newborns were continuously recorded from the first oral cue until infants attained a total of 2

Table 17–2
PARENT-INFANT NURSING RESEARCH ON BEHAVIORAL ORGANIZATION

DESCRIPTIVE
Descriptions of Behavioral Organization
Anderson & Vidyasagar (1979), sucking in ill preterm infants
Anderson et al. (1982), sucking in normal infants
Duxbury et al. (1984), sleep in ill infants
Gill et al. (1984), cry of normal newborns
Krueger (1970), cry of 2-mo-old infant
Neal (1979), heart rate in preterm infants
Neal & Nauen (1968), temperature in preterm infants
Differences and Changes in Behavioral Organization
Becker (1987), adolescent vs. adult mothers
Brown (1979), high- vs. low-contact parents of preterm infants
Choi & Hamilton (1986), American Korean vs. American Caucasian infants
Ellison et al. (1979), LBW vs. normal infants
Kang & Barnard (1979), term vs. preterm infants
Medoff-Cooper (1986), preterm infants at 6 and 12 months
Medoff-Cooper (1988), infants with vs. without BPD
Medoff-Cooper et al. (1989), preterm vs. term infants
Medoff-Cooper & Schraeder (1982), VLBW infants vs. normative sample
Schraeder & Medoff-Cooper (1983), VLBW toddlers vs. normative sample
Updike et al. (1985), preterm infants over 24 hours
RELATIONS AMONG VARIABLES/PREDICTIVE MODELS
Relations to Behavioral Organization
Blackburn & Barnard (1985)
Maloni et al. (1986)
Relations to Sleep, Sucking
Duxbury et al. (1984)
Weaver & Anderson (1988)
Relations to Temperament
Houldin (1987)
Jones & Parks (1983)
Koniak-Griffin & Rummell (1988)
INTERVENTION RESEARCH
Barnard (1973), auditory and kinesthetic stimulation
Barnard & Bee (1983), three patterns of stimulation
Boyer & Vidyasagar (1987), early feeding after birth
Britton (1980), postbirth skin-to-skin contact
Brown & Grunfeld (1980), nonsweetened baby food
Burroughs et al. (1978), nonnutritive sucking
Chapman (1978, 1979), tape of mother's voice or lullaby

Table 17–2
PARENT-INFANT NURSING RESEARCH ON BEHAVIORAL ORGANIZATION *(Continued)*

INTERVENTION RESEARCH (Continued)
Collinge et al. (1982), demand feeding of preterm infants
Gardner (1979), maternal holding after birth
Gill et al. (1988), nonnutritive sucking
Grauer (1989), intermittent lighting
Jay (1982), passive tactile contact
Keefe (1987, 1988), nighttime rooming-in
Koniak-Griffin & Ludington-Hoe (1987, 1988), unimodal and multimodal stimulation
Lambesis et al. (1979), postbirth surrogate mothering
Measel & Anderson (1979), nonnutritive sucking
Meier (1988), breast-feeding preterm infants
Meier & Anderson (1987), breast-feeding preterm infants
Neeley (1979), nonnutritive sucking
Newport (1984), skin-to-skin contact
Oliver & Oliver (1978), modified Leboyer birth
Rausch (1981), rubbing and passive exercise
Salter (1978), Leboyer birth
Schwartz, Moody, Yarandi, & Anderson (1987), meta-analysis of nonnutritive sucking
Segall (1972), tape recording of mother's voice
Whitner & Thompson (1970), warm bath at birth

minutes of crying. In addition, infant cries were rated for level of crying. The most frequent first oral cue emitted was hand-to-mouth behavior. The average longest cry was 24.7 seconds. The average interval between cries was 2.2 minutes. The average time from first oral cue to 2 minutes of total crying was 30.9 minutes. The most frequent momentary behavior recorded was tonguing. The most frequent continuous behavior recorded was intrinsic mouthing. Infants engaged in some level of crying 13 percent of the time. There were no significant associations between perinatal variables and duration from first oral cue to cry.

Duxbury, Henley, Broz, Armstrong, & Wachdorf (1984) described sleep in 48 critically ill infants observed during 74 3-hour occasions. Infants ranged from 25 to 44 weeks' gestation at birth. Infants' sleep episodes averaged 38 minutes with an average of 3.55 awakenings over 3 hours. Two of these awakenings were in response to caregiving. The average span between caregiving episodes was 30 minutes. There was a trend for more acutely ill infants to sleep more, but for shorter intervals.

Descriptions of Temperature and Heart Rate

Neal and Nauen (1968) investigated the capability of premature infants to maintain adequate axillary temperature (36.5 to 37°) after transfer from incubator to crib. Temperatures of 16 infants weighing 1450 to 1750 g were measured prior to transfer and every 3 hours thereafter until adequate axillary temperature was attained. Temperature monitoring also included measurement of infants' temperatures at nine body sites. Seven of nine infants with gestational ages of 31 weeks or less had achieved adequate axillary temperatures within 24 hours after transfer; in comparison, only two of seven infants with gestational ages of 32 weeks or more did so. After transfer to cribs, sites of highest body temperatures were rectal, axillary, and back near scapular region. On average, infants gained 25.9 g per day after transfer to cribs.

Neal (1979) reported heart rate responses to auditory stimuli in preterm infants from 31 to 36 weeks gestation. At 31 weeks, deceleration was shown in response to auditory stimulation. At 32 to 36 weeks, responses to stimulation showed acceleration with subsequent deceleration.

Descriptions of Sucking

Anderson and Vidyasagar (1979) sought to document development of sucking responses in critically ill preterm infants. Ten preterm infants (mean gestation of 31 weeks, mean birth weight of 1271 g) were observed from a mean age of 6.3 hours. Infants were provided finger sucking (investigator's finger) opportunities twice a day and quality of sucking was scored. All infants made sucking responses. On a sucking scale with scores ranging from 0 to 12, the mean sucking score for infants on the day of birth was 6.0. Sucking scores were unrelated to gestational age or weight, but they did correlate with pH and pCO_2. Sucking scores increased progressively over a 7-day period except for a drop on the third day.

In a related study, Anderson et al. (1982) described the development of sucking responses in 30 normal, term infants. Two dimensions of sucking, suction and expression, were measured at birth and repeatedly thereafter with a suckometer until the infants were 4 hours old. First feedings, given at 4 hours, were rated by observers for feeding quality. Mean suction was 5 mm Hg shortly after birth; it increased progressively to 103 mm Hg at 90 minutes; and it then declined regressively to 65 mm Hg at 4 hours. Mean expression, in contrast, was 12 mm Hg shortly after birth; it increased to 29 mm Hg at 15 minutes; and it remained at that level during the majority of the subsequent measurements. On over half of the occasions, suction and expression were positively related. Expression, but not suction, was correlated with feeding quality.

Differences and Changes in Behavioral Organization

Kang and Barnard (1979) reported differences between term and preterm infants in behavioral organization. Infants were assessed on the NBAS as well as supplementary items tailored to the response repertoire of preterm infants. In the first comparison, 193 infants from an extant database (182 term and 11 preterm infants) were compared with 30 preterms with a mean age of 34 weeks gestation (postconceptual age). Comparing the 182 term with the 30 preterm infants, 36.3 percent of term and 73.3 percent of preterm infants were classified as deficit in interactive processes and 13.7 percent of term and 26.7 percent of preterm infants were classified as deficit in state control. At 1 month after discharge (equivalent to 40 weeks' gestation), preterm infants had reduced the percent of deficit classifications in interactive processes and state control to 33.3 and 3.3 percent, respectively.

Kang and Barnard (1979) also reported a second set of comparisons involving 42 term infants and 123 preterm infants at comparable postconceptual age in which differences on NBAS supplementary items (focused on preterms' behavioral repertoire) were tested. Overall, term and preterm infants differed significantly in interactive processes and state control with differences favoring term infants. Of 15 comparisons on specific items, 10 showed no differences, 3 favored term infants, and 2 favored preterm infants. Specifically, preterms had briefer and less spontaneous alert states, had less self-quieting, and less often responded to the bell stimulus than term infants. Term infants less often responded to the light stimulus and also had more variable response to it compared to preterm infants.

Medoff-Cooper (1988) compared physiologic distress of 9 very low birth weight (VLBW) infants with bronchopulmonary dysplasia (BPD) to 23 VLBW infants without BPD. Neurobehavioral assessments that included common and subtle signs of distress were done weekly from birth to hospital discharge. Infants with BPD displayed significantly greater tachycardia, tachypnea, and bradycardia during assessments than the comparison group without BPD. Further, infants with BPD continued to have distress signs, such as tachycardia, at significantly later postconceptual ages than the comparison group. Infants with BPD also showed subtle distress cues, such as facial grimacing and avoidance gazing, more often than the comparison group.

To assess the influence of culture, Choi and Hamilton (1986) compared 21 American Caucasian mother-infant pairs with 18 American Korean mothers and their infants. Based on data gathered on the 2nd to 3rd postpartum days, the following differences in infant behavioral organization were identified: American Korean infants habituated more quickly; American Causasian infants had better state regulation. No group differences were found in five other areas.

Circadian Rhythms

Updike, Accurso, and Jones (1985) studied circadian rhythms in six preterm infants' physiological parameters. Variables of interest were transcutaneous oxygen, pulse rate, respiratory rate, respiratory pauses, and skin temperature. Infants were monitored for 24 hours at a postnatal age of 10 to 20 days. Five of six infants evidenced a circadian pattern for skin temperature. From 2 to 3 infants showed evidence of circadian rhythms on the other four variables.

Differences and Changes in Sucking

In a comparison of sucking in term and preterm infants, Medoff-Cooper, Weininger, and Zukowsky (1989) measured nutritive sucking in 42 term infants at 1 to 2 days after birth. Nutritive sucking of 44 preterm infants was assessed at mean postconceptual age of 35 weeks. By use of a technological apparatus, six dimensions of sucking were measured while investigators gave infants their formula feeding. Term infants demonstrated greater sucking vigor than preterm infants in four of six dimensions of nutritive sucking: maximum pressure, suck width, suck/burst, and volume consumed. No suck width and interburst width differences were found.

Ellison, Vidyasagar, and Anderson (1979) studied two properties of nonnutritive sucking, suction pressure and expression pressure, in 13 low-birth-weight (LBW) and 17 normal-birth-weight (NBW) infants during the first hour of life. Using a suckometer and special nipple, sucking was measured at 5, 15, 30, 45, and 60 minutes after birth. The range of suction pressure of NBW and LBW infants was 0 to 230 and 0 to 132 mm Hg, respectively. NBW infants showed progressive increases in suction pressure over the first hour after birth; LBW infants did not show comparable progressive increases over the first hour. The range of expression pressure of NBW and LBW infants was 0 to 36 and 0 to 43 mm Hg, respectively. Overall, expression pressures increased over trials for NBW infants and decreased for LBW infants. Although the overall association of suction and expression pressures was direct and positive for NBW infants, the association was an inverse one for LBW infants.

Differences and Changes in Temperament

In a study of 26 VLBW infants, Medoff-Cooper and Schraeder (1982) completed infant assessments at 7.9 months corrected age. With regard to the distribution of infant temperament classifications, VLBW infants did not differ significantly from the standardization sample. However, there were significant differences between the two groups in the proportion of VLBW infants classified as having easy and difficult temperaments. For example, 38 percent of VLBW infants were classified as difficult compared to 10 percent in the standardization sample. Further, two characteristics of infants, distractability and mood, were negatively correlated with characteristics of the home environment.

In a follow-up study of 20 of the original 26 VLBW infants, Schraeder and Medoff-Cooper (1983) reassessed infants at 19 months (mean age corrected for prematurity). The overall distribution of toddler temperament classifications of the VLBW toddlers did not differ significantly from the standardization sample. However, VLBW toddlers did differ from the standardization sample on two of nine subscales of the temperament inventory: rhythmicity and persistence. VLBW toddlers were arrhythmic and low in persistence. The proportion of VLBW children with difficult temperaments decreased from 38 percent to 10 percent from the first to the second year. One temperament dimension, activity, was significantly negatively related to characteristics of the home environment.

In another longitudinal study of VLBW infants, Medoff-Cooper (1986) assessed 41 infants at 6 and 12 months of age corrected for prematurity. When VLBW infants' scores on nine dimensions of temperament were compared to those of the normative sample, differences in adaptability and intensity were found at 6 months and in persistence at 12 months. In comparing the distribution of temperament classifications of VLBW infants to the normative sample, significant differences were found. In particular, there were more difficult and fewer easy infants at 6 months within the VLBW sample. At 12 months there was no significant difference between the two samples. No consistent pattern of relations between nine temperament subscales and characteristics of the home environment was found.

Differences in Maternal Perceptions of Behavior, Parental Concerns

In a comparison of 23 adolescent and 22 adult mothers, Becker (1987) assessed mothers' perceptions of their newborn infants' behavior. Adolescent mothers' rated their babies as less capable of regulating state than adult mothers. No differences were found in four other areas: orientation, motoric processes, range of state, and autonomic stability. Further, no consistent pattern of relations between measures of stress and perception of infant behaviors was found.

Brown (1979) explored parental concerns about behavioral organization of 35 preterm infants. Parents were divided into high- and low-contact groups based on frequency of contact with health professionals during a 4-month period. Contacts included visits (home, hospital, and clinic) and telephone calls. Parental concerns were recorded by health professionals during contacts. High- and low-contact groups did not differ on obstetric or postnatal complications, but they did differ on parity. Further, the two groups differed significantly with regard to three areas of behavioral organization: concerns about feeding, crying, and sleep-wake cycles. The high-contact group had a greater number of concerns.

RELATIONAL/PREDICTIVE RESEARCH

Relations to Behavioral Organization

Blackburn and Barnard (1985) examined the relation between caregiving events and activity in preterm infants in incubators. Activity data from 102 infants enrolled in a larger study of infant stimulation were used in this study. By use of time-lapse videotaping, infant behaviors and caregiving were coded at the equivalent of every minute of real time for a 24-hour period at six time points during the study. Mean activity levels for 24 hours were compared with mean activity levels 5 minutes before and after four caregiving activities (diapering/feeding, miscellaneous/technical, out of incubator, and social stroking). Except for social stroking, mean infant activity before caregiving events was higher than the 24-hour average. However, only after miscellaneous/technical events was infant activity higher than the 24-hour average. When caregiving events and infant activity were examined longitudinally across a 24-hour period, there was evidence of phase synchronization with infant activity rising and falling in concert with rises and falls in occurrence of caregiving events.

In an investigation of the correspondence between nurses' clinical judgments about infants and NBAS scores, Maloni, Stegman, Taylor, and Brownell (1986) studied two groups of infants, one judged by nurses as suspect (n = 55) and a matched group of nonsuspect (normal) infants (n = 55). Both groups were 2 to 5 days old, medically normal, full-term infants. Nurses identified infants about whom they felt concerned (i.e., suspect), described what they saw as different about the infants, and selected which of the four dimensions of the NBAS they thought were problematic. Infants in both groups were assessed on the NBAS by an examiner unaware of infants' classifications. Suspect infants scored significantly lower on the NBAS than normal infants. Suspect infants were most often lower on interactive processes and state organization. Nurses named such characteristics as physical appearance and infant cry as among the cues that were the basis for their concern. However, when NBAS dimensions identified as problematic by nurses were compared with actual NBAS outcomes, nurses underidentified suspect infants on the interactive dimension and overidentified them on the motor and state organization dimensions.

Relations to Infant Sleep and Sucking

Duxbury et al. (1984) examined the relations between caregiving disruptions and sleep characteristics of 48 critically ill infants observed over 74 3-hour intervals. Number of caregiving disruptions, total duration of disruptions, and average interval between disruptions were significantly related to three of four infant sleep characteristics such as average duration of sleep periods. One sleep variable, total sleep time, was unrelated to any caregiving variables.

Weaver and Anderson (1988) examined the relation of nonnutritive sucking pressures to feeding quality of 30 preterm infants at first bottle feeding. Using a suckometer, sucking pressures were measured before the first feeding. Then feedings were administered and scored for quality of feeding on two alternative scales. Although scores on both feeding scales were highly related, there were no significant correlations between feeding scores and nonnutritive sucking pressures (peak or mean suction or peak or mean expression).

Relations to Temperament

In a study examining convergence among measures related to infant temperament, Jones and Parks (1983) followed 19 term, healthy infants over the first year. The observers tested infants on the NBAS at 2 to 3 days after birth, and fathers also rated their perceptions of the infants at that time. When the infants were 1 year old, mothers and fathers separately rated infants' temperaments. Results showed that more than one item (of 26) on the NBAS was correlated with fathers' 1-year rating of activity (one of five temperament dimensions) and with mothers' 1-year ratings of adaptability and approachability. However, of five temperament dimensions, mothers' and fathers' ratings were significantly correlated in only one, rhythmicity. In addition, of 30 correlations between fathers' neonatal perceptions and 1-year temperament ratings, only three significant correlations were found.

To investigate relations of infant temperament and the environment, Houldin (1987) studied mothers of 20 healthy, term, 5-month-old infants. Mothers provided ratings and perceptions of their children's temperament, and an observer rated characteristics of the home environment. The distribution of temperament classifications for the study sample differed significantly from that of the sample with which the temperament inventory was standardized. Findings varied with the method of configuring temperament data and partitioning of the sample. Overall, the total characteristics of the home environment correlated negatively with three of nine dimensions of temperament: activity, rhythmicity, and mood; that is, higher temperament scores were related to less responsive home environments.

To clarify the relations of temperament to neonatal behavior and developmental status, Koniak-Griffin and Rummell (1988) studied 81 normal, term infants from birth. Data gathered at one month included the NBAS and maternal perceptions of the infants. Seventy-nine mother-infant pairs were available for follow-up at 4 months and 75 at 8 months. Both temperament and developmental status were assessed at 4 and 8 months. The median correlation between temperament dimensions at 4 and 8 months was

.31. Temperament classifications were not associated differentially with mothers' neonatal perceptions of infants. Of 90 correlations between NBAS items and 4- and 8-month temperament dimension scores, only two significant correlations were found. Of 54 correlations between temperament dimension scores and developmental status indices, only one significant correlation was found.

INTERVENTION RESEARCH

Because of their number, intervention studies related to infant behavioral organization are presented in Table 17–3 for easier display. Because research subjects were not randomly assigned to conditions in many studies and because a number of studies included small sample sizes, it is difficult to draw definitive conclusions from the studies. Of particular note are studies of nonnutritive sucking, which generally show some favorable effects. Also, the three studies of early mother-infant contact are consistent in regard to no adverse effects on infant temperature. Promising areas of research include interventions related to feeding of preterm infants (e.g., Meier, 1988). The studies of infant stimulation suggest that benefits attained by preterm infants may not occur in full-term infants.

FUTURE RESEARCH DIRECTIONS

It is troubling that some studies reviewed in this chapter contained samples of 20 or fewer subjects. If rare, special populations (such as VLBW infants) are being studied, a sample of that size may be all that can reasonably be expected. However, when normal, term infants are involved, it is unwise to accept such small samples—especially for phenomena such as temperament—as a basis for scientific generalizations in future nursing research. (See Clarke-Stewart, VanderStoep, and Killian [1979] for empirical data pertinent to this issue.)

Another shortcoming of several studies reviewed in this chapter was failure to cite published nursing research on the same topic. In a small number of studies, although virtually identical instrumentation was used, replications failed to cite the important preceding studies. This suggests that more thorough searches of scientific literature sources prior to submitting manuscripts for publication are in order. Of note, this omission was most likely to occur when authors were employed outside key research universities or when authors did not hold doctoral degrees. It may seem pedantic to suggest that manuscript reviewers should carefully check submissions for basic documentation of extant research, but the documentation is critical to informed and cumulative building of parent-infant nursing science. Several of the studies reviewed, however, were exemplary in their thoroughness and precision.

Table 17–3
INTERVENTIONS RELATED TO BEHAVIORAL ORGANIZATION

Citation: Group/Population	Independent Variable(s)	Dependent Variable(s) and Study Outcomes*
Whitner & Thompson (1970): One hundred sixteen normal newborn infants: 54 in experimental (bath) and 62 in control (no bath) groups	Randomization to bath in 105° F water after birth	Immediately after bath, axillary temperature of experimental group about 1° F less than controls (−) From 3 to 6 h after bath, axillary temperature of experimental group exceeded controls by about 0.5° F (+)
Segall (1972): Sixty preterm infants: 30 in experimental and 30 in control groups	Randomization to conditions; experimental group had a tape recording of mother's voice played for a total of 30 min/d until 36 wk gestational age	At 36 wk gestation: in quiescent state, overall greater cardiac acceleration in response to white noise (+); in aroused state, greater cardiac deceleration to sound of mother's voice (+); in aroused state, greater cardiac deceleration to sound of strange woman's voice (+)
Barnard (1973): Fifteen normal preterm infants: seven in experimental and eight in control groups	Method of assignment to conditions not described; auditory (heart beat sound) and kinesthetic (rocker bed) stimulation every hour for 15 min during 33 to 34 wk postconceptual age	After birth weight regained, changes in weight from 32 to 35 wk postconceptual age (0) Changes in gestational age (total score, neurological score) from 32 to 35 wk postconceptual age (0) For observations of sleep-awake states at 33, 34, and 35 wk postconceptual age: two of three differences were significant for quiet sleep (+); one of three differences was significant for active alert & transitional sleep (+, direction assumed to be positive); zero of three differences was significant for active sleep, drowsy, and quiet alert (0).

Burroughs et al. (1978): Diverse group of 11 preterm infants with regard to respiratory status; all received intervention	From one to three 8-min sessions of nonnutritive sucking given to infants while in high-risk nursery	For infants breathing room air, no significant difference in transcutaneous oxygen tension during 8 min of intervention and 8 min thereafter compared to baseline (0) For infants with assisted ventilation, increased transcutaneous oxygen tension during 8 min of intervention and 8 min thereafter compared to baseline (+)
Oliver & Oliver (1978): Thirty-seven newborns from a clinic population: 20 in experimental and 17 in control groups	Method of assignment to conditions not described; experimental group delivered by means of modified Leboyer method	Rectal temperature at admission to nursery (0) Hematocrit on day after birth (0) Of 18 newborn behaviors, significant differences occurred on 5 (+)
Salter (1978): Twelve normal, full-term newborn infants: six in experimental and six in control groups	Method of assignment to conditions not stated; experimental group delivered by means of Leboyer method	Amount of time in alert inactive state during 15-min observations in delivery room, in nursery 1 h after birth, and 24 to 30 h after birth (+) (*Note:* No test statistics reported)
Chapman (1978, 1979): One hundred fifty-three preterm infants; 50 in experimental group (mother's voice), 51 in experimental group (lullaby), and 52 in control group	Randomization to conditions: (1) Had tape of mother's voice played for 5 min six times per day from 5th day of life until reached at least 1843 g, (2) had tape of Brahms' lullaby played for 5 min six times per day from 5th day of life until reached at least 1843 g, (3) no tapes for control group	Age at which criterion weight achieved favored music group over control group (+) During 48 h after discontinuation of treatment: infant activity (0); upper limb activity predominant over lower limb (0); right or left limb predominance (0)

Table 17–3
INTERVENTIONS RELATED TO BEHAVIORAL ORGANIZATION *(Continued)*

Citation: Group/Population	Independent Variable(s)	Dependent Variable(s) and Study Outcomes*
Gardner (1979): Nineteen normal newborns; 10 in experimental and 9 in control groups	Method of assignment to conditions not described; after delivery, experimental nude infants held on mothers' bare chest for 15 min with both covered with blanket	Rectal temperature at 2 min into holding (0) Rectal temperature at end of 15 min of holding (0)
Lambesis et al. (1979): Sixteen term, healthy infants: eight in experimental and eight in control groups	Randomization to conditions; experimental group given surrogate mothering (e.g., rocking, interacting, and giving nonnutritive sucking) during first hours of life	During first 4 h: mean temperature (0); mean respiratory rate (0); mean heart rate differed on only one of nine occasions (0); frequency of heart murmurs (+); absence of acrocyanosis (0); passage of urine and meconium (0); total duration of crying (+) At end of 4 h: mean suction pressure of infant suck (+); mean expression pressure of infant suck (0); amount of water consumed (+)
Measel & Anderson (1979): Fifty-nine preterm infants weighing greater than 1000 g a birth; 29 in experimental and 30 in control groups	Assigned to conditions by alternate sequential series and other criteria; nonnutritive sucking given during feeding and 5 min after, begun when infant in room air and fed 10 mL of full-strength formula by tube and ended when totally bottle-fed	Experimental group began bottle feedings 3.4 d earlier than controls (+) Daily weight gain (0) Length of hospitalization (+) Number of tube feedings (+) Evaluation of initial bottle feeding (0)

Neeley (1979): Twenty full-term, healthy infants: 10 in experimental and 10 in control groups	Assigned alternatively to conditions with consideration of gender balance also; experimental group received nonnutritive sucking to satiation at 1, 4, and 8 h after birth	Sleep between 1 and 8 h was less for experimental group (+) Wakefulness between 1 and 8 h was greater for experimental group (+) Irritability between 1 and 8 h was less for experimental group (+) Of four measures of first feeding at 12 h, one was significant (+)
Britton (1980): Thirty-four healthy mother-infant pairs: 19 in control and 15 in experimental groups	Nonrandomization to conditions; skin-to-skin contact between mother and baby for 1 h after birth	Infants' axillary temperature 1 h after admission (0) Infants' rectal temperature 1 h after admission (0)
Brown & Grunfeld (1980): Forty healthy infants: 20 in experimental and 20 in control groups	Nonrandomization to use of nonsweetened (experimental group) or sweetened (control group) baby food for 3 mo after solid foods were initiated	Preference for sweetened over nonsweetened baby food during 4th month after initiating solid baby food (0) Grams of baby food consumed during 4th month after initiating solids was greater for experimental group (+)
Rausch (1981): Forty preterm infants: 20 in experimental and 20 in control groups	Matched groups with use of historical controls; experimental group received 15 min of gentle rubbing and passive exercise of extremities once daily from postnatal days 1 to 10	Weight gain on 10th day of treatment (0) Mean feeding intake during treatment (+) Mean frequency of stooling during treatment (+)

Table 17–3
INTERVENTIONS RELATED TO BEHAVIORAL ORGANIZATION *(Continued)*

Citation: Group/Population	Independent Variable(s)	Dependent Variable(s) and Study Outcomes*
Collinge et al. (1982): Thirty-six preterm infants all over 1800 g at start of study: 18 in experimental and 18 in control groups	Randomization to conditions; experimental group given bottle feedings on demand; control group given bottle feedings on schedule	From start of study until ready for discharge: amount of formula consumed orally per day (0); number of feedings per day (less for experimental) (+); number of gavage feedings (more for control group) (+); proportion of total nutrition given by bottle (+); total number of gavages (+); length of time until feeding adequate for discharge (+)
Jay (1982): Twenty-six mechanically ventilated infants born from 28 to 32 wk gestation: 13 in experimental and 13 in control groups	Experimental group compared to matched historical controls; the experimental group received 12 min of tactile contact (nonstroking) four times per day for 10 d	Based on measurement during the 10 d of treatment: weight gain/loss (0); temperature stability (0); oxygen requirements (0); hematocrit (+); tolerance of oral feedings (0)
Barnard & Bee (1983): Eighty-eight preterm infants: 26 in fixed-interval condition, 23 in self-activating condition, 10 in quasi-self-activating condition, and 28 in control condition (*Note:* Sum of numbers reported by authors equal 87).	Assigned to conditions based on modified random assignment with blocking for three variables (*Note:* Quasi-self-activating formed inadvertently via a technical error) The three intervention conditions were given from mean age of 7 d until mean age of 21 d: (1) fixed interval had 15 min of stimulation (rocking and heartbeat sound) each hour; (2) self-activitating had stimulation for 15 min after each 90 s period of inactivity; (3) quasi-self-activating had stimulation for 15 min after being inactive 90 s but not more than once per hour	Overall, of 109 comparisons only 15 were significant (weak + to 0) Fixed-interval and self-activating had lower activity levels in four of six comparisons (+) About one-third of scores on NBAS were significant (+) Two differences in length of activity cycles were significant (?)

Newport (1984): Seventy-six healthy infants: 37 in experimental and 39 in control groups	Randomization to conditions; experimental group received 15 min of skin-to-skin contact with mother after birth	Postbirth measures taken on five occasions: axillary temperature (0); pulse rate (0); respiratory rate (0); weight loss (0); presence of diarrhea or ketouria (0)
Boyer & Vidyasagar (1987): Thirty normal, full-term newborn infants: 10 in each of three groups	Sequential assignment to conditions: (1) fed sterile water at 1, 2, and 3 h of life; (2) fed formula at 1, 2, and 3 h; (3) fed sterile water at 4 h and formula at 8 h (control group)	Time of initial meconium passage (+) Serum indirect bilirubin at 48 h of life (0) Observed jaundice at 48 h of life (+) Total calories ingested in first 48 h of life (0) Weight loss at 48 h (0)
Keefe (1987, 1988): Twenty-one full-term, healthy infants and their mothers: 11 in experimental and 10 in control groups	Nonrandomization to conditions; experimental infants stayed in mothers' rooms at night on first two nights following birth; control infants returned to nursery at night	During two 8 h nights after birth: illumination in room (+); noise level in room (+); amount of caregiver contact (+); response time of caregiver to cry (+); contingent care (+); proportion of time infant in quiet sleep (+); proportion of time crying (+); hours of maternal sleep at night (0); quality of maternal sleep (0)
Meier & Anderson (1987) & Meier (1988): Five preterm infants weighing less than 1500 g at the time oral feedings were started	Infants served as own controls; experimental condition was breastfeeding, control condition was bottle feeding; for first 1 to 2 wk of study, one bottle feeding and one breastfeeding were given on alternate days—subsequently, both given on same day	Compared to bottle feedings: feeding behaviors were more coordinated during breast feeding; less bradycardia during breast feeding; less decline in transcutaneous oxygen tension with breast feeding; increased skin temperature during breast feeding; longer duration of feeding with breast feeding.

Table 17–3
INTERVENTIONS RELATED TO BEHAVIORAL ORGANIZATION *(Continued)*

Citation: Group/Population	Independent Variable(s)	Dependent Variable(s) and Study Outcomes*
Schwartz et al. (1987): Five studies of nonnutritive sucking in preterm infants	Nonnutritive sucking (meta-analysis)	Days to first bottle feeding (+) Days of hospitalization (+) Weight gain (0)
Gill et al. (1988): Twenty-four preterm infants during first 48 h of bottle feedings: 12 in experimental and 12 in control groups	Randomized to conditions; experimental group received 5 min of nonnutritive sucking prior to first 16 bottle feedings	Prior to feedings, experimental group was less often in restless states (+) and more often in wakeful states than control group (+) Prior to feedings, both groups were less often in sleep states (0)
Koniak-Griffin & Ludington-Hoe (1987, 1988): Eighty-one healthy, full-term infants; numbers in each of three experimental groups and one control group not given	Randomization to conditions which began on 3 to 4 d after birth and ended at 3 mo; experimental conditions were (1) daily stroking of infant for 5–7 min or (2) placement in multisensory hammock during sleep, or (3) a combination of (1) and (2); control (placebo) condition used a bicolored sheet for sleeping	Of nine temperament dimensions compared at 4 mo, two (mood and distractibility) generally favored the control group (−) Of nine temperament dimensions compared at 8 mo, three (mood, distractability, and approach) generally favored the control group (−) Weight and weight gain at 1 mo (0) Maternal perception of infant at 1 mo (0) Three of six NBAS clusters (range of state, autonomic stability, and reflexes) (0) NBAS orientation cluster (−) NBAS motor cluster significantly lower in multisensory hammock group; others not significantly different (−/0)

		NBAS state regulation lower in multisensory hammock and combined stimulation groups than in stroking and control groups (−/0)
Grauer (1989): Ninety-nine healthy newborns—49 in experimental and 50 in control groups with blocking for state predominance (sleep vs. awake)	Assigned to conditions initially by randomization and then sequentially; experimental group received intermittent lighting in nursery for two nights	Changes in salivary cortisol at 7 a.m. after 2 nights in study: Main effect for treatment = (0) Main effect for state predominance = (0) Interaction effect of treatment and state predominance = (+), i.e., both state groups changed in opposite directions in intermittent lighting.

**Note:* A (+) indicates outcomes favored group(s) that received treatments hypothesized to enhance behavioral organization over comparison/control groups; a (0) indicates no difference between treated and comparison/control groups; and a (−) indicates outcomes favored comparison/control group(s) that did not receive treatment over groups that received treatments hypothesized to enhance behavioral organization.

A more fundamental issue threaded through the research on behavioral organization in infants is the connections between biological (particularly neurological) and behavioral phenomena. Researchers who study infants are confronted with a subject who is undergoing rapid maturational changes and does not yet have language. Thus, research involves observing behavior and measuring physiological events—both moving targets. Many studies surveyed a number of biological and behavioral variables, but careful rationales for the selections were often absent. Future research would be strengthened by explicitly proposing the linkages between and among behavioral and biological phenomena.

In regard to future interventive studies, special effort should be taken to design them carefully. In only about a quarter of the studies reviewed in this chapter were subjects assigned to conditions randomly. Random assignment should be used in most future studies except perhaps in early pilot work. In addition, power analyses should serve as the basis for determining sample sizes so that true experimental effects can be detected. Most important, though, care should be taken to locate and critically analyze all pertinent studies before beginning an intervention study. Every effort should be made to ensure that new studies not only build on past knowledge but also extend that knowledge. Careful thinking about how to advance what is known about a phenomenon is as important as or perhaps more important than adding another data point to an already researched area.

Finally, it is critical that nurses continue to study the dimensions of behavioral organization in order to shape care environments in ways that enhance the organizational processes of infants. To do so, investigators must maintain programs of research that build cumulatively and provide a training ground for clinicians as well as new investigators entering the field. The nonnutritive sucking studies by G. Anderson and associates (Anderson et al., 1982; Anderson & Vidyasagar, 1979; Burroughs, et al., 1978; Ellison, et al., 1979; Gill, et al., 1988; Measel & Anderson, 1979; Weaver & Anderson, 1988) reported in this chapter illustrate that type of program.

REFERENCES

Anderson, C. J. (1981). Enhancing reciprocity between mother and neonate. *Nursing Research, 30,* 89–93.

Anderson, G. C., McBride, M. R., Dahm, J., Ellis, M. K., & Vidyasagar, D. (1982). Development of sucking in term infants from birth to four hours postbirth. *Research in Nursing and Health, 5,* 21–27.

Anderson, G. C., & Vidyasagar, D. (1979). Development of sucking in premature infants from 1 to 7 days post birth. In G. C. Anderson, B. Raff, M. Duxbury, & P. Carroll (Eds.), *Newborn behavioral organization: Nursing research and implications.* New York: Liss. March of Dimes Birth Defects Foundation. *Birth Defects, Original Article Series, 15*(7), 145–171.

Bacon, C. J., Mucklow, J. C., Saunders, A., Rawlins, M. D., & Webb, J. K. G. (1978). A method for obtaining saliva samples from infants and young children (Letter). *British Journal of Clinical Pharmacology, 5*(1), 89–90.

Bakeman, R., & Gottman, J. M. (1986). *Observing interaction: An introduction to sequential analysis.* Cambridge, England: Cambridge University Press.

Barnard, K. (1973). The effect of stimulation on the sleep behavior of the premature infant. In M. V. Batey (Ed.), *Communicating nursing research: Collaboration and competition* (Vol. 6, 12–33). Boulder, CO: Western Interstate Commission for Higher Education.

Barnard, K. E., & Bee, H. L. (1983). The impact of temporally patterned stimulation on the development of preterm infants. *Child Development, 54,* 1156-1167.

Barnard, K. E., & Eyres, S. J. (1979). *Child health assessment: 2. The first year of life.* (DHEW Publication No. HRA 79-25). Hyattsville, MD: U.S. Dept. of Health, Education, & Welfare, Public Health Service, HRA, Bureau of Health Manpower, Division of Nursing.

Barnard, K. E., Hammond, M. A., Sumner, G. A., Kang, R., Johnson-Crowley, N., Snyder, C., Spietz, A., Blackburn, S., Brandt, P., & Magyary, D. (1987). Helping parents with preterm infants: Field test of a protocol. *Early Child Development and Care, 27,* 255–290.

Bayley, N. (1969). *Bayley Scales of Infant Development: Birth to Two Years.* New York: Psychological Corporation.

Becker, P. T. (1987). Sensitivity to infant development and behavior: A comparison of adolescent and adult single mothers. *Research in Nursing & Health, 10,* 119–127.

Becker, P. T., Lederman, R. P., & Lederman, E. (1989). Neonatal measures of attention and early cognitive status. *Research in Nursing & Health, 12,* 381–388.

Bee, H. L., Bernard, K. E., Eyres, S. J., Gray, C. A., Hammond, M. A., Spietz, A. L., Snyder, C., & Clark, B. (1982). Prediction of IQ and language skill from perinatal status, child performance, family characteristics, and mother-infant interaction. *Child Development, 53,* 1134–1156.

Blackburn, S. T., & Barnard, K. E. (1985). Analysis of caregiving events relating to preterm infants in the special care unit. In A. W. Gottfried & J. L. Gaiter (Eds.), *Infant stress under intensive care* (pp. 113–129). Baltimore: University Park Press.

Blank, D. M. (1986). Relating mothers' anxiety and perception to infant satiety, anxiety, and feeding behavior. *Nursing Research, 35,* 347–351.

Bowen, S. M., & Miller, B. C. (1980). Paternal attachment behavior as related to presence at delivery and preparenthood classes: A pilot study. *Nursing Research, 29,* 307–311.

Boyer, D. B., & Vidyasagar, D. (1987). Serum indirect bilirubin levels and meconium passage in early fed normal newborns. *Nursing Research 36,* 174–178.

Brazelton, T. B. (1973). *Neonatal behavioral assessment scale.* London: Heinemann.

Brazelton, T. B. (1984). *Neonatal behavioral assessment scale* (2nd ed.). Philadelphia: Lippincott.

Britton, G. R. (1980). Early mother-infant contact and infant temperature stabilization. *Journal of Obstetric, Gynecologic and Neonatal Nursing, 9,* 84–86.

Brown, M. M. (1979). Parental concerns about infant behavioral organization from term to 4 months. In G. C. Anderson, B. Raff, M. Duxbury, & P. Carroll (Eds.), *Newborn behavioral organization: Nursing research and implications.* New York: Liss. March of Dimes Birth Defects Foundation. *Birth Defects, Original Article Series, 15*(7), 27–42.

Brown, M. S., & Grunfeld, C. G. (1980). Taste preferences of infants for sweetened or unsweetened foods. *Research in Nursing and Health, 3,* 11–17.

Burroughs, A. K., Asonye, U. O., Anderson-Shanklin, G. C., & Vidyasagar, D. (1978). The effect of nonnutritive sucking on transcutaneous oxygen tension in noncrying, preterm neonates. *Research in Nursing and Health, 1,* 69–75.

Carey, W., & McDevitt, S. (1978). A revision of the infant temperament questionnaire. *Pediatrics, 61,* 735–738.

Chapman, J. S. (1978). The relationship between auditory stimulation and gross motor activity of short-gestation infants. *Research in Nursing and Health, 1,* 29–36.

Chapman, J. S. (1979). Influence of varied stimuli on development of motor patterns in the premature infant. In G. C. Anderson, B. Raff, M. Duxbury, & P. Carroll (Eds.), *Newborn behavioral organization: Nursing research and implications.* New York: Liss. March of Dimes Birth Defects Foundation. *Birth Defects, Original Article Series, 15*(7), 61–80.

Choi, E. S. C., & Hamilton, R. K. (1986). The effects of culture on mother-infant interaction. *Journal of Obstetric, Gynecologic and Neonatal Nursing, 15,* 256–261.

Clarke-Stewart, K. A., VanderStoep, L. P., & Killian, G. A. (1979). Analysis and replication of mother-infant relations at two years of age. *Child Development, 50,* 777–793.

Collinge, J. M., Bradley, K., Perks, C., Rezny, A., & Topping, P. (1982). Demand vs. scheduled feedings for premature infants. *Journal of Obstetric, Gynecologic and Neonatal Nursing, 11,* 362–367.

Dreyfus-Brisac, C. (1974). Organization of sleep in prematures: Implications for caregiving. In M. Lewis & L. Rosenblum (Eds.), *The effect of the infant on its caregiver* (pp. 123–140). New York: Wiley.

Dubowitz, L. M. S., Dubowitz, V., & Goldberg, C. (1970). Clinical assessment of gestational age in the newborn infant. *Journal of Pediatrics, 77,* 1–10.

Duxbury, M. L., Henly, S. J., Broz, L. J., Armstrong, G. D., & Wachdorf, C. M. (1984). Caregiver disruptions and sleep of high-risk infants. *Heart & Lung, 13*(2), 141–147.

Ellison, S. L., Vidyasagar, D., & Anderson, G. C. (1979). Sucking in the newborn infant during the first hour of life. *Journal of Nurse-Midwifery, 24,* 18–25.

Field, T. M., Dempsey, J. P., Hallock, N. H., & Shuman, H. H. (1978). The mother's assessment of the behavior of her infant. *Infant Behavior and Development, 1,* 156-167.

Flagler, S. (1988). Maternal role competence. *Western Journal of Nursing Research, 10,* 274–290.

Fullard, W., McDevitt, S., & Carey, W. (1984). Assessing temperament in one- to three-year-old children. *Journal of Pediatric Psychology, 9,* 205–217.

Gardner, S. (1979). The mother as incubator—after delivery. *Journal of Obstetric, Gynecologic and Neonatal Nursing, 8,* 174–176.

Gill, N. E., Behnke, M., Conlon, M., McNeely, J. B., & Anderson, G. C. (1988). Effect of nonnutritive sucking on behavioral state in preterm infants before feeding. *Nursing Research, 37,* 347–350.

Gill, N. E., White, M. A., & Anderson, G. C. (1984). Transitional newborn infants in a hospital nursery: From first oral cue to first sustained cry. *Nursing Research, 33,* 213–217.

Grauer, T. T. (1989). Environmental lighting, behavioral state, and hormonal response in the newborn. *Scholarly Inquiry for Nursing Practice, 3*(1), 53–66.

Houldin, A. D. (1987). Infant temperament and the quality of the childrearing environment. *Maternal-Child Nursing Journal, 16,* 131–143.

Jay, S. S. (1982). The effects of gentle human touch on mechanically ventilated very-short-gestation infants. [Monograph]. *Maternal-Child Nursing Journal, 11,* 199–256.

Jones, C. (1981). Father to infant attachment: Effects of early contact and characteristics of the infant. *Research in Nursing and Health, 4,* 193–200.

Jones, C., & Parks, P. (1983). Mother-, father-, and examiner-reported temperament across the first year of life. *Research in Nursing and Health, 6,* 183–189.

Jones, L. C., & Lenz, E. R. (1986). Father-newborn interaction: Effects of social competence and infant state. *Nursing Research, 35,* 149–153.

Kang, R., & Barnard, K. (1979). Using the neonatal behavioral assessment scale to evaluate premature infants. In G. C. Anderson, B. Raff, M. Duxbury, & P. Carroll (Eds.), *Newborn behavioral organization: Nursing research and implications.* New York: Liss. March of Dimes Birth Defects Foundation. *Birth Defects, Original Article Series, 15*(7), 119–144.

Keefe, M. R. (1987). Comparison of neonatal nighttime sleep-wake patterns in nursery versus rooming-in environments. *Nursing Research, 36,* 140–144.

Keefe, M. R. (1988). The impact of infant rooming-in on maternal sleep at night.

Journal of Obstetric, Gynecologic and Neonatal Nursing, 17, 122–126.

Keefe, M. R., Kotzer, A. M., Reuss, J. L., & Sander, L. W. (1989). Development of a system for monitoring infant state behavior. *Nursing Research, 38,* 344–347.

Koniak-Griffin, D., & Lundington-Hoe, S. M. (1987). Paradoxical effects of stimulation on normal neonates. *Infant Behavior and Development, 10,* 261–277.

Koniak-Griffin, D., & Ludington-Hoe, S. M. (1988). Developmental and temperament outcomes of sensory stimulation in healthy infants. *Nursing Research, 37,* 70–76.

Koniak-Griffin, D., & Rummell, M. (1988). Temperament in infancy: Stability, change, and correlates. *Maternal-Child Nursing Journal, 17,* 25–40.

Kron, R., & Litt, M. (1971). Fluid mechanics of nutritive sucking behavior: The sucking infant's oral apparatus analyzed as a hydraulic pump. *Medical Biologic Engineering, 9,* 45–60.

Krueger, J. M. (1970). A spectrographic analysis of the differing cries of a normal two-month-old infant. *Nursing Research, 19,* 459–463.

Lambesis, C. C., Vidyasagar, D., & Anderson, G. C. (1979). Effects of surrogate mothering on physiologic stabilization in transitional newborns. In G. C. Anderson, B. Raff, M. Duxbury, & P. Carroll (Eds.), *Newborn behavioral organization: Nursing research and implications.* New York: Liss. March of Dimes Birth Defects Foundation. *Birth Defects, Original Article Series, 15*(7), 201–223.

Lawson, K. R., & Turkewitz, G. (1985). Relationship between the distribution and diurnal periodicities of infant state and environment. In A. W. Gottfried & J. L. Gaiter (Eds.), *Infant stress under intensive care* (pp. 157–170). Baltimore: University Park Press.

Levine, M. (1967). The four conservation principles of nursing. *Nursing Forum, 6,* 45–59.

Maloni, J. A., Stegman, C. E., Taylor, P. M., & Brownell, C. A. (1986). Validation of infant behavior identified by neonatal nurses. *Nursing Research, 35,* 133–138.

Measel, C. P., & Anderson, G. C. (1979). Nonnutritive sucking during tube feedings: Effect on clinical course in premature infants. *Journal of Obstetric, Gynecologic and Neonatal Nursing, 8,* 265–272.

Medoff-Cooper, B. (1986). Temperament in very low birth weight infants. *Nursing Research, 35,* 139–143.

Medoff-Cooper, B. (1988). The effects of handling on preterm infants with bronchopulmonary dysplasia. *Image, 20,* 132–134.

Medoff-Cooper, B., & Brooten, D. (1987). Relation of the feeding cycle to neurobehavioral assessment in preterm infants: A pilot study. *Nursing Research, 36,* 315–317.

Medoff-Cooper, B., & Schraeder, B. D. (1982). Developmental trends and behavioral styles in very low birth weight infants. *Nursing Research, 31,* 68–72.

Medoff-Cooper, B., Weininger, S., & Zukowsky, K. (1989). Neonatal sucking as a clinical assessment tool: Preliminary findings. *Nursing Research, 38,* 162–165.

Meier, P. (1988). Bottle- and breast-feeding: Effects on transcutaneous oxygen pressure and temperature in preterm infants. *Nursing Research, 37,* 36–41.

Meier, P., & Anderson, G. C. (1987). Responses of small preterm infants to bottle- and breast-feeding. *MCN, The American Journal of Maternal-Child Nursing, 12,* 97–105.

Mitchell, S. K., Bee, H. L., Hammond, M. A., & Barnard, K. E. (1985). Prediction of school and behavior problems in children followed from birth to age eight. In W. K. Frankenburg, R. N. Emde, & J. W. Sullivan (Eds.), *Early identification of children at risk* (pp. 117–132). New York: Plenum.

Neal, M. V. (1979). Organizational behavior of the premature infant. In G. C. Anderson, B. Raff, M. Duxbury, & P. Carroll (Eds.), *Newborn behavioral organization: Nursing research and implications.* New York: Liss. March of Dimes Birth Defects Foundation. *Birth Defects, Original Article Series, 15*(7), 43–60.

Neal, M. V., & Nauen, C. M. (1968). Ability of premature infant to maintain his own body temperature. *Nursing Research, 17,* 396–402.

Neeley, C. A. (1979). Effects of nonnutritive sucking upon the behavioral arousal of the newborn. In G. C. Anderson, B. Raff, M. Duxbury, & P. Carroll (Eds.), *Newborn behavioral organization: Nursing research and implications.* New York: Liss. March of Dimes Birth Defects Foundation. *Birth Defects, Original Article Series, 15*(7), 173-200.

Newport, M. A. (1984). Conserving thermal energy and social integrity in the newborn. *Western Journal of Nursing Research, 6,* 175-190.

Oliver, C. M., & Oliver, G. M. (1978). Gentle birth: Its safety and its effect on neonatal behavior. *Journal of Obstetric, Gynecologic and Neonatal Nursing, 7,* 35-40.

Perry, S. E. (1983). Parents' perceptions of their newborn following structured interactions. *Nursing Research, 32,* 208-212.

Pohlman, S., & Beardslee, C., (1987). Contacts experienced by neonates in intensive care environments. *Maternal-Child Nursing Journal, 16,* 207-226.

Poley-Strobel, B. A., & Beckmann, C. A. (1987). The effects of a teaching-modeling intervention on early mother-infant reciprocity. *Infant Behavior and Development, 10,* 467-476.

Pollack, M. M., Yeh, T. S. Ruttiman, U. E., Holbrook, P. R., & Fields, A. I. (1984). Evaluation of pediatric intensive care. *Critical Care Medicine, 12*(4), 376-383.

Rausch, P. B. (1981). Effects of tactile and kinesthetic stimulation on premature infants. *Journal of Obstetric, Gynecologic and Neonatal Nursing, 10,* 34-37.

Reisch, S. K. (1979). Enhancement of mother-infant and social interaction. *Journal of Obstetric, Gynecologic and Neonatal Nursing, 8,* 242-246.

Riesch, S. K. (1984). Occupational commitment and the quality of maternal infant interaction. *Research in Nursing and Health, 7,* 295-503.

Roberts, F. B. (1983). Infant behavior and the transition to parenthood. *Nursing Research, 32,* 213-217.

Rothbart, M. K. (1978). Infant behavior questionnaire. (Available from M. K. Rothbart, Department of Psychology, University of Oregon, Eugene, OR 97403.)

Rothbart, M. K., & Goldsmith, H. H. (1985). Three approaches to the study of infant temperament. *Developmental Review, 5,* 237-260.

Salter, A. (1978). Birth without violence: A medical controversy. *Nursing Research, 27,* 84-88.

Sander, L. (1969). Regulation and organization in the early infant-caretaker system. In R. J. Robinson (Ed.), *Brain and early behavior* (pp. 311-333). London: Academic Press.

Schraeder, B. D., & Medoff-Cooper, B. (1983). Development and temperament in very low birth weight infants—the second year. *Nursing Research, 32,* 331-335.

Schwartz, R., Moody, L., Yarandi, H., & Anderson, G. C. (1987). A meta-analysis of critical outcome variables in nonnutritive sucking in preterm infants. *Nursing Research, 36,* 292-295.

Segall, M. E. (1972). Cardiac responsivity to auditory stimulation in premature infants. *Nursing Research, 21,* 15-19.

Snyder, C., Eyres, S. J., & Barnard, K. (1979). New findings about mothers' antenatal expectations and their relationship to infant development. *MCN, The American Journal of Maternal/Child Nursing, 4,* 354-357.

Tomlinson, P. S. (1987). Spousal differences in marital satisfaction during transition to parenthood. *Nursing Research, 36,* 239-243.

Updike, P. A., Accurso, F. J., & Jones, R. H. (1985). Physiologic circadian rhythmicity in preterm infants. *Nursing Research, 34,* 160-163.

Ventura, J. N. (1982). Parent coping behaviors, parent functioning, and infant temperament characteristics. *Nursing Research, 31,* 269-273.

Ventura, J. N. (1986). Parent coping: A replication. *Nursing Research, 35,* 77-80.

Walker, R. F., Riad-Fahmy, D., & Read, G. F. (1978). Adrenal status assessed by direct radioimmunoassay of cortisol in whole saliva or parotid saliva. *Clinical Chemistry, 24*(9), 1460-1463.

Weaver, K. A., & Anderson, G. C. (1988). Relationship between integrated sucking pressures and first bottle-feeding scores in premature infants. *Journal of Obstetric,*

Gynecologic and Neonatal Nursing, 17, 113–120.

Whitner, W., & Thompson, M. C. (1970). The influence of bathing on the newborn infant's body temperature. *Nursing Research, 19,* 30–36.

Wolff, P. H. (1966). *The causes, controls, and organization of behavior in the neonate.* (*Psychological Issues* Monograph No. 17, Vol. 5, No. 1.) New York: International Universities Press.

Zahr, L. K., & Khoury, M., & Nugent, K. (1988). Neonatal behavior of prenatally stressed Lebanese infants. *Image, 20,* 200–202.

CHAPTER 18

Parent-Infant Nursing Research on Behavioral Interaction in Infancy and Parenting

DEFINITIONS AND DESCRIPTIONS OF BEHAVIORAL INTERACTION

DEFINING BEHAVIORAL INTERACTION

Most studies have not defined behavioral interaction; instead, they have identified its positive dimensions. For example, Censullo, Lester, and Hoffman (1985) stressed the rhythmicity and synchrony of interaction, and Anderson (1981) emphasized the reciprocity as a dimension of early parent-infant adaptation. Alternatively, Holaday (1987) described her view of interaction as "a behavioral dialogue or conversation, with communicative acts consisting of vocal and visual dialogues between the pair" (p. 30). Further, most investigators started out with the premise that infants are preadapted for interaction with adults. To illustrate, Jones and Thomas (1989) stated: "Human infants are biologically predisposed to emit signals to which adults are biologically predisposed to respond" (p. 237).

THEORETICAL MODELS OF BEHAVIORAL INTERACTION

Although most studies did not include elaborate theoretical frameworks, several provided explicitly stated frameworks for the study. For example, Blank (1986) based her study on two theorems from the work of Sullivan (1953), Holaday (1982) used Johnson's (1980) behavioral system model, Jones & Lenz (1986) incorporated Goldberg's (1977) contingency model of interaction into their research, and Magyary (1983) employed social exchange theory as her conceptual framework.

MEASUREMENT

GENERAL STRATEGIES

Data about parent-infant interaction can be gathered at two levels of analysis: macrolevel rating of interaction or microlevel coding of discrete behavioral events. Although both methods have been used in parent-infant nursing research, macrolevel ratings are probably more common. In some instruments an attempt is made to blend the two approaches by basing ratings on occurrences of certain momentary events.

Most macrolevel ratings can be statistically analyzed with commonly used test statistics, but aggregating and analyzing data gathered at a microlevel requires special computational procedures, for example, see Hansen, Pridham, Stephenson, and Tsui (1987) and Booth, Lyons, and Barnard (1984).

SPECIFIC TOOLS

A variety of rating scales and coding systems have been used in parent-infant nursing research. The most widely used rating scales in nursing at the time of writing were the Nursing Child Assessment Feeding Scale and the Nursing Child Assessment Teaching Scale (Barnard et al., 1989) (Table 18–1).

METHODOLOGICAL STUDY

One methodological study was conducted to assess the convergence of three measures of mother-infant interaction. Flick and McSweeney (1987) observed 136 adolescent mothers of infants aged 8 to 27 months. The three measures included a scale for interaction during teaching, 14 global rating scales of maternal care, and a 100-item inventory of maternal attachment and child response. All interaction measures were completed during a home observation of unspecified duration. Data from the teaching

Table 18–1
MEASURES/TOOLS FOR THE CONCEPT OF BEHAVIORAL INTERACTIONS

Tool	Source Described in	Studies Using Tool
Feeding Interaction Scales: Twenty-one items for rating mother-infant interaction during feeding	Bee et al. (1982)	Bee et al. (1982) Barnard & Bee (1983) Barnard et al. (1984)
Nursing Child Assessment Feeding Scale: Seventy-six binary items for rating mother-infant interaction	Barnard et al. (1989)	Capuzzi (1989) Barnard, Booth, et al. (1988) Barnard, Magyary, et al. (1988) Barnard et al. (1987) Booth, Mitchell, Barnard, & Spieker (1989) Ruff (1987) Furr & Kirgis (1982) White-Traut & Nelson (1988)
Teaching Interaction Scales: Twenty-four items for rating mother-infant interaction during teaching tasks	Bee et al. (1982)	Bee et al. (1982) Barnard & Bee (1983) Barnard et al. (1984) Booth, Johnson-Crowley, & Barnard (1985)
Nursing Child Assessment Teaching Scale: Seventy-three binary items for rating mother-infant interaction	Barnard, et al. (1989)	Dormire, Strauss, & Clarke (1989) Barnard, Booth, et al. (1988) Barnard, Magyary, et al. (1988) Barnard et al. (1987) Booth et al. (1989)
Maternal-Infant Rating Scale: A checklist of eight categories of maternal or infant behavior during feeding	Schroeder-Zwelling & Hock (1986)	Schroeder-Zwelling & Hock (1986)
Dyadic Interaction Code: Coding system of six levels of engagement for rating dyad behavior changes of at least 2 s duration	Censullo et al. (1985)	Censullo et al. (1985)

Dyadic Mini Code: Six-item index of synchrony in infant-adult interaction	Censullo et al. (1987)	—
Method of Observation of Mother and Infant Behavior: Protocol for coding feeding interaction	deChateau (1976) as cited in Julian (1983)	Julian (1983)
Premature Infant Activity Schedule: Codes for time sampling of preterm infant behavior and caretaker activities	Chamorro, Davis, Green, & Kramer (1973)	Kramer, Chamorro, Green, & Knudtson (1975)
Maternal-Infant Adaptation Scale: Rating scale for feeding interaction; revised as the Assessment of Mother-Infant Sensitivity (AMIS)	Price (1977) as cited in Walker, Crain, & Thompson (1986) Price (1983) Price (1977) as cited in Harrison & Twardosz (1986)	Walker et al. (1986) Harrison & Twardosz (1986) Riesch (1984) Anderson (1981) Poley-Strobel & Beckmann (1987) Choi & Hamilton (1986)
Mother-Infant Play Interaction Scale: Scale for rating early mother-infant interaction	Walker & Thompson (1982)	Choi & Hamilton (1986)
Interpersonal Behavior Construct system: Coding system for analysis of interaction	Kogan et al. (1975) as cited in Booth et al. (1985)	Booth et al. (1985)
Paternal-Newborn Interactional Behavior: Codes for infant state and four father behaviors	Jones & Lenz (1986)	Jones & Lenz (1986)
Father-infant interaction codes: Coding scheme for verbal and nonverbal behavior and infant state	Jones & Thomas (1989)	Jones & Thomas (1989)

Table 18–1
MEASURES/TOOLS FOR THE CONCEPT OF BEHAVIORAL INTERACTIONS *(Continued)*

Tool	Source Described in	Studies Using Tool
Behavioral Checklist: Checklist of neonatal and maternal social behaviors and interview questions	Riesch et al. (1978) as cited in Riesch & Munns (1984)	Riesch & Munns (1984)
Coding categories: Behavioral codes for caregiver behavior in newborn nursery	Karraker (1986)	Karraker (1986)
Maternal expectations and observations of infant interactive capacities: Interview schedules	Riesch (1979)	Riesch (1979)
Prenatal expectations for interaction and self-report of parent-infant interaction	Humenick & Bugen (1981)	Humenick & Bugen (1981)
Cardiovascular measures during interaction: Heart rate and blood pressure	—	Jones & Thomas (1989)

scale were aggregated into six a priori subscales, and data from the attachment inventory were reduced by factor analysis to four maternal factors and three child factors. Analysis of the global rating scales did not yield reliable factors. Next, the teaching subscales, attachment inventory factors, and individual global rating scales were factor-analyzed as two sets: one using maternally focused variables and one using child-focused variables. For maternal variables, four interpretable factors were extracted, and they accounted for 62 percent of the variance. Internal consistencies of these factors were questionable, however; the range was from 0.27 to 0.58. For child variables, three factors were extracted, but they were uninterpretable and failed to have adequate internal consistency. Some evidence of convergence was found at the level of correlations among global ratings, teaching subscales, and attachment inventory factors. The authors concluded that "the three measures are not associated with a shared set of underlying factors" (p. 136).

SUMMARY OF RESEARCH

SCOPE OF BEHAVIORAL INTERACTION RESEARCH

Compared to behavioral organization, less research in nursing has addressed behavioral interaction. Most of the existing research is descriptive; much less of it is relational or predictive (Table 18–2). Intervention studies, though few in number, have been a continued focus of research. (*Note:* Research on behavioral interaction during labor is contained in Chapter 12. Additional studies of postpartum interventions can be found in Chapter 13, and studies of the hospital caregiving environment can be found in Chapters 17 and 20.)

DESCRIPTIVE RESEARCH

Interaction Dimensions Identified

In a descriptive study of mothers' awareness of infant interactive capacities, Riesch (1979) questioned 30 new mothers about their expectations for and subsequent observations of infant behavioral capacities. Infant behaviors were also assessed by the investigator. Overall, mothers expected and observed most of the habituation, orientation, and stimulus-control behaviors of infants. Mothers' assessments of their infants' best behaviors, however, were at variance with infants' actual performance. Most mothers rated their infants as best at orientation, whereas most infants performed best at either habituation or stimulus control. Most mothers,

Table 18–2
PARENT-INFANT NURSING RESEARCH ON BEHAVIORAL INTERACTION

DESCRIPTIVE
Descriptions of Behavioral Interaction
Dzik (1979), mothers and infants during immunizations
Holaday (1987), mothers and chronically ill infants
Karraker (1986), newborns and nursery personnel
Magyary (1983), mothers and preterm infants
Riesch (1979), new mothers and infants
Patterns of Behavioral Interaction
Holaday (1982), crying in chronically ill infants
Changes in Behavioral Interaction
Ruff (1987), from birth to 6 to 12 weeks
Differences in Behavioral Interaction
Barnard et al. (1984), mothers of term vs. preterm infants
Capuzzi (1989), mothers of handicapped vs. nonhandicapped infants
Censullo et al. (1985), mothers of term vs. preterm infants
Choi & Hamilton (1986), American Korean vs. American Caucasian mothers
Schroeder-Zwelling & Hock (1986), diabetic vs. nondiabetic mothers
RELATIONS TO BEHAVIOR INTERACTION
Blank (1986), maternal perceptions and anxiety
Humenick & Bugen (1981), prenatal, intrapartal, and postpartal correlates
Jones & Lenz (1986), behavioral competence, infant state
Jones & Thomas (1989), cardiovascular correlates
Riesch (1984), job commitment
INTERVENTION RESEARCH
Anderson (1981), demonstration or verbal teaching about infant capabilities
Barnard et al. (1987), clinical protocol on infant behaviors, health concerns, and resources
Perry (1983), structured interaction
Poley-Strobel & Beckmann (1987), teaching-modeling about interaction
Riesch & Munns (1984), audiotape about interaction
Turley (1985), meta-analysis of interventions about informing parents about infant capabilities
White-Traut & Nelson (1988), sensorimotor stimulation

although aware of infant behavior, failed to understand the function of behavior in infant-environment interactions.

In a study of interactions between five mothers and their chronically ill infants, Holaday (1987) quantitatively described behavioral "dialogue states" that occurred when infants were 4 to 5 months old. Dialogue states were based on visual and vocal communicative acts. Four dialogue states included mother acting alone, infant acting alone, coacting (both acting), and quiescent (neither acting). Using transition probabilities, that is, "the ratio of the frequency of a specific transition from state 'A' to state 'B' to the total frequency of state 'A' within an observation period" (p. 36), mothers were identified as the controlling partner in initiating both vocal and visual interactions. For example, the transition probability of going from quiescent to mother acting alone was .91, and the probability of going from quiescent to infant acting alone was .09 for visual behavior. However, the infant was more likely to be the partner to end interactions. For visual interaction, the probability of going from coacting to mother acting alone was .82 and the probability of going from coacting to infant acting alone was .18.

In a related study, Magyary (1983) measured dialogue states (termed "social exchange units") in visual interactions of 16 mothers and their preterm infants at hospital discharge and at 4 and 8 months. With regard to duration of each dialogue state, the least amount of time was spent in a state of infant gazing with mother not attending, and the most amount of time was spent in a state of mother gazing and infant not attending. Mutual gazing, that is, coacting, was an infrequent state; infants were unlikely to initiate gazing and were likely to end mutual gazing. Within this overall pattern, some differences were associated with infant age and type of situation (caregiving or play). For example, infants initiated gaze more often during caregiving than play at 4 and 8 months.

In a study of the social interactions that normal infants experience in the newborn nursery, Karraker (1986) conducted six 3-hour observations of caregiving and related interactions received by 67 newborns. No infant was observed more than once. The majority of infants received some attention from an adult while in the nursery, the average amount being just under 8 minutes. The two most frequent forms of attention received by infants from nurse's aides in the nursery were having diapers or clothes changed or rearranged and having bassinets moved. Fifty-four of 67 infants cried while in the nursery and averaged over 6 minutes of crying. The amount of crying was correlated with the amount of adult attention. The lag between when crying initiated and when adult attention subsequently occurred was just over 8 minutes. Among infants who received attention from nurse's aides, the amounts of various types of attention were related to such infant characteristics as age, sex, race, prematurity, and physical attractiveness. (Less attention was paid to attractive infants.)

Dzik (1979) studied mother-infant interaction during infant immunization at a clinic. Thirty mothers and their 2-, 4-, or 6-month-old infants were observed. The frequency of "satisfying behaviors" (i.e., comforting and caretaking) was 16 percent of maternal behaviors. Comforting was more common than caretaking. Comforting after the immunization took the form of patting, rocking, or cuddling. Two mothers, both adolescents, were unable to successfully terminate their infants' cries triggered by the immunizations. Primiparas sometimes were observed to engage in affectionate behavior in response to infant distress if infants were 2 or 4 months old. Six-month-old infants cried less and also received less comforting.

Qualitative Patterns of Interaction

In a qualitative study of mother-infant interaction, Holaday (1982) observed six mothers with their chronically ill infants. Home observations, supplemented by interviews, were made every 3 weeks when infants were 4 to 6 months old. Infant cries and maternal response patterns were the units of analysis. By use of a behavioral system framework, three stages of maternal response were proposed: (1) inadequate conceptual set, (2) developing conceptual set, and (3) sophisticated conceptual set. These stages parallel mothers' shifts from simple, fixed rules to eventual flexible cognitive processes in responding to cries of their chronically ill infants.

Changes in Parent-Infant Interaction

To assess adolescent mothers' interaction patterns, Ruff (1987) examined the feeding interaction of 95 adolescent mothers and their infants shortly after birth and 6 to 12 weeks later. Mothers' scores at the second observation were lower than scale norms on four of four maternal subscales, particularly those related to fostering cognitive and socioemotional growth of the infant. Infant scores on two of two subscales approximated those of normative samples. With regard to changes in interaction that occurred between the two observations, adolescents remained unchanged in sensitivity to cues, decreased in responsiveness to infant distress, and increased in both cognitive and socioemotional growth-fostering behaviors. Infants, in turn, increased in both their clarity of cues and responsiveness to their mothers. Maternal age was correlated with maternal interaction at both observations.

Differences in Interaction

In a study of the effects of high-risk pregnancy, Schroeder-Zwelling and Hock (1986) compared 20 diabetic women (14 with chronic diabetes and 6 with gestational diabetes) to 20 nondiabetic, low-risk women. Mother-infant interaction was observed twice in the immediate postpartum period and once at 6 weeks. Of eight categories of maternal or infant behavior observed during feeding interactions, only one—maternal facial expression—differed significantly. Differences favored nondiabetic mothers.

In a study comparing mothers of handicapped (n = 15) and nonhandicapped infants (n = 21), Capuzzi (1989) used mother-infant interaction as a measure of maternal attachment. Ages of infants at the time of postnatal observations at 1, 6, and 12 months were corrected for gestational age. At 1 month, mothers of handicapped infants scored lower in their interaction than mothers of nonhandicapped infants. At 6 and 12 months, the two groups did not differ in their interactions.

Barnard, Bee, and Hammond (1984) compared interaction patterns between 166 mothers and their term infants and between 88 mothers and their preterm infants. Feeding interactions were assessed at 4 and 8 months and teaching interactions at 4, 8, and 24 months. Also, home environment was assessed at 24 months. All observations except those of term infants at 4 and 8 months took place in a clinic setting. Group differences were found for mothers during teaching interaction and for infants during feeding interaction. All favored the term dyads. Further, group by age interactions were significant in five of six comparisons. For example, mothers of preterm infants showed more precipitous declines in positive messages after 4 months than mothers of term infants. The preterm infants increased markedly in involvement in teaching interactions after 4 months. As for home environment, mothers of preterm infants rated themselves as providing less stimulating environments than mothers of term infants.

In another study comparing term and preterm mother-infant dyads, Censullo, Lester, and Hoffman (1985) examined rhythmic patterning and synchrony in the interactions of both groups. Fifteen term infants and their mothers were videotaped at 36 to 72 hours after birth in 3-minute, face-to-face interactions. Similarly, preterm infants and their mothers were videotaped at 40 weeks postconceptual age. Videotapes were coded on a moment-by-moment basis for level of engagement in the dyads. Analysis of spectral density of interactions showed no significant difference between the two groups supporting similar rhythmic patterning in both. Further, analysis of the amount of time in mutual regard showed no significant group differences supporting similar levels of synchrony in both groups.

To assess the influence of culture, Choi and Hamilton (1986) compared 21 American white mother-infant pairs with 18 American Korean mothers and their infants. Based on data gathered at 2 to 3 days after delivery, American Korean mothers viewed infants as more passive than American white mothers. However, no differences were found in the sensitivity or reciprocity of mother-infant interaction during feeding or play.

RELATIONAL/PREDICTIVE RESEARCH

In a study to test Sullivan's (1953) theorems about tenderness and anxiety in the mother-infant relationship, Blank (1986) examined relations between maternal perceptions and anxiety and infant satiety, anxiety, and feeding. Using 65 healthy, low-socioeconomic mother-infant dyads, Blank assessed maternal perceptions of infants on the first postpartum day. On the second postpartum day Blank assessed maternal state anxiety before and after a feeding and trait anxiety 1 hour after the feeding. Immediately before and after the same feeding, each infant's serum glucose and cortisol levels were measured as indicators of infant satiety and anxiety, respectively. Also, amount of formula consumed was noted. Maternal prefeed state anxiety, postfeed state anxiety, trait anxiety and perceptions were used as independent variables, and their effects on infant variables (amount of formula taken, differences in cortisol from prefeed to postfeed, and differences in glucose from prefeed to postfeed) were assessed. Contrary to Sullivan's theorems, analyses revealed that mothers with very low prefeed state anxiety had infants with greater cortisol values compared to mothers with slight state anxiety. Slightly more anxious mothers at postfeed had infants who consumed more formula than very low anxiety mothers' infants. (*Note:* No mothers met criteria for high anxiety.)

In a study of occupational commitment and mother-infant interaction, Riesch (1984) studied 50 mothers from the latter half of pregnancy to 6 weeks postpartum. The majority of the members of the sample were in professional or semiprofessional positions. Job satisfaction, measured prenatally, was correlated with mother-infant feeding interaction at 3 days, but not at 6 weeks, after delivery. In addition, the following factors were associated with less positive mother-infant interactions: (1) The mother's mother worked during the mother's childhood, (2) female infant, (3) bottle feeding, (4) nonattendance at childbirth classes, and (5) intent to return to work before 4 months postpartum.

Jones and Lenz (1986) examined the relation between paternal and infant competence and between infant state and paternal interactive behaviors. Infant competence was indexed by the orientation and range of state clusters on the Neonatal Behavioral Assessment Scale administered when infants were about 60 hours old. At 2 to 4 days postpartum, fathers rated their perceived competence as fathers and were videotaped while holding their infants for 10 minutes. Videotapes were analyzed at 10-second intervals for four father behaviors (touch-stimulate, touch-affection, talk-stimulate, and talk-affection) and infant state. Along with socioeconomic status and infant sex as control variables, infant competence, infant state, and paternal competence explained less than 20 percent of the variance in touch-stimulate and talk-stimulate but 29 percent of the variance in touch-affection and 40 percent of the variance in talk-affection. Infant state during interaction was the most consistent predictor of paternal interactive behaviors.

In an investigation of cardiovascular correlates of father-infant interaction, Jones and Thomas (1989) studied 148 first-time fathers during interaction with their newborn infants. Fathers' blood pressure and heart rate were measured for 6 minutes before, during, and after interaction. In controlling for preinteraction levels, heart rate and diastolic and systolic blood pressure were found to be higher during rather than after interaction. Nonverbal behavior was unrelated to blood pressure and heart rate, but verbal behavior was negatively related to blood pressure and positively related to heart rate. Further, the amount of infant crying during interaction was related to diastolic blood pressure.

In a longitudinal study of correlates of parent-infant interaction, Humenick and Bugen (1981) studied 66 parents from late in pregnancy to 3 weeks postpartum. Mothers and fathers rated their prenatal expectations for the amount of interaction with infants and reported their actual interaction at 3 weeks. In addition, trait anxiety, masculinity, femininity, and a number of antenatal, intrapartal, and postpartal variables were measured. In regression analyses, men's and women's self-reported interactions were significantly predicted by prenatal expectations for interaction. In addition, trait anxiety was a significant predictor for fathers but not for mothers.

INTERVENTION RESEARCH

Behavioral interaction has served as both an independent and a dependent variable in nursing intervention studies. Using structured interaction as the independent variable, Perry (1983) randomly assigned 57 couples to three intervention groups and a control group. The intervention consisted of having mother, father, or both parents (depending on group assignment) assess behavioral capabilities of their infants in the hospital. The investigator provided a structured format for the assessment. The dependent variable, parents' perceptions of their infants, was measured before intervention and at 1 week and 1 month after birth. Mothers in the three intervention groups demonstrated a significant increase in their perceptions of their infants at 1 week compared to mothers in the control group. No significant differences were found at 1 month for mothers, nor were any significant differences found for fathers at either 1 week or 1 month. In addition, no relation was found between actual infant behaviors, measured at the hospital or at 1 week, and parental perceptions of the infants.

In two studies of the effect of a teaching intervention on maternal awareness of interactive behaviors, Riesch and Munns (1984) tested the intervention with two different samples. In the first study, 108 mothers and their term infants were randomly assigned to intervention ($n = 54$) and control ($n = 54$) groups, and the intervention was conducted in the hospital within 48 hours after delivery. In the second study, 32 mothers and their healthy preterm infants were similarly assigned to intervention ($n = 16$) and control ($n = 16$) groups, and the intervention was conducted within 5 days of delivery. The intervention, provided by audiotape and printed material, covered newborn infant behaviors and maternal strategies to elicit or complement them. On the 2nd or 3rd day in the hospital or on the 2nd or 4th day at home after discharge, respectively, mothers of term infants and preterm infants were observed for 10 minutes during feedings. After a feeding, the mother was asked to report infant behavior that occurred as well as their own behavior. Mothers in both the term and preterm intervention groups reported more infant and maternal behaviors than their control counterparts. Further, intervention-group mothers' reports of behaviors were more consistent with the observations made by the investigators than with the control group mothers' reports.

Two other studies investigated the impact on mother-infant interaction of teaching mothers about behavioral capabilities of infants. In the first study, Anderson (1981) randomly assigned 30 mothers of healthy term infants to three groups (10 per group): teaching about infant behaviors with demonstration on own infant, teaching only with infant not present, and a placebo group comprised of teaching about infant furnishings. Administered in the hospital, the intervention was preceded by assessment of mother-infant interaction for each group; interaction was again assessed at 10 to 12 days after delivery. In comparing the teaching-with-demonstration (group III) and control (group I) groups, significantly greater gains occurred for maternal behaviors in group III, gains in infant behaviors for group III approached significance, and no differences were found for dyadic behaviors. Comparison of the teaching-only (group II) and control (group I) groups showed significantly greater gains in infant behaviors for group II, but not in maternal or dyadic behaviors. Comparing the teaching-with-demonstration (group III) and the teaching-only (group II) groups, significantly greater gains in maternal behavior occurred for group III, but no significant gains occurred in infant or dyadic behaviors.

In the second study, Poley-Strobel and Beckmann (1987) tested a related teaching-modeling intervention on 20 black, low-income, new mothers. Mothers were assigned randomly to intervention ($n = 10$) and control ($n = 10$) groups. The intervention, administered in the home at 1 to 3 days after hospital discharge, focused on ways caregivers can elicit infant responsiveness and facilitate infant behavioral capabilities. Impact of the intervention was assessed by measures of mother-infant interaction, maternal perceptions of infant behaviors, and maternal self-confidence taken during hospitalization and at 10 to 14 days after birth. Significant increases favoring the intervention group were found in maternal and dyadic interactive behaviors but not infant behaviors. No significant increases in maternal perceptions of infant behaviors or in maternal self-confidence occurred.

Two other studies focused on interventions with preterm infants. First, Barnard et al. (1987) reported on a field test of a protocol for public health nurse visits to families with premature and low birth weight infants. The protocol, Nursing Systems Toward Effective Parenting-Premature (NSTEP-P), was used by 23 nurses on a total of 76 families. The protocol consisted of structured content on state regulation, behavioral responsiveness, health concerns, and family and community resources presented over eight home visits from 37 to 60 weeks' conceptual age. Various parent, infant, and parent-infant interaction measures were taken during the eight sessions of the protocol. Analysis of changes over the duration of the protocol revealed no significant alterations in social support and family functioning. Significant increases occurred in infant weight, height, and head circumference during the field test. Amount of daytime sleep decreased significantly, and amount of daytime wakefulness increased significantly during the protocol. With regard to developmental delays, 6.2 percent of the NSTEP-P infants were suspect compared with 6.8 percent in a normative sample. Maternal interactive behaviors during feeding increased significantly in two areas: cognitive growth fostering and social-emotional growth fostering. Infant behaviors during feeding also increased significantly in two of two areas. However, for maternal interactive behaviors during teaching, a significant increase occurred in only one area (cognitive growth fostering); no significant increases in infant behaviors during teaching emerged. Further, significant increases were found in three areas of assessing quality of the home environment: responsivity of mother, provision of appropriate play materials, and opportunities for variety of daily stimulation. Finally, compared to normative sample data available on feeding interaction, teaching interaction, and the home environment, the NSTEP-P sample in general fared as well or better.

Second, White-Traut and Nelson (1988) randomly assigned 33 mothers and their preterm infants to three groups: control, talking-only, and the Rice Infant Sensorimotor Stimulation Technique (RISS) (Rice, 1977) of massage and rocking. Infants were between 28 and 35 weeks' gestation age at birth and were not on assisted ventilation. The control group received routine care and, in addition, a discussion of infant clothing. The talking-only group received the discussion of infant clothing and instruction about talking or singing to their infants for 15 minutes at four intervals during the mothers' postpartum hospitalization. Those in the RISS group were instructed to massage their infants for 10 minutes and rock them for 5 minutes according to a set protocol at four intervals during maternal hospitalization. On the day preceding infants' hospital discharge, mother-infant interaction was rated during feeding. Overall, significant differences among the three groups were found for maternal interactive behavior as well as infant behavior. Pairwise comparisons between groups with regard to infant behavior revealed no significant differences. As for maternal behavior, group differences specifically occurred in the areas of sensitivity to infant cues (favoring the RISS group over the control group) and cognitive growth fostering (favoring the RISS group over both the talking-only and control groups).

The remaining study concerned with interaction-related interventions was a meta-analysis conducted by Turley (1985). Twenty studies that tested the effects on parent-infant interaction of giving parents information about infants' sensory and related capabilities were found. Across the studies, overall effect size was 0.44, indicating that the overall effects of interventions favored intervention groups over control groups. A significantly larger effect size occurred if interventions were provided in the home setting rather than in the hospital. Further, interventions provided after 4 weeks postdischarge had the greatest effect size. (See Worobey [1985] for a related review.)

FUTURE RESEARCH DIRECTIONS

Threaded through studies on behavioral interaction is the supposition that early parent-infant interaction forms a base for the further development of the infant and for the quality of the parent-infant relationship. (See Chapter 20 for studies that link the parenting environment to children's development.) Although not directly opposing the hypothesis about the importance of early contact, studies of interaction provide a more dynamic and evolving view of the parent-infant relationships. Further, studies of behavioral interaction between parents and infants reveal the intimate aspects of the day-to-day interchanges that shape the relationship. For this reason, research on behavioral interaction is essential to the field of parent-infant nursing—for understanding basic processes, for assessment, and for focusing intervention.

The importance to nursing of the early parent-infant relationship is revealed in concern with such phenomena as attachment and role attainment (Chapters 9, 13, and 14). The preverbal nature of the infant, however, makes the study of relational phenomena accessible largely through observational methods and specifically through those focused on behavioral interaction. Thus, it is important that conceptual and empirical bridges be built between behavioral interaction and the other prevailing construct systems in parent-infant nursing.

Because measuring behavioral interaction involves careful observation and specialized training, it is time-intensive. Fortunately, a variety of observational protocols to aid investigators are available. Noteworthy among them are the teaching and feeding scales developed by Barnard and associates (1989). They and other ratings scales are of special interest because of their utility in capturing early interactional phenomena (Parke & Tinsley, 1987). Also, ratings scales, in contrast to microanalytic approaches, often lend themselves to clinical applications such as assessment protocols.

Finally, to build effectively on what is already known about interaction (Osofsky & Conners, 1979; Parke, 1979; Parke & Tinsley, 1987; Field, 1987), it is important that programs of nursing research that emphasize behavioral interaction emerge. To date, too few nurse investigators have made behavioral interaction a continuing central focus of their research. Such a focus is needed in order to further develop nursing knowledge about how best to intervene: (1) with dyads showing interactive deficits, (2) with subpopulations known to deviate from normative patterns of interaction—such as preterm infants, and (3) with culturally diverse populations in ways that are culturally sensitive.

REFERENCES

Anderson, C. J. (1981). Enhancing reciprocity between mother and neonate. *Nursing Research, 30,* 89-93.

Barnard, K. E., & Bee, H. L. (1983). The impact of temporally patterned stimulation on the development of preterm infants. *Child Development, 54,* 1156-1167.

Barnard, K. E., Bee, H. L., & Hammond, M. A. (1984). Developmental changes in maternal interactions with term and preterm infants. *Infant Behavior and Development, 7,* 101-113.

Barnard, K. E., Booth, C. L., Mitchell, S. K., & Telzrow, R. W. (1988). Newborn nursing models: A test of early intervention to high-risk infants and families. In E. D. Hibbs (Ed.), *Children and families: Studies in prevention and intervention* (pp. 63-81). Madison: International Universities Press.

Barnard, K. E., Hammond, M. A., Booth, C. L., Bee, H. L., Mitchell, S. K., & Spieker, S. J. (1989). Measurement and meaning of parent-child interaction. In F. J. Morrison, C. Lord, & D. P. Keating (Eds.), *Applied developmental psychology* (Vol. 3, pp. 39-80). New York: Academic Press.

Barnard, K. E., Hammond, M. A., Sumner, G. A., Kang, R., Johnson-Crowley, N., Snyder, C., Spietz, A., Blackburn, S., Brandt, P., & Magyary, D. (1987). Helping parents with preterm infants: Field test of a protocol. *Early Child Development and Care, 27,* 255-290.

Barnard, K. E., Magyary, D., Sumner, G., Booth, C. L., Mitchell, S. K., & Spieker, S. (1988). Prevention of parenting alterations for women with low social support. *Psychiatry, 51*(3), 248-253.

Bee, H. L., Barnard, K. E., Eyres, S. J., Gray, C. A., Hammond, M. A., Spietz, A. L., Snyder, C., & Clark, B. (1982). Prediction of IQ and language skill from perinatal status, child performance, family characteristics, and mother-infant interaction. *Child Development, 53,* 1134-1156.

Blank, D. M. (1986). Relating mothers' anxiety and perception to infant satiety, anxiety, and feeding behavior. *Nursing Research, 35,* 347-351.

Booth, C. L., Johnson-Crowley, N., & Barnard, K. E. (1985). Infant massage and exercise: Worth the effort? *MCN, The American Journal of Maternal/Child Nursing, 10,* 184-189.

Booth, C. L., Lyons, N. B., & Barnard, K. E. (1984). Synchrony in mother-infant interaction: A comparison of measurement methods. *Child Study Journal, 14*(2), 95-114.

Booth, C. L., Mitchell S. K., Barnard, K. E., & Spieker, S. J. (1989). Development of maternal social skills in multiproblem families: Effects on the mother-child relationship. *Developmental Psychology, 25,* 403-412.

Capuzzi, C. (1989). Maternal attachment to handicapped infants and the relationship to social support. *Research in Nursing and Health, 12,* 161-167.

Censullo, M., Bowler, R., Lester, B., & Brazelton, T. B. (1987). An instrument for the measurement of infant-adult synchrony. *Nursing Research, 36,* 244-248.

Censullo, M., Lester, B., & Hoffman, J. (1985). Rhythmic patterning in mother-newborn interaction. *Nursing Research, 34,* 342-346.

Chamorro, I. L., Davis, M. L., Green, D., & Kramer, M. (1973). Development of an instrument to measure premature infant behavior and caretaker activities: Time-sampling methodology. *Nursing Research, 22,* 300-309.

Choi, E. S. C., & Hamilton, R. K. (1986). The effects of culture on mother-infant interaction. *Journal of Obstetric, Gynecologic and Neonatal Nursing, 15,* 256-261.

Dormire, S. L., Strauss, S. S., & Clarke, B. A. (1989). Social support and adaptation to the parent role in first-time adolescent mothers. *Journal of Obstetric, Gynecologic and Neonatal Nursing, 18,* 327-337.

Dzik, M. A. (1979). Maternal comforting of the distressed infant. *Maternal-Child Nursing Journal, 8,* 163-171.

Field, T. (1987). Affective and interactive disturbance in infants. In J. D. Osofsky (Ed.), *Handbook of infant development* (2nd ed., pp. 972-1005). New York: Wiley.

Flick, L. H., & McSweeney, M. (1987). Measures of mother-child interaction: A comparison of three methods. *Research in Nursing & Health, 10,* 129–137.

Furr, P. A., & Kirgis, C. A. (1982). A nurse-midwifery approach to early mother-infant acquaintance. *Journal of Nurse-Midwifery, 27,* 10–14.

Goldberg, S. (1977). Social competence in infancy: A model of parent-infant interaction. *Merrill-Palmer Quarterly, 23,* 165–177.

Hansen, M. F., Pridham, K. F., Stephenson, G. R., & Tsui, P. (1987). The clinically focused descriptive study: A method of graphic summary of complex observational data. *Computers in Nursing, 5*(2), 50–58.

Harrison, L. L., & Twardosz, S. (1986). Teaching mothers about their preterm infants. *Journal of Obstetric, Gynecologic and Neonatal Nursing, 15,* 165–172.

Holaday, B. (1982). Maternal conceptual set development: Identifying patterns of maternal response to chronically ill infant crying. *Maternal-Child Nursing Journal, 11,* 47–59.

Holaday, B. (1987). Patterns of interaction between mothers and their chronically ill infants. *Maternal-Child Nursing Journal, 16,* 29–45.

Humenick, S. S., & Bugen, L. A. (1981). Correlates of parent-infant interaction: An exploratory study. In R. P. Lederman, B. S. Raff, & P. Carroll (Eds.), *Perinatal parental behavior: Nursing research and implications for newborn health.* New York: Liss. March of Dimes Birth Defects Foundation. *Birth Defects, Original Article Series, 17*(6), 181–199.

Johnson, D. (1980). The behavioral system model for nursing. In J. Riehl & C. Roy (Eds.), *Conceptual models for nursing practice* (2nd ed., pp. 207–216). New York: Appleton-Century-Crofts.

Jones, L. C., & Lenz, E. R. (1986). Father-newborn interaction: Effects of social competence and infant state. *Nursing Research, 35,* 149–153.

Jones, L. C., & Thomas, S. A. (1989). New fathers' blood pressure and heart rate: Relationships to interaction with their newborn infants. *Nursing Research, 38,* 237–241.

Julian, K. C. (1983). A comparison of perceived and demonstrated maternal role competence of adolescent mothers. *Issues in Health Care of Women, 4,* 223–236.

Karraker, K. H. (1986). Adult attention to infants in a newborn nursery. *Nursing Research, 35,* 358–363.

Kramer, M., Chamorro, I., Green, D., & Knudtson, F. (1975). Extra tactile stimulation of the premature infant. *Nursing Research, 24,* 324–334.

Magyary, D. (1983). Cross-time and cross-situational comparisons of mother-preterm infant interactions. (Proceeding of Western Society for Research in Nursing Conference). *Western Journal of Nursing Research, 5,* 15–25.

Osofsky, J. D., & Connors, K. (1979). Mother-infant interaction: An integrative view of a complex system. In J. D. Osofsky (Ed.), *Handbook of infant development* (pp. 519–548). New York: Wiley.

Parke, R. D. (1979). Perspectives on father-infant interaction. In J. D. Osofsky (Ed.), *Handbook of infant development* (pp. 549–590). New York: Wiley.

Parke, R. D., & Tinsley, B. J. (1987). Family interaction in infancy. In J. D. Osofsky (Ed.), *Handbook of infant development* (2nd ed., pp. 579–641). New York: Wiley.

Perry, S. E. (1983). Parents' perceptions of their newborn following structured interactions. *Nursing Research, 32,* 208–212.

Poley-Strobel, B. A., & Beckmann, C. A. (1987). The effects of a teaching-modeling intervention on early mother-infant reciprocity. *Infant Behavior and Development, 10,* 467–476.

Price, G. M. (1983). Sensitivity in mother-infant interactions: The AMIS scale. *Infant Behavior and Development, 6,* 353–360.

Rice, R. D. (1977). Neurophysical development in premature infants following stimulation. *Developmental Psychology, 13,* 69–76.

Riesch, S. (1979). Enhancement of mother-infant social interaction. *Journal of Obstetric, Gynecologic and Neonatal Nursing, 8,* 242–246.

Riesch, S. K. (1984). Occupational commitment and the quality of maternal infant interaction. *Research in Nursing and Health, 7,* 295–503.

Riesch, S. K., & Munns, S. K. (1984). Promoting awareness: The mother and her baby. *Nursing Research, 33,* 271-276.

Ruff, C. C. (1987). How well do adolescents mother? *MCN, The American Journal of Maternal/Child Nursing, 12,* 249-253.

Schroeder-Zwelling, E., & Hock, E. (1986). Maternal anxiety and sensitive mothering behavior in diabetic and nondiabetic women. *Research in Nursing & Health, 9,* 249-255.

Sullivan, H. S. (1953). *The interpersonal theory of psychiatry.* New York: Norton.

Turley, M. A. (1985). A meta-analysis of informing mothers concerning the sensory and perceptual capabilities of their infants: The effects on maternal-infant interaction. *Maternal-Child Nursing Journal, 14,* 183-197.

Walker, L. O., Crain, H., & Thompson, E. (1986). Mothering behavior and maternal role attainment during the postpartum period. *Nursing Research, 35,* 352-355.

Walker, L. O., & Thompson, E. T. (1982). Mother-infant play interaction scale. In S. S. Humenick (Ed.), *Analysis of current assessment strategies in the health care of young children and childbearing families* (pp. 191-201). Norwalk, CN: Appleton-Century-Crofts.

White-Traut, R. C., & Nelson, M. N. (1988). Maternally administered tactile, auditory, visual, and vestibular stimulation: Relationship to later interactions between mothers and premature infants. *Research in Nursing & Health, 11,* 31-39.

Worobey, J. (1985). A review of Brazelton-based interventions to enhance parent-infant interaction. *Journal of Reproductive and Infant Psychology, 3,* 64-73.

PART SIX

Person-Environment Interaction and Development

CHAPTER 19

The Paradigm of Person-Environment Interaction and Development

OVERVIEW OF THE PARADIGM

The paradigm of person-environment interaction and development (PEID) focuses on mutual influence of individuals and their environments that shape human development. Barnard has referred to such a perspective as the ecology of human development (Barnard, Eyres, Lobo, & Snyder, 1983). This paradigm was heavily influenced by Sameroff and Chandler's (1975) pivotal review concluding that, except in the most severe cases, biological risk alone was insufficient to predict later child development. Instead, it was the mutual influence of biological risk in the context of certain environments that most profoundly affected children's later development. Thus, the concepts of person, environment, and development (1) provide abstract ways of modeling how children arrive at differing levels on outcomes and (2) aid in identifying risk factors that signal potential for compromised outcomes. Further, the concepts attempt to account for instances wherein individuals overcome or fail to succumb to manifestly difficult circumstances.

KEY CONCEPTS AND RELATIONSHIPS

PERSON

The concept of person refers broadly to the individual parent and infant with their inherent genetic and acquired characteristics. Key attributes of adult persons include personality variables, such as intelligence, self-concept, trait anxiety, and social competence, as well as biological condition. In infants, biological condition is a key variable. Within a PEID paradigm, the concept of person in particular represents factors residing within the individual, which increase (risk factors) or decrease (protective factors) the likelihood of compromised outcomes. Although personal factors that increase the risk of compromised development are widely known, for example, preterm birth, a few investigators have studied protective factors, such as self-esteem (Garmezy, 1985), that reduce risk. With regard to the infant in particular, it is important to note that person characteristics and developmental level are not fixed properties of an entity but instead are changing attributes of the same individual, views that Sameroff (1978) has called the mechanical object and living subject, respectively.

ENVIRONMENT

The concept of environment is one of the most broad and difficult concepts to define. At its simplest, it is everything that stands outside the individual. During infancy, environment has particular salience because, like other primates, humans bear altricial, not precocial, young. Because a long period of specialized care is required before maturation is complete, environment can be contrasted with such concepts as heredity. It also has more restricted meanings. In regard to parents, it often refers to context—particularly the social context. Social support and social network often are used to index parents' social context. In regard to the infant's context, environment typically has still broader meaning. It includes not only the social environment provided by parents or caregivers and the physical or inanimate surroundings in which the infant lives but also the socioeconomic context.

The environment may increase risk or compensate for personal risk factors. It may pose direct risk for an infant or may increase risk because it adds a needed ingredient to a complex combination of person variables that lead to increased incidence of compromised development. One of the most global environmental variables associated with risk and compromised outcomes is low socioeconomic status. Despite its predictive power, socioeconomic status is only a summary variable and represents a complex combination of other variables that enhance or inhibit healthy development (Sameroff, Seifer, Barocas, Zax, & Greenspan, 1987).

The environment may also operate correctively or preventively in the face of risk factors (Cohen, Sigman, Parmelee, & Beckwith, 1982). Sameroff (1985) proposed that the caretaking environment may have norms for parental or others' behavior that aid in self-righting after biological insults or risks to infants. Some of the environmental factors that operate to protect children in the face of insults are family warmth and cohesiveness and available support systems (Garmezy, 1985).

DEVELOPMENT

The concept of development, as often used in parent-infant nursing research, has to do with the unfolding of age-related competencies—physical, mental, and social—in the infant and child through interaction with the environment. Development shares meaning with maturation. Although maturation may emphasize the emergence of age-related normative changes and changes in the direction of greater complexity, development also reflects plasticity with respect to the manner in which maturational changes are manifest. Views of development may, alternatively, see it as goal-directed (organismic) or simply as a description of age-related behaviors (behavioristic). (For an analysis of organismic and behavioristic definitions of development, see Reese and Overton, 1970.)

Sameroff (1985) summarized the research about early developmental functioning and later outcomes by using the principles of convergent and divergent development. Simply stated, a common developmental outcome may ensue from differing beginning points, whereas one developmental point may be associated with different end points. These principles underlie the complex and dynamic relations between environment and development addressed below.

THE INTERRELATIONS OF PERSON, ENVIRONMENT, AND DEVELOPMENT

The key characteristic about the relations of person, environment, and development is that they are not fixed but fluid during infancy. Thus, Barnard et al. (1983) have noted: "The low predictive validity of assessments during the first year of life has been consistent with the highly dynamic interplay between the developing child and the changing styles of the environment" (p. 199). Where continuity is found, however, it is usually not a simple relation. For example, Barnard et al. (1983) have described patterning within the caregiving environment as it relates to developmental outcomes as follows:

When a child's cues are difficult to interpret or if the parent perceives very little positive feedback when trying to interact with the child, then the parent-child adaptive process is interrupted, and eventually the child's developmental progress will be influenced. Conversely, if the parent does not respond to the infant's cues or if the parent fails to alleviate the child's distress or to provide growth fostering situations, then the parent-child interaction system does not support the environment necessary for a positive developmental course." (p. 209)

The dynamic interplay of person, environment, and development renders simple linear models of development of limited utility. The structural relations in linear and dynamic models in the context of infancy are presented in Figure 19–1. Dynamic models of development parallel the adoption of field models for describing developmental shifts in infancy (Emde, Gaensbauer, and Harmon, 1976).

More generally, concern about the relations between person and environment have been evident in nursing. Clarke and Driever (1983) proposed that the construct of vulnerability be understood in terms of the perceived transactions between individual capabilities and environmental situations. Clarke and Driever's construct of vulnerability is congruent with a dynamic model of development, but it is limited in its application to young infants because it requires a level of perceptual awareness not present at early ages.

Overall, the link between developmental outcomes and infant behavior and experience is not strong (Rutter, 1987). That may be true because (1) infancy constitutes only a small part of total development, (2) later biological changes such as puberty are not linked to preceding stages, and (3) with new maturational competencies, individuals may reprocess past experiences (Rutter, 1987). In turn, when continuities between infancy and later development are found, Rutter (1987) has outlined possible mechanisms responsible for them: structural changes, habits, attitudes, and self-concepts, vulnerabilities and sensitivities, environmental links, and person-environment transactions. Of these, links between early environments and later ones are the major source of continuities.

METHODOLOGY

Studies of person-environment interaction as they pertain to development must necessarily be done longitudinally. That is because cross-sectional and retrospective studies may be misleading due to confusion about cause and effects or sampling biases, to mention only two examples. Although longitudinal studies are costly, they must be well done to be informative. To compare alternative sources of influence over time, large numbers of variables are typically sampled and analyzed by using multi-

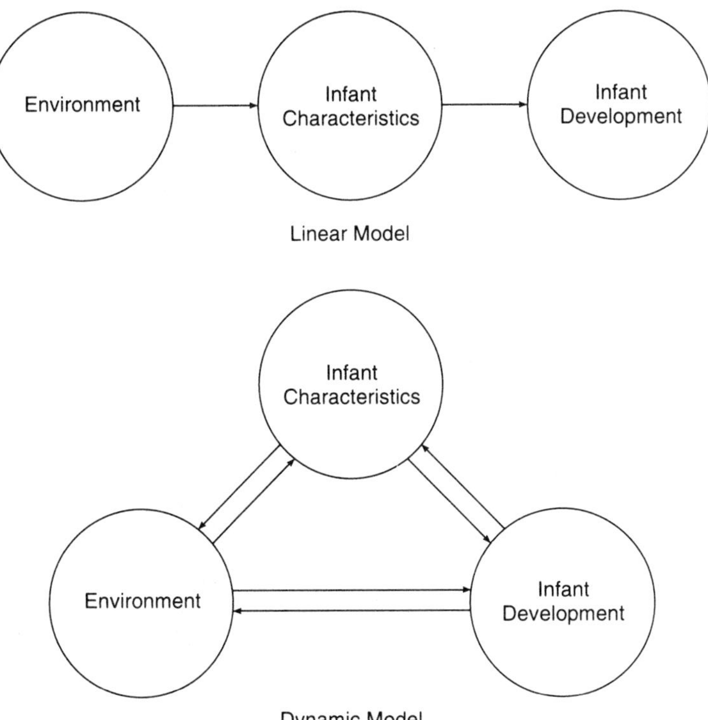

Figure 19–1
Models of development.

variate statistical procedures. That, in turn, necessitates a sample size sufficiently large for reliable findings. Finally, conducting quality longitudinal research is contingent on maintaining the sample size across the duration of the study to avoid differential attrition of such subgroups as low-income parents (Zahr, Parker, Cole, & Engler, 1989). All these considerations dictate that longitudinal research be carefully planned conceptually and operationally if it is to be successful (Magnusson & Bergman, 1990). For example, Zahr et al. (1989) suggest specific strategies, such as collaboration with public health nurses, to aid in preventing attrition of low socioeconomic families.

Selection of predictive measures is a major consideration in longitudinal research. One of the prevailing views in predictive studies of development is that single risk factors, except perhaps for socioeconomic status, are seldom powerful predictors (Sameroff et al., 1987). Instead, it is the accumulation or number of risk factors that is associated with compromised child outcomes. For example, Sameroff et al. (1987) showed that 10 risk factors (maternal mental health, maternal anxiety, parental perspectives, maternal interactive behavior, maternal education, occupation of head of household, minority status, family social support, family size, and stressful life events) accounted for more variance in children's intelligence than socioeconomic status. A related consideration is *when* predictors and outcomes measures should be sampled. For example, not all environmental features are equally salient at differing points in development. Sensitivity to when specific features of the environment may interact with particular characteristics of the child is important in timing data collection points.

REFERENCES

Barnard, K., Eyres, S., Lobo M., & Snyder, C. (1983). An ecological paradigm for assessment and intervention. In T. B. Brazelton & B. M. Lester (Eds.), *New approaches to developmental screening of infants* (pp. 199–218). New York: Elsevier.

Clarke, H. F., & Driever, M. J. (1983). Vulnerability: The development of a construct for nursing. In P. L. Chinn (Ed.), *Advances in nursing theory development* (pp. 207–220). Rockville, MD: Aspen.

Cohen, S. E., Sigman, M., Parmelee, A. H., & Beckwith, L. (1982). Perinatal risk and developmental outcome in preterm infants. *Seminars in Perinatology, 6,* 334–339.

Emde, R. N., Gaensbauer, T. J., & Harmon, R. J. (1976). Emotional expression in infancy: A biobehavioral study [Monograph 37]. *Psychological Issues, 10*(1), 3–198. New York: International Universities Press.

Garmezy, N. (1985). Broadening research on developmental risk. In W. K. Frankenburg, R. N. Emde, & J. W. Sullivan (Eds.), *Early identification of child at risk: An international perspective* (pp. 45–58). New York: Plenum.

Magnusson, D., & Bergman, L. R. (Eds.) (1990). *Data quality in longitudinal research.* Cambridge, England: Cambridge University Press.

Reese, H. W., & Overton, W. F. (1970). Models of development and theories of development. In L. R. Goulet & P. B. Baltes (Eds.), *Life-span developmental psychology* (pp. 115–145). New York: Academic Press.

Rutter, M. (1987). Continuities and discontinuities in infancy. In J. D. Osofsky (Ed.), *Handbook of infant development* (2nd ed., pp. 1256–1296). New York: Wiley.

Sameroff, A. J. (1978). Caretaking or reproductive casualty? Determinants in developmental deviancy. In F. D. Horowitz (Ed.), *AAAS Selected Symposia Series, 19,* 79–101. Boulder, CO: Westview Press.

Sameroff, A. J. (1985). Environmental factors in the early screening of children at risk. In W. K. Frankenburg, R. N. Emde, & J. W. Sullivan (Eds.), *Early identification of children at risk: An international perspective* (pp. 21–44). New York: Plenum.

Sameroff, A. J., & Chandler, M. (1975). Reproductive risk and the continuum of caretaking casualty. In F. D. Horowitz, M. Hetherington, S. Scarr-Salapatek, & G. Siegel (Eds.), *Review of child development research* (Vol. 4, pp. 187–244). Chicago: University of Chicago Press.

Sameroff, A. J., Seifer, R., Barocas, R., Zax, M., & Greenspan, S. (1987). Intelligence quotient scores of 4-year-old children: Social-environmental risk factors. *Pediatrics, 79*(3), 343–350.

Zahr, L., Parker, S., Cole, J., & Engler, C. (1989). Follow-up of premature infants of low socioeconomic status. *Nursing Research, 38,* 246–247.

CHAPTER 20

Parent-Infant Nursing Research on Person-Environment Interaction and Development

DEFINITIONS AND DESCRIPTIONS OF DEVELOPMENT AND ENVIRONMENT

In this chapter two elements of the person-environment interaction and development paradigm are considered: environment and development. The element of person or personal characteristics is subsumed in preceding chapters, for example, behavioral organization and health status. Because of their interdependent nature, this chapter considers the two phenomena of development and environment simultaneously. In infants, development is critically shaped by the environment. In turn, aspects of the environment become salient only as they shape developmental processes. Further, the concept of environment has a broader meaning in relation to infants. Whereas parental environments are typically described in terms of social support or other sociodemographic parameters, the dependent nature of the infant extends the concept of environment to include the many external influences affecting early development.

DEFINING DEVELOPMENT AND ENVIRONMENT

Schraeder (1986) depicted "developmental progress" as the "product of interrelated medical, biological, and environmental spheres of influence" (p. 237). Schraeder (1986) also defined the concept of canalization pertinent to early development as "the tendency of all members of a species to follow a single path . . . under typical environmental conditions" (p. 241).

THEORETICAL MODELS OF DEVELOPMENT AND ENVIRONMENT

Although most studies did not use a highly elaborated theoretical framework, several predictive studies explicitly stated broad views of the dynamic nature of the relations between children and their environment (e.g., Schraeder, 1986; Schraeder, Rappaport, & Courtwright, 1987). Intervention studies of the effects of stimulation on infant growth and development provided rationales for potential effects based on environmental deprivation of preterm infants (e.g., Malloy, 1979; Kramer, Chamorro, Green, & Knudtson, 1975; Nelson, Heitman, & Jennings, 1986) or need for temporal patterning (Barnard & Bee, 1983).

MEASUREMENT

GENERAL STRATEGIES

Assessment of the environment may take many forms. Observational rating scales comprise one way to measure the stimulus properties and organization of the infant's immediate environment. A broad summary variable pertinent to the environment is socioeconomic status.

Measures of child development fall into two classifications: (1) assessments suitable for developmental screening and (2) tests that require extensive training and administration time so that their use is limited to research or in-depth child assessment. For a review of screening tools, see Castiglia and Petrini (1985).

SPECIFIC TOOLS

Table 20–1 presents tools related to measuring properties of development and the environment. It is clear from Table 20–1 that the most widely used measure of infant development is the Bayley Scales of Infant Development (Bayley, 1969). Caregiving environments of infants most often have been assessed with the Home Observation for Measurement of the Environment (HOME) (Caldwell & Bradley, 1978; Bradley & Caldwell, 1979).

Table 20–1
MEASURES/TOOLS FOR THE CONCEPTS OF DEVELOPMENT AND ENVIRONMENT

Tool	Source Described in	Studies Using Tool
	TOOLS MEASURING DEVELOPMENT	
Mother's Expectations about Baby's Age for Specified Activities: Five-item scale for maternal expectations	Barnard & Eyres (1979) Snyder et al. (1979)	Becker (1987) Snyder et al. (1979) Bee et al. (1982) Mitchell et al. (1985)
Physical and Adaptive Social Development: Scales for assessing developmental status	Ross Laboratories 625 Cleveland Ave. Columbus, OH 43215	Mercer et al. (1984b) Mercer (1986) Mercer et al. (1984a)
Graham/Rosenblith Behavioral Examination: Test of general maturation for newborns with scores for motor and other neurological areas	Rosenblith (1961) Rosenblith (1979)	Neal (1969) Katz (1971) Malloy (1979)
Bayley Scales of Infant Development: Standardized scales of mental and motor development	Bayley (1969)	Barnard, Booth, Mitchell, & Telzrow (1988) Barnard, Magyary, et al. (1988) Becker et al. (1989) Koniak-Griffin & Rummell (1988) Koniak-Griffin & Ludington-Hoe (1988) Barnard & Bee (1983) Trotter et al. (1982) Snyder et al. (1979) Bee et al. (1982) Barnard et al. (1984b) Mitchell et al. (1985) Booth et al. (1985) Kramer et al. (1975) Malloy (1979) Rice (1979)

Table 20–1
MEASURES/TOOLS FOR THE CONCEPTS OF DEVELOPMENT AND ENVIRONMENT *(Continued)*

Tool	Source Described in	Studies Using Tool
	TOOLS MEASURING DEVELOPMENT (Continued)	
Gesell Development Schedules: Multiple-component test of developmental status	Gesell & Amatruda (1947)	Porter (1972) Kramer et al. (1975)
Stanford-Binet Intelligence Scale: Test of mental development	Terman & Merrill (1973)	Bee et al. (1982) Barnard et al. (1984b) Mitchell et al. (1985)
McCarthy Scales of Children's Abilities: Test for mental and motor development	McCarthy (1972)	Bee et al. (1982) Mitchell et al. (1985)
Sequenced Inventory of Communication Development: Test of receptive and expressive language	Hedrick et al. (1975)	Bee et al. (1982) Mitchell et al. (1985)
Fluharty Speech and Language Screening Test: Test of receptive and expressive language	Fluharty (1974)	Bee et al. (1982) Mitchell et al. (1985)
Preschool Behavior Questionnaire: Scale for assessment of socioemotional development	Behar & Stringfield (1974)	Bee et al. (1982) Mitchell et al. (1985)
Minnesota Child Development Inventory: Three hundred twenty item inventory completed by parent to assess for developmental delay	Ireton & Thwing (1974)	Schraeder (1986) Schraeder et al. (1987)
Peabody Individual Achievement Test: Test of academic achievement	Dunn & Markwardt (1970)	Mitchell et al. (1985)
Wechsler Intelligence Scale for Children-Revised: Test of general intelligence	Wechsler (1974)	Mitchell et al. (1985)
Pupil Rating Scale: Scale for classroom behavior problems	Myklebust (1981)	Mitchell et al. (1985)

McDaniel-Piers Young Children's Self-Concept Scale: Scale for self-concept of children	McDaniel & Piers (1973)	Mitchell et al. (1985)
Denver Developmental Screening Test: Screening test for risk of developmental delay	Frankenburg & Dodds (1977) Frankenberg, Goldstein, & Camp (1971)	Medoff-Cooper & Schraeder (1982) Schraeder & Medoff-Cooper (1983) Schraeder (1986) Bee et al. (1982) Mitchell et al. (1985)
Denver Prescreening Developmental Questionnaire: Brief screening tool for developmental status	Frankenburg, van Doornick, Liddell, & Dick (1976)	Barnard et al. (1987)
Phylogenetic reflexes	—	Rice (1979)
Mature reflexes	—	Rice (1979)
Head circumference	—	Whiteman et al. (1985) Rice (1979)
Height or length gain	—	Whiteman et al. (1985) Porter (1972) Rice (1979)
Weight or weight gain	—	Whiteman et al. (1985) Neal (1969) Nelson et al. (1986) Porter (1972) Malloy (1979) Rice (1979)
Plasma cortisol	—	Kramer et al. (1975)

Table 20–1
MEASURES/TOOLS FOR THE CONCEPTS OF DEVELOPMENT AND ENVIRONMENT *(Continued)*

Tool	Source Described in	Studies Using Tool
	TOOLS MEASURING ENVIRONMENT	
Home Observation for Measurement of the Environment (HOME): Observer and interview-based assessment of the home environment (infancy and preschool versions)	Caldwell & Bradley (1978) Bradley & Caldwell (1979)	Bee, Hammond, Eyres, Barnard, & Snyder (1986) Barnard, Booth et al. (1988) Barnard et al. (1987) Harrison & Twardosz (1986) Medoff-Cooper & Schraeder (1982) Schraeder & Medoff-Cooper (1983) Medoff-Cooper (1986) Houldin (1987) Schraeder (1986) Schraeder et al. (1987) Snyder et al. (1979) Bee et al. (1982) Barnard et al. (1984b) Mitchell et al. (1985)
Modification of HOME scale: Adapted for clinic setting	Barnard & Bee (1983)	Barnard & Bee (1983) Barnard et al. (1984a) Bee et al. (1982) Barnard et al. (1984b)
Time-sampling tool for caregiving activities in neonatal intensive care	Orsuto (1985) as cited in Pohlman & Beardslee (1987)	Pohlman & Beardslee (1987)

Not cited in the list, because of their pervasive nature, are indicators of socioeconomic status. For a review of indices of socioeconomic status, see Mueller and Parcel (1981).

SUMMARY OF RESEARCH

SCOPE OF DEVELOPMENTAL AND ENVIRONMENT RESEARCH

Table 20–2 presents studies of development and the environment. The studies include descriptive, correlational, and interventive investigations of infants' developmental outcomes and their environments. (For additional studies of caregiving environments as they relate to infant behavioral organization and interaction, see Chapters 17 and 18. For additional studies on the relations of social support to developmental outcomes, see Chapter 5. For a summary of effects of stimulation programs on premature infants, see the Appendix.)

DESCRIPTIVE RESEARCH

Descriptions of Caregiving Environments

Thomas (1989) examined sound levels associated with receiving care in a Level III neonatal intensive care unit. A sound meter located inside an incubator placed in the center of the nursery indicated sound levels for various environmental events. Although average sound levels for the events studied did not exceed 90 decibels, peak decibel levels of several events did. Examples are tapping hood of incubator with fingers, shutting incubator cabinet, placing plastic bottle on top of incubator, shutting solid plastic port, and dropping head of mattress.

A study conducted by Duxbury, Henly, Broz, Armstrong, and Wachdorf (1984) provides evidence of caregiving events experienced by infants in neonatal intensive care units. Over 74 three-hour-long observations made on 48 infants, the duration of caregiving events, person providing care/contact, and type of care were recorded along with related infant data (Chapter 17). The frequency of occurrence of caregiving events was as follows: activities of daily living/comfort (28 percent), observation/monitoring (38 percent), and medications and treatments (34 percent). The number of caregiving events occurring over a 3-hour period ranged from 1 to 15. Infants averaged 14 minutes of caregiving events per hour. The mean interval between events was just over 30 minutes. Nurses were most often the ones who performed caregiving events. Shift and day of week were not associated with differences in frequency and duration of care-

Table 20–2
PARENT-INFANT NURSING RESEARCH ON DEVELOPMENT AND THE ENVIRONMENT

DESCRIPTIVE
Descriptions of the Environment
Blackburn & Barnard (1985), caregiving events in intensive care
Duxbury et al. (1984), caregiving events in intensive care
Pohlman & Beardslee (1987), contact with infants in intensive care unit
Thomas (1989), sound levels in intensive care unit
Descriptions of Development
Medoff-Cooper & Schraeder (1982), very low birth weight infants
Schraeder & Medoff-Cooper (1983), very low birth weight infants
Differences in Development
Barnard et al. (1984b), infants of high- vs. low-education mothers
Becker (1987), adolescent vs. adult mothers' developmental expectations
Mercer et al. (1984a), infants of mothers in three age groups
Whiteman et al. (1985), infants with vs. without NEC
RELATIONSHIPS AMONG VARIABLES/PREDICTIVE MODELS
Barnard et al. (1984b), predictors of developmental outcomes at 12, 24, and 48 months
Bee et al. (1982), predictors of developmental outcomes at 36 and 48 months
Mitchell et al. (1985), predictors of development outcomes at 8 years
Schraeder (1986), predictors of developmental outcomes at 6 and 12 months
Schraeder et al. (1987), predictors of development outcomes at 36 months
Snyder et al. (1979), predictors of development outcomes at 12 and 24 months
Trotter et al. (1982), predictors of developmental outcomes at 12 months
INTERVENTION RESEARCH
Barnard & Bee (1983), three patterns of infant stimulation
Booth et al. (1985), infant message
Katz (1971), tape recording of mother's voice
Koniak-Griffin & Ludington-Hoe (1988), unimodal and multimodal stimulation
Kramer et al. (1975), stroking
Malloy (1979), tape recording of mother's voice or lullaby
Neal (1969), swinging hammock
Nelson et al. (1986), pile decubitus ulcer pad
Porter (1972), passive motion exercises
Rice (1979), stroking/massage & rocking

giving events. Severity of illness, as expected, was associated with frequency and duration of caregiving events.

In the context of a larger study, Blackburn and Barnard (1985) studied caregiving events experienced by preterm infants in the intensive care unit. Infants' mean postbirth age was 6.8 days. Using 24-hour time-lapse videotaping, caregiving events at six time points were recorded for 102 infants. Just over 14 percent of the 24-hour cycle was comprised of caregiving events. The mean duration of events over 24 hours was as follows: out of incubator for 86 minutes, diapering/feeding for 56.7 minutes, miscellaneous/technical for 47.4 minutes, and social stroking for 18.6 minutes.

Pohlman and Beardslee (1987) conducted a descriptive study to identify types of contact experienced by 16 infants in intensive care units (pediatric and neonatal). Infants' ages ranged from 2 to 26 days. By using time sampling during 2-hour observation periods, direct and indirect contacts were tabulated. Of 3840 observational points, 2205 involved either direct (61 percent) or indirect (39 percent) contacts with one or more caretakers. The proportion of direct contacts was distributed as follows: highly intrusive procedures (11 percent); moderately intrusive procedures (49 percent); minimally intrusive procedures (9 percent); activities of daily living (15 percent); and comforting touch (16 percent). Most direct contacts (60 percent) were from registered nurses. Infants on assisted ventilation received three times less comforting touch than infants not on assisted ventilation. Among other findings, intrusive contacts were similar regardless of physiological stability of infants. However, comforting touch was virtually absent in the case of the most seriously ill infants.

Descriptions of Developmental Status

In a study of 26 very low birth weight (VLBW) infants, Medoff-Cooper and Schraeder (1982) completed infant assessments at 7.9 months corrected age. On a developmental screening test, 88 percent of the infants met criteria for being at risk for developmental delay using uncorrected age. Based on use of age corrected for prematurity, 42 percent met criteria for being at risk. Infants were most often delayed in the areas of gross motor development. Scores on the developmental screening test were unrelated to overall characteristics of the home environment.

In a further study of 20 of the original 26 VLBW infants, Schraeder and Medoff-Cooper (1983) reassessed infants at 19 months (mean age corrected for prematurity). Based on corrected age, 20 percent of the VLBW sample was at risk for developmental delay. This was a significant reduction from the 42 percent at risk during the first year. Again, developmental status was unrelated to characteristics of the home environment.

Differences in Development

In an investigation of differences among three maternal-age groups (15 to 19, 20 to 29, and 30 to 42), Mercer, Hackley, and Bostrom (1984a) compared 294 new mothers and their infants over a 12-month period. Infants of teenaged mothers showed evidence of more advanced motor and social development in the first 6 months postnatally compared to infants of older mothers. That advance disappeared in the second half of the first year. The loss of advanced development paralleled declines in assistance provided by the mothers of teen mothers.

In a comparison of 23 adolescent and 22 adult mothers, Becker (1987) assessed developmental expectations of infants. As compared to adult mothers, adolescents consistently underestimated the age at which infants attained capabilities. Accuracy of expectations also was greater for adult than adolescent mothers. Further, stress was unrelated to expectations in adult mothers; stress in adolescent mothers was related to expectations, but in the direction opposite from that predicted.

Whiteman, Wuethrich, and Egan (1985) compared outcomes of children who were born prematurely and had necrotizing enterocolitis (NEC) with matched controls (premature infants without NEC). Each group included 19 children from 1 to 4 years of age. Data were collected from parents by mail questionnaire. Growth of the two groups was compared by using head circumference, height, and weight. Significantly more children who had had NEC were at the third percentile for weight compared to matched controls. NEC children averaged 1 month behind controls for onset of walking and sitting. NEC children more often had food intolerances and averaged more physician contacts and rehospitalizations than controls. No significant differences were found in such other areas as temperament.

Barnard, Bee, and Hammond (1984b) contrasted mental development in children with mothers who had high or low education levels. Using data from the Nursing Child Assessment Project, children's mental development was compared to 12, 14, and 48 months. No differences in mental development were found at 12 months, but at both 24 and 48 months, children of high-education mothers performed more favorably than those of low-education mothers.

RELATIONAL/PREDICTIVE RESEARCH

In a retrospective study of developmental outcomes of preterm infants admitted to the neonatal intensive care unit, Trotter, Chang, and Thompson (1982) analyzed outcomes on 101 of 262 surviving infants. Developmental delays were measured by infants' performance on the Bayley Scales of Infant Development (Bayley, 1969) at 12 months postconceptual age. Relations of perinatal variables to outcomes were also explored. Overall, 18 percent of the infants demonstrated developmental delays. Among infants with respiratory distress syndrome (RDS), the incidence of delay was 24 percent, but the incidence of delay did not differ among groups differing in severity of RDS. Associations between development outcomes and the following were not significant: weight for gestational age, neonatal mortality, and high-risk pregnancy scores.

In a longitudinal follow-up of VLBW infants, Schraeder (1986; Schraeder et al., 1987) examined developmental outcomes. Subjects were

41 infants with a mean birth weight of 1203 g. Data were collected from hospital charts and during home visits at 6 and 12 months corrected age (Schraeder, 1986). For this sample, 16 percent of the infants had scores consistent with suspect or delayed development at 12 months corrected age. Predictor variables accounted for 68 percent of the variance in developmental outcomes as measured by the Minnesota Child Development Inventory. Measures of the environment accounted for 67 percent of the variance, and biological and medical variables accounted for the least variance. Furthermore, contemporaneous measures of home environment and developmental level were significantly correlated at both 6 and 12 months. However, the correlation between 6-month home environment and 12-month development exceeded that of 6-month development and 12-month home environment.

At 36 months' corrected age, Schraeder et al. (1987) assessed 40 of the original 41 VLBW children. In a regression analysis including five predictors (days in intensive care, degree of intraventricular hemorrhage, birth weight, days of mechanical ventilation, and total score for home environment), 27 percent of the variance in developmental outcomes was accounted for, and home environment was most important. Of the home environment subscales, language stimulation was foremost in accounting for developmental level. Again, the correlation between 6-month home environment and 36-month developmental level was significantly greater than that between 6-month developmental level and 36-month home environment.

In a follow-up study on an even larger scale, the Nursing Child Assessment Project (NCAP), Barnard and associates (Snyder, Eyres, & Barnard, 1979; Bee et al., 1982; Barnard et al., 1984b; Mitchell, Bee, Hammond, & Barnard, 1985) charted the development of 193 newborns over time. Beginning in the eighth month of pregnancy, the NCAP sample was followed at birth and at 1, 4, 8, 12, 24, 36, and 48 months (Bee et al., 1982; Barnard et al., 1984b). Subsequently, additional follow-up occurred when children were 8 years old (Mitchell et al., 1985). The NCAP sample, recruited from a health maintenance organization, consisted of primiparous mothers who varied with regard to education and perinatal risk. For the most part, the sample was healthy and reflected working and middle-class families (Bee et al., 1982).

In the first publication examining the role of prenatal expectations on infant development, Snyder et al. (1979) reported on mothers' expectations concerning when infants developed certain sensory and learning capacities. Mothers who had later developmental expectations had lower education, income, and psychosocial assets, among other variables. Mothers' prenatal developmental expectations were unrelated to actual newborn behaviors, gestational age, or neurological status. Mothers with later development expectations provided less stimulating home environments to infants during the first year and had infants with less favorable development at 12 and 24 months than mothers with earlier expectations.

In the second publication, Bee et al. (1982) reported a comprehensive analysis of assessments completed from birth through age 4. Variables were grouped into four clusters: (1) perinatal and early infant physical status, (2) family ecology and maternal perceptions, (3) parent-infant interaction and environment, and (4) children's mental, language, and interpersonal developmental levels. Developmental outcomes were mental development at 48 months and receptive and expressive language at 36 months. Only one of 17 variables in the perinatal and infant status cluster was significantly related to any outcome. Overall, the three clusters of family ecology and perception (particularly mother's education and support), parent-infant interaction and environment, and earlier developmental levels each predicted approximately 20 percent to 50 percent of the variance in children's mental and receptive language outcomes. Additional analyses focused on predictors gathered at specific time points; among variables assessed at birth, maternal education, maternal perceptions of infants, and social support were significant predictors of developmental outcomes. Generally, measures of children's performance on developmental tests before 24 months were poor predictors of later outcomes compared to those measured at 24 months or later.

In a third publication (Barnard et al., 1984b), relations between the environmental assessment scale, HOME, and developmental and contextual variables were further explored. HOME subscale scores at 4, 8, 12, and 24 months showed either no or weak relations to mental development at 12 months. However, a number of significant relations occurred between HOME scores, regardless of time measured, and mental development at 24 and 48 months. Overall, when correlations between HOME scores and mental development were examined separately by gender and mother's educational level, few differences were found. In analyses designed to determine at what age certain HOME subscales may be most important for mental development, the following emerged: provision of appropriate play materials at 8 months, opportunity for variety of stimulation at 8 months, maternal involvement at 8 and 12 months, and avoidance of restriction and punishment at 24 months. Further, even when maternal education and socioeconomic class were controlled for, most relations between HOME subscales and mental development still remained significant.

At age 8, children were tested for the presence of learning and behavior problems (Mitchell et al., (1985). Data were analyzed by clusters, by age periods, and finally by combining periods and clusters. Overall discriminant function analyses identified variables associated with learning problems and behavior problems at age 8 years. For learning problems, at least one variable from each of the four clusters was a significant predictor of later problems. In this analysis, nine variables (sex, birth weight, IQ at 48 months, motor development at 36 months, expressive language at 24 months, accidents requiring medical attention at 48 months, years with only one parent, infant-feeding interaction at 12 months, and home environment at 48 months) resulted in a canonical correlation of .64 with learning problems. For behavior problems, no perinatal or infant status variables were among those discriminating between children. Ten variables (expressive language at 12 months, IQ at 48 months, receptive language at 12 months, motor development at 12 months, accidents requiring medical attention at 48 months, years with only one parent, prenatal social support, life change at 24 months, maternal feeding interaction at 12 months, and infant feeding interaction at 4 months) resulted in a canonical correlation of 0.70 with behavior problems.

INTERVENTION RESEARCH

Because there are a number of intervention studies investigating different types of environmental stimulation and developmental outcomes, they are summarized in Table 20–3 for easier display. These studies provided various forms of stimulation to preterm or term infants in hospital or home settings and assessed effects on growth and development. (*Note:* Additional interventions that assessed effects on infant behavior are included in Chapter 17.) Among preterm infants, more studies report increases in weight gain with stimulation in home or hospital settings (Neal, 1969; Malloy 1979; Rice, 1979) than report no increases compared to controls (Kramer et al., 1975; Nelson et al., 1986). Results of stimulation of preterm infants show widely varying effects on developmental outcomes ranging from no effects (Malloy, 1979) to effects on about 80 percent of areas assessed (Katz, 1971). These differences may stem from differences in time of outcome assessment, differences in samples, or intensity of the interventions. In regard to stimulation of term infants in home settings in the United States, results show either no effect on developmental outcomes (Booth, Johnson-Crowley, & Barnard 1985) or negative effects (Koniak-Griffin & Ludington-Hoe, 1988). One study of term infants in the Philippines showed extensive effects of stimulation in the form of passive exercise (Porter, 1972). These differing outcomes may reflect cultural or sample differences or differences in the stimulation given to infants. (See Harrison [1985] [summary in Appendix] and Blackburn [1983] for additional reviews of effects of infant stimulation on growth and development.)

FUTURE RESEARCH DIRECTIONS

Because the infant's environment includes social, temporal, and other contextual aspects of that environment, research about the interaction between the infant, the environment, and developmental outcomes embraces aspects of most other paradigms used to study parents and infants. That is

Table 20–3
INTERVENTIONS RELATED TO ENVIRONMENTAL INFLUENCE ON DEVELOPMENT

Citation: Group/Population	Independent Variable(s)	Dependent Variable(s) & Study Outcomes*
Neal (1969): Sixty-two preterm infants: 31 in experimental and 31 in control groups	Randomization to conditions; experimental group placed in swinging hammock for 30 min three times per day from 5th day of life until 36 wk postconceptual age	At the 36th week postconceptual age: general maturation (+); motor maturation (+); tactile adaptive behavior (0); auditory functioning (+); visual functioning (+); muscle tension (0); irritability (0); weight gain (+); edema (+)
Katz (1971): Sixty-two preterm infants: 31 in experimental and 31 in control groups	Systematically assigned to conditions; experimental group had recording of mothers' voice played for 5 min six times per day from 5th day of life until 252 postconceptual day	At 36 wk postconceptual age: motor development (+); tactile adaptive behavior (+); auditory functioning (+); visual functioning (+); muscle tension (+); irritability (0)
Porter (1972): Ninety-four term Philippine infants aged 4 to 40 wk: 47 in experimental and 47 in control groups	Randomization (?) to conditions; passive motion exercises to extremities for 5 min four times per day for 6 d/wk for 2 mo	After 1 mo of treatment: weight gain (0); length gain (+); motor development (+); adaptive development (+); language development (+); personal-social development (+) After 2 mo of treatment: weight gain (+); length gain (+); motor development (+); adaptive development (+); language development (+); personal-social development (+)
Kramer et al. (1975): Fourteen preterm infants: 8 in experimental and 6 in control groups	Alternatively assigned to conditions; experimental group was hand-stroked for a total of 48 min/day for at least 2 wk while in incubator	Weight gain at hospital discharge (0). Of six comparisons of rate of mental and motor development from time moved to crib to 3 mo later, none were significant (0)

		Rate of social development from 6 wk to 3 mo after transfer to crib (+) Of five comparisons of degree of social development, none were significant (0) Of 30 comparisons of mental & motor development, 5 were significant for motor development (0/+) Production of serum cortisol during stress (0)
Malloy (1979): One hundred twenty-seven preterm infants: 40 in mother's voice group, 44 in Brahms' lullaby group, and 43 in control group	Randomization to conditions: (1) had tape of mother's voice played for 5 min six times per day from 5th day of life till reached 2000 g; (2) had tape of Brahms' lullaby played for 5 min six times per day from 5th day of life till reached 2000 g; (3) no tapes played for control group	At time of hospital discharge: age at discharge (music group significantly younger than control group (+); auditory & visual functioning (0); irritability (0); muscle tension (0); general maturation (0) Rate of weight gain in hospital (+) Mental and motor development at 9 mo of age (0)
Rice (1979): Twenty-nine preterm infants: 15 in experimental and 14 in control group	Randomization to conditions; experimental group received stroking and massaging for 15 min and rocking for 5 min four times per day for 1 mo beginning just after infant's hospital discharge	At 4 mo postnatal age: weight gain (+); length (0); head circumference (0); mature reflexes (+); mental development (+); motor development (0)
Barnard & Bee (1983): Eighty-eight preterm infants: 26 in fixed-interval condition, 23 in self-activating condition, 10 in quasi-self-activating condition, and 28 in control condition (*Note:* Sum of numbers reported by authors equals 87).	Assigned to conditions based on modified random assignment with blocking for three variables (*Note:* Quasi-self-activating formed inadvertently via a technical error)	For 109 variables assessed during hospitalization to age 24 mo, only 15 significant differences were found overall (0) On HOME subscales at 24 mo, two of six were significant (+)

Table 20–3
INTERVENTIONS RELATED TO ENVIRONMENTAL INFLUENCE ON DEVELOPMENT *(Continued)*

Citation: Group/Population	Independent Variable(s)	Dependent Variable(s) & Study Outcomes*
	The three intervention conditions were given from mean age of 7 d until mean age of 21 d: (1) fixed interval had 15 min of stimulation (rocking and heart beat sound) each hour; (2) self-activating had stimulation for 15 min after each 90-s period of inactivity; (3) quasi-self-activating had stimulation for 15 min after being inactive 90 s but not more than once per hour	On teaching interaction at 8 mo, 1 of 4 was significant (−) Mental development at 8 mo (0) Mental development at 24 mo (+) Psychomotor development at 8 and 24 mo (0)
Booth et al. (1985): Thirty-four primiparous mothers and their term infants: 11 in each experimental group and 12 in control group	Sequential assignment to conditions: (1) powder massage or (2) nonpowder massage groups in which mothers massaged infants twice daily for 15 min from 4 wk to 16 wk; or (3) control group	At 16 wk: infant development (0); mother-infant teaching interaction (0); mother-infant free-play interaction (0)
Nelson et al. (1986): Thirty preterm infants in stable condition: 15 in experimental and 15 in control groups	Randomization to conditions; experimental group placed on pile decubitus ulcer pad for 5 d	Weight gain during 5 d on pad (0)
Koniak-Griffin & Ludington-Hoe (1988): Eighty-one healthy, full-term infants; numbers in each of three experimental groups and one control group not given	Randomization to conditions that began 3 to 4 d after birth and ended at 3 mo; experimental conditions were (1) daily stroking of infant for 5 to 7 min, (2) placement in multisensory hammock during sleep, or (3) a combination of (1) and (2); in control (placebo) condition a bicolored sheet was used for sleeping	Weight gain at 4 and 8 mo (0) Psychomotor development at 4 and 8 mo (0) Mental development at 4 mo (0) Mental development at 8 mo: control group had higher scores than stroked group (−)

Note: A *(+) indicates outcomes favored group(s) that received treatments hypothesized to enhance attachment over comparison/control groups; a (0) indicates no differences between treated and comparison/control groups; a (−) indicates outcomes favored comparison/control group(s) that did not receive treatment over groups that received treatments hypothesized to enhance development.

evident in studies that test long-term effects of neonatal intervention to enhance behavioral organization (Barnard & Bee, 1983). It is also evident in long-term prospective studies of developmental outcomes (Bee et al., 1982). Thus, one of the most noteworthy additions to future research projects in nursing would be to extend them into longitudinal programs of research that consider developmental outcomes also. Although improved developmental outcome is not relevant to all studies undertaken in parent-infant nursing, in many cases it could contribute a significant perspective to existing investigations. For example, do studies that test interventions aimed at easing the transition to parenthood also enhance infants' developmental outcomes? Because parents are critical factors in infants' environments, it is not unreasonable to expect that aiding parents may also aid infants. Studies of prenatal stress and emotional disequilibrium during pregnancy (Norbeck & Tilden, 1983) provide a base for subsequent exploration of child outcomes in diverse socioemotional environments (Gross, 1989). Still another emerging area of interest is intergenerational studies of parenting and development (Fox & Fogelman, 1990).

If future research in parent-infant nursing does include extensions of short-term correlational and intervention studies, several methodological considerations are pertinent. First, setting up methods for tracking families over time is needed. At the outset, it should include obtaining alternatives for locating families in the event of moves, for example, names, addresses, and telephone numbers of relatives. Second, families should be informed of the potential of long-term follow-up and should be willing to engage in such an endeavor. Third, a comprehensive plan for each project phase of the overall longitudinal research program should be developed. Critical decisions in such a plan are when measurements will be taken, what those measures will be, how contact and motivation of families will be maintained, and how financing in each phase will be approached. Ideally, a plan of alternative sources of funding for each phase of the program should be in place. Fourth, the commitment of the investigator to undertaking a longitudinal investigation is critical to maintaining the integrity of the study and data quality. The complexity of longitudinal research requires meticulous attention to operational and methodological matters (Magnusson & Bergman, 1990).

Longitudinal studies trace pathways of influence related to children's development. As a result, from them we learn information essential for understanding how development proceeds and how and when intervention should be offered. For that reason, longitudinal studies of children's development should receive high priority in parent-infant nursing.

REFERENCES

Barnard, K. E., & Bee, H. L. (1983). The impact of temporally patterned stimulation on the development of preterm infants. *Child Development, 54,* 1156–1167.

Barnard, K. E., Bee, H. L., & Hammond, M. A. (1984a). Developmental changes in maternal interactions with term and preterm infants. *Infant Behavior and Development, 7,* 101–113.

Barnard, K. E., Bee, H. L., & Hammond, M. A. (1984b). Home environment and cognitive development in a healthy, low-risk sample: The Seattle study. In A. W. Gottfried (Ed.), *Home environment and early cognitive development* (pp. 117–149). Orlando: Academic Press.

Barnard, K. E., Booth, C. L., Mitchell, S. K., & Telzrow, R. W. (1988). Newborn nursing models: A test of early intervention to high-risk infants and families. In E. D. Hibbs (Ed.), *Children and families: Studies in prevention and intervention* (pp. 63–81). Madison: International Universities Press.

Barnard, K. E., & Eyres, J. (1979). *Child health assessment: 2. The first year of life.* DHEW Publication No. HRA 79-25.

Barnard, K. E., Hammond, M. A., Sumner, G. A., Kang, R., Johnson-Crowley, N., Snyder, C., Spietz, A., Blackburn, S., Brandt, P., & Magyary, D. (1987). Helping parents with preterm infants: Field test of a protocol. *Early Child Development and Care, 27,* 255–290.

Barnard, K. E., Magyary, D., Sumner, G., Booth, C. L., Mitchell, S. K., & Spieker, S. (1988). Prevention of parenting alterations for women with low social support. *Psychiatry, 51*(3), 248–253.

Bayley, N. (1969). *Bayley Scales of Infant Development: Birth to Two Years.* New York: Psychological Corporation.

Becker, P. T. (1987). Sensitivity to infant development and behavior: A comparison of adolescent and adult single mothers. *Research in Nursing & Health, 10,* 119–127.

Becker, P. T., Lederman, R. P., & Lederman, E. (1989). Neonatal measures of attention and early cognitive status. *Research in Nursing & Health, 12,* 381–388.

Bee, H. L., Barnard, K. E., Eyres, S. J., Gray, C. A., Hammond, M. A., Spietz, A. L., Snyder, C., & Clark, B. (1982). Prediction of IQ and language skill from perinatal status, child performance, family characteristics, and mother-infant interaction. *Child Development, 53,* 1134–1156.

Bee, H. L., Hammond, M. A., Eyres, S. J., Barnard, K. E., & Snyder, C. (1986). The impact of parental life change on the early development of children. *Research in Nursing & Health, 9,* 65–74.

Behar, L., & Stringfield, S. (1974). A behavior rating scale for the preschool child. *Developmental Psychology, 10,* 601–610.

Blackburn, S. T. (1983). Fostering behavioral development of high-risk infants. *Journal of Obstetric, Gynecologic and Neonatal Nursing, 12,* 76s–86s.

Blackburn, S. T., & Barnard, K. E. (1985). Analysis of caregiving events relating to preterm infants in the special care unit. In A. W. Gottfried & J. L. Gaiter (Eds.), *Infant stress under intensive care* (pp. 113–129). Baltimore: University Park Press.

Booth, C. L., Johnson-Crowley, N., & Barnard, K. E. (1985). Infant massage and exercise: Worth the effort? *MCN, The American Journal of Maternal/Child Nursing, 10,* 184–189.

Bradley, R. H., & Caldwell, B. (1979). Home observation for measurement of the environment: A revision of the preschool scale. *American Journal of Mental Deficiency, 84,* 234–244.

Caldwell, B. M., & Bradley, R. H. (1978). *Manual for the home observation for measurement of the environment.* Little Rock, AK: University of Arkansas.

Castiglia, P. T., & Petrini, M. A. (1985). Selecting a developmental screening tool. *Pediatric Nursing, 11*(1), 8–17.

Dunn, L. M., & Markwardt, F. C. (1970). *Manual for Peabody individual achievement test.* Circle Pines, MN: American Guidance Service.

Duxbury, M. L., Henly, S. J., Broz, L. J., Armstrong, G. D., & Wachdorf, C. M. (1984). Caregiver disruptions and sleep of high-risk infants. *Heart & Lung, 13*(2), 141–147.

Fluharty, N. B. (1974). The design and standardization of a speech and language screening test for use with preschool children. *Journal of Speech and Hearing Disorders, 39,* 75–88.

Fox, J., & Fogelman, K. (1990). New possibilities for longitudinal studies of intergenerational factors in child health and development. In D. Magnusson & L. R. Bergman (Eds.), *Data quality in longitudinal research* (pp. 233–248). Cambridge, England: Cambridge University Press.

Frankenberg, W. K., & Dodds, J. (1977). *Manual: Denver developmental screening test.* Denver: University of Colorado Medical Center.

Frankenberg, W. K., Doorninck, W. J. van, Liddell, T. N., & Dick, N. P. (1976). The Denver prescreening developmental questionnaire (PDQ). *Pediatrics, 57,* 744–753.

Frankenburg, W. K., Goldstein, A., & Camp, B. (1971). The revised Denver developmental screening test: Its accuracy as a screening instrument. *Journal of Pediatrics, 79,* 988–995.

Gesell, A. L., & Amatruda, C. S. (1947). *Developmental diagnosis* (2nd ed.). New York: Paul B. Hoeber.

Gross, D. (1989). Implications of maternal depression for the development of young children. *Image, 21,* 103–107.

Harrison, L. L. (1985). Effects of early supplemental stimulation programs for premature infants: Review of the literature. *Maternal-Child Nursing Journal, 14,* 69–90.

Harrison, L. L., & Twardosz, S. (1986). Teaching mothers about their preterm infants. *Journal of Obstetric, Gynecologic, and Neonatal Nursing, 15,* 165–172.

Hedrick, D. L., Prather, E. M., & Tobin, A. R. (1975). *Sequenced inventory of communication development.* Seattle: University of Washington.

Houldin, A. D. (1987). Infant temperament and the quality of the childrearing environment. *Maternal-Child Nursing Journal, 16,* 131–143.

Ireton, H., & Thwing, E. (1974). *Manual for Minnesota child development inventory.* Minneapolis: Behavior Science Systems.

Katz, V. (1971). Auditory stimulation and developmental behavior of the premature infant. *Nursing Research, 20,* 196–201.

Koniak-Griffin, D., & Ludington-Hoe, S. M. (1988). Developmental and temperament outcomes of sensory stimulation in healthy infants. *Nursing Research, 37,* 70–76.

Koniak-Griffin, D., & Rummell, M. (1988). Temperament in infancy: Stability, change, and correlates. *Maternal-Child Nursing Journal, 17,* 25–40.

Kramer, M., Chamorro, I., Green, D., & Knudtson, F. (1975). Extra tactile stimulation of the premature infant. *Nursing Research, 24,* 324–334.

Magnusson, D., & Bergman, L. R. (Eds.). (1990). *Data quality in longitudinal research.* Cambridge, England: Cambridge University Press.

Malloy, G. B. (1979). The relationship between maternal and musical auditory stimulation and the developmental behavior of premature infants. In G. C. Anderson, B. Raff, M. Duxbury, & P. Carroll (Eds.), *Newborn behavioral organization: Nursing research and implications.* New York: Liss. March of Dimes Birth Defects Foundation. *Birth Defects, Original Article Series, 15*(7), 81–98.

McCarthy, D. (1972). *Manual for the McCarthy scales of children's abilities.* New York: Psychological Corporation.

McDaniel, E. D., & Piers, E. V. (1973). *McDaniel-Piers young children's self-concept scale.* West Lafayette, IN: Purdue Educational Research Center.

Medoff-Cooper, B. (1986). Temperament in very low birth weight infants. *Nursing Research, 35,* 139–143.

Medoff-Cooper, B., Schraeder, B. D. (1982). Developmental trends and behavioral styles in very low birth weight infants. *Nursing Research, 31,* 68–72.

Mercer, R. T. (1986). Predictors of maternal role attainment at one year postbirth. *Western Journal of Nursing Research, 8,* 9–25.

Mercer, R. T., Hackley, K. C., & Bostrom, A. (1984a). Adolescent motherhood. *Journal of Adolescent Health Care, 5*(1), 7–13.

Mercer, R. T., Hackley, K. C., & Bostrom, A. (1984b). Social support of teenage mothers. In K. E. Barnard, P. A. Brandt, B. S.

Raff, & P. Carroll (Eds.), *Social support and families of vulnerable infants.* White Plains, NY: March of Dimes Birth Defects Foundation. *Birth Defects, Original Article Series, 20*(5), 245–272.

Mitchell, S. K., Bee, H. L., Hammond, M. A., & Barnard, K. E. (1985). Prediction of school and behavior problems in children followed from birth to age eight. In W. K. Frankenburg, R. N. Emde, & J. W. Sullivan (Eds.), *Early identification of children at risk* (pp. 117–132). New York: Plenum.

Mueller, C. W., & Parcel, T. L. (1981). Measures of socioeconomic status: Alternatives and recommendations. *Child Development, 52,* 13–30.

Myklebust, H. R. (1981). *The pupil rating scale revised: Screening for learning disabilities.* New York: Grune & Stratton.

Neal, M. V. (1969). The relationship between a regimen of vestibular stimulation and developmental behavior of the small premature infant. Paper presented at American Nurses Association Fifth Nursing Research Conference, Louisiana.

Nelson, D., Heitman, R., & Jennings, C. (1986). Effects of tactile stimulation on premature infant weight gain. *Journal of Obstetric, Gynecologic and Neonatal Nursing, 15,* 262–267.

Norbeck, J. S., & Tilden, V. P. (1983, March). Life stress, social support, and emotional disequilibrium in complications of pregnancy: A prospective, multivariate study. *Journal of Health and Social Behavior, 24,* 30–46.

Pohlman, S., & Beardslee, C., (1987). Contacts experienced by neonates in intensive care environments. *Maternal-Child Nursing Journal, 16,* 207–226.

Porter, L. S. (1972). The impact of physical-physiological activity on infants' growth and development. *Nursing Research, 21,* 210–219.

Rice, R. D. (1979). The effects of the Rice infant sensorimotor stimulation treatment on the development of high-risk infants. In G. C. Anderson, B. Raff, M. Duxbury, & P. Carroll (Eds.), *Newborn behavioral organization: Nursing research and implications.* New York: Liss. March of Dimes Birth Defects Foundation. *Birth Defects, Original Article Series, 15*(7), 7–26.

Rosenblith, J. F. (1961). The modified Graham behavior test for neonates: Test-retest reliability, normative data and hypotheses for future work. *Biology for the Neonate, 3,* 174–192.

Rosenblith, J. F. (1979). The Graham/Rosenblith behavioral examination for newborns: Prognostic value and procedural issues. In J. D. Osofsky (Ed.), *Handbook of infant development* (pp. 216–249). New York: Wiley.

Schraeder, B. D. (1986). Developmental progress in very low birth weight infants during the first year of life. *Nursing Research, 35,* 237–242.

Schraeder, B. D., & Medoff-Cooper, B. (1983). Development and temperament in very low birth weight infants—the second year. *Nursing Research, 32,* 331–335.

Schraeder, B. D., Rappaport, J., & Courtwright, L. (1987). Preschool development of very low birthweight infants. *Image, 19,* 174–177.

Snyder, C., Eyres, S. J., & Barnard, K. (1979). New findings about mothers' antenatal expectations and their relationship to infant development. *MCN, The American Journal of Maternal/Child Nursing, 4,* 354–357.

Terman, L. M., & Merrill, M. A. (1973). *Stanford-Binet intelligence scale-manual for the third revision form L-M.* Boston: Houghton Mifflin.

Thomas, K. A. (1989). How the NICU environment sounds to a preterm infant. *MCN, The American Journal of Maternal/Child Nursing, 14,* 249–251.

Trotter, C. W., Chang, P., & Thompson, T. (1982). Perinatal factors and the developmental outcome of preterm infants. *Journal of Obstetric, Gynecologic, and Neonatal Nursing, 11,* 83–89.

Wechsler, D. (1974). *Manual for the Wechsler intelligence scale for children—revised.* New York: Psychological Corporation.

Whiteman, L., Wuethrich, M., & Egan, E. (1985). Infants who survive necrotizing entercolitis. *Maternal-Child Nursing Journal, 14,* 123–133.

CHAPTER 21

Conclusion

"Rather than there being a fixed set of methodological standards for evaluating theories, science evolves new methods and standards as it advances, and these standards are formed by what has been learned" (Suppe & Jacox, 1985, p. 258). Similarly, our understanding of nursing science evolves and is transformed by the advances and experiences of nurse scientists.

This book captures the science of the field of parent-infant nursing at a point in time. The research and theoretical work reported here will serve as the base for both advancing and transforming our ideas about future directions for parent-infant nursing as a specialized area of nursing knowledge. What are some of the lessons to be learned?

First, because the field of parent-infant nursing is young and diverse, some areas are considerably more developed than others. Some of the most actively researched phenomena include stress, social support, health status, postpartal role attainment experiences, and infant behavioral organization. Particularly noteworthy is the accumulating research relative to (1) the effects of stress and social support on parent-infant well-being and (2) the effects of the environment (generally) and stimulation (specifically) on infant development. Many other areas of parent-infant nursing research provide promising insights into phenomena, but they lack the volume of research needed to formulate strong research-based conclusions. *Thus, the field of parent-infant nursing science has much room for growth and is far from saturated.*

Second, at present all the phenomena covered in this book offer promise for understanding nursing's contribution to the health and well-being of parents and infants. *The critical hubs for parent-infant nursing research are the phenomena of parental role attainment and infant behavioral organization.* My reason for saying this is twofold. First, both role attainment and behavioral organization focus on the person, the metaparadigm concept inherent in each recurring theme (Fawcett, 1984) identified by Donaldson and Crowley (1978). Second, role attainment and behavioral organization form the base for future development. If one of the goals of parent-infant nursing is to assist parents and infants in being in the very best position for future development, then understanding role attainment and behavioral organization is critical to nurses. At the same time, it would be a mistake to view these phenomena in isolation from other important phenomena such as the environment. The phenomena of parent-infant nursing are multifaceted and interconnected.

Third, apparent in some facets of this book is the shared nature of the knowledge embedded in parent-infant nursing science. Nurses participate, along with members of other disciplines, in advancing the knowledge about health and well-being of parents and infants. Nurses also use theories originated in other fields to study aspects of parent-infant nursing, particularly with regard to phenomena such as stress, social support, and developmental outcomes. Contributing to the development of shared knowledge does not mean that the scientific contribution of nurses is not unique. *Parent-infant nursing science draws on its own sources as well as those from other disciplines for its theoretical understanding.* Those sources include nursing conceptual models, midrange nursing theories such as role attainment and identity, and theories originated by health- and development-related disciplines. In this regard, parent-infant nursing is a unique intersection of nursing perspectives with the health and developmental needs of parents and infants.

If parent-infant nurses use knowledge or theories from outside nursing in their research, is their research really nursing research? The answer is "yes" because the nursing metaparadigm provides a broad rubric, not a narrow one, for nursing research. Concern for the person, health, environment, and nursing, and the recurring themes, for example, laws governing health and well-being (Donaldson & Crowley, 1978; Fawcett, 1984), invite a broad, complex, and comprehensive perspective. That perspective is held together by a focus on the person and one or more of the metaparadigm concepts (see Newman, 1983; Fawcett, 1984). Because theories from other disciplines aid in elaborating aspects of nursing's metaparadigm should not detract from the unique perspective of nursing as a field of study. Would not many sciences be paralyzed without knowledge from mathematics and logic? The more important issue for nursing science is how well theories from any field, including nursing, successfully elaborate the nursing metaparadigm. *At this stage of parent-infant nursing science, it is not necessarily the origin of a theory, but rather its creative use by nursing investigators to solve scientific problems, that determines its merit.*

Fourth, it was apparent in preparing this book that many nurse investigators still work in isolation. This isolation takes many forms. Some are isolated from existing literature because of limited access to libraries and computerized literature retrieval systems. Others are intellectually isolated from others who are simultaneously engaging in similar work. Still others conduct research in isolation from theorists whose work could potentially offer substance and dimensionality to the research. *More forums are needed to bring parent-infant nurse investigators and theorists together. Because science is a communal enterprise, parent-infant nurse investigators need more avenues for participating in their emerging scientific community.*

REFERENCES

Donaldson, S. K., & Crowley, D. M. (1978). The discipline of nursing. *Nursing Outlook, 26*(2), 113–120.

Fawcett, J. (1984). The metaparadigm of nursing: Present status and future refinements. *Image, 16*, 84–87.

Newman, M. A. (1983). The continuing revolution: A history of nursing science. In N. L. Chaska (Ed.), *The nursing profession: A time to speak* (pp. 385–393). New York: McGraw-Hill.

Suppe, F., & Jacox, A. K. (1985). Philosophy of science and the development of nursing theory. *Annual Review of Nursing Research, 3*, 241–267.

Appendix

Preterm

Infants

Table A–1
STUDIES OF TACTILE STIMULATION OF PRETERM INFANTS

Investigator	Subjects	Type of Stimulation	Results
Solkoff, Yaffe, Weintraub, & Blase, 1969	5 E, 5 C,* 1190- to 1590-g birthweight	Stroked 5 min/h during first 10 d	E more active; regained birth weight faster; and had fewer developmental abnormalities
Powell, 1974	12 E_1, 12 E_2 †, 12 C; 1000–2000 g	E_1—maternal handling (varied) E_2—extra handling by nurse 20 min bid E_1&$_2$—started at age 3 d and continued throughout hospital stay	Increased Bayley scores at 4 mo for handled infants in E_1 and E_2
Kattwinkel, Nearman, Fanaroff, Katona, & Klaus, 1975	6 E_1, 12 E_2; 620- to 1600-g birthweight 26- to 31-wk gestational age	E_1—rubbing extremities 5 out of each 15 min for 3 h E_2—nasal CPAP Age at time of study 2—35 d	E_1 and E_2 had decreased apnea compared to control periods
Kramer, Chamorro, Green, & Knudtson, 1975	8E, 6C; birthweights: E = 1441 g C = 1418 g Gestational age E and C=33 wk	48 min of stroking qd for 2 wk (2–3 min before and after each feeding)	No difference in weight gain or plasma cortisol levels in response to stress; increased rate of social dev. in E's
Jay, 1982	13E, 13C; birthweights: E = 1287 g C = 1323 g; Gestational age: E = 29.53 wk C = 29.69 wk	12 min of "gentle human touch," 4 times each day for 10 d	No difference in weight gain, temperature stability, apnea, tolerance of oral nutrients, or incidence of neonatal complications E infants had higher hematocrits and required less oxygen

*E = experimental group;
†E_1 = experimental group 1
C = control group
E_2 = experimental group 2
Source: L. Harrison (1985). Effects of early supplemental stimulation programs for preterm infants. *Maternal Child Nursing Journal, 14,* pp. 72–73. Copyright 1985 by the Graduate Programs of Maternity Nursing and Nursing Care of Children at the University of Pittsburgh. Reprinted by permission.

Table A–2
STUDIES OF AUDITORY STIMULATION OF PRETERM INFANTS

Investigator	Subjects	Type of Stimulation	Results
Katz, 1971	31 E, 31 C; 28–32 wk	Starting at age 5 d, ending at 36 wk postconception age; tape of mother's voice × 5 min, six times per day at 2-h intervals	E's had greater auditory and visual function at 36 wk
Segall, 1971	30 E, 30 C; 28–32 wk	E—mother's recorded voice 30 min/d until 36 wks postconception age	E—showed greater increase in heart rate when exposed to "white noise" at 36 wk during quiet period and greater decrease in heart rate when exposed to tape of mother's voice while crying
Chapman, 1979	50 E_1, 51 E_2, 52 C; 26–33 wk gestation	E_1—tape recording of mother's voice E_2—tape of Brahm's lullaby starting at age 5 d, continuing to 1800 g (average duration = 34 d)	E_2 had faster weight gain than E_1 or C; no differences in limb movements
Malloy, 1979	40 E_1, 44 E_2, 43 C; 26–33 wks	Same as Chapman, 1979	E_1 and E_2 discharged 6–9 d sooner; E's had lower scores on Bayley at 9 mo

Source: L. Harrison (1985). Effects of early supplemental stimulation programs for preterm infants. *Maternal Child Nursing Journal, 14,* p. 74. Copyright 1985 by the Graduate Programs of Maternity Nursing and Nursing Care of Children at the University of Pittsburgh. Reprinted by permission.

Table A–3
STUDIES OF VESTIBULAR STIMULATION OF PRETERM INFANTS

Investigator	Subjects	Type of Stimulation	Results
Neal, 1969	31E 31C; 28–32 wk gestation, 800–1700 g	Vestibular stimulation in oscillating hammock, beginning at age 5 d continuing until infant reached 36 wk postconceptual age. Stimulation was provided for 30-min periods three times a day.	E's had increased weight gain, motor and general maturity, and auditory and visual functioning and were less irritable than C infants
Korner, Kraemer, Haffner, & Cosper, 1975	10 E, 11 C; 1050–1920 g 27–34 wk	E—placed on oscillating water bed before age 6 d; remained on for 7 d	E had less apnea; better results if placed before age 4 d
Korner, Guilleminault, Van den Hoed, & Baldwin, 1978	Eight infants with apnea; 1270–1650 g 27–32 wk	24 h on oscillating water beds during alternate 6-h periods between ages 7 and 28 d	Decreased apnea while on water beds
Korner, 1981 (letter to editor)	No specific details of study mentioned	12 h each on oscillating and nonoscillating water beds compared with two 12-h control periods	Response of very sick infants was unpredictable; some actually had increased apnea and bradycardia on water beds
Jones, 1981	14 infants with apnea; (some receiving theophylline) 930–1470 g 27- to 33-wk gestation	23 h on water bed, alternating 4 h with and 4 h without oscillations; postnatal age at treatment ranged from 1 to 32 d	Nonoscillating bed associated with less prolonged apnea as compared to oscillating and control periods
Tuck, Monin, Duvivier, May, & Vert, 1982	12 preterm infants with recurrent, idiopathic apnea 800–1700 g 26–32 wk	Bed rocking for 3–4 h compared to control period; postnatal age at treatment ranged from 2 to 45 d	All infants had decreased apnea, bradycardia, and hypoxia when bed was rocking
Korner & Schneider, 1983	12 E, 8 C; 22–33 wks; severe RDS on ventillators Mean birth weights = 1309 g (E) and 1149 g (C)	E placed on oscillating water bed starting at age 4 d and ending at 34- to 35-wk conceptional age	At 34 to 35 wk postconception, E's had better orientation and motor maturity and less irritability and wakefulness

Source: L. Harrison (1985). Effects of early supplemental stimulation programs for preterm infants. *Maternal Child Nursing Journal, 14,* pp. 76–77.

Table A–4
EFFECTS OF GUSTATORY STIMULATION OF PRETERM INFANTS

Investigator	Subjects	Type of Stimulation	Results
Measel & Anderson, 1979	59 infants; 24–34 wks; NG feeding at least 10 ml full-strength formula per feeding; randomly assigned to E or C	Pacifier during and 5 min after feeding for E group	E had increased readiness for bottle; increased weight gain; earlier hospital discharge

Source: L. Harrison (1985). Effects of early supplemental stimulation programs for preterm infants. *Maternal Child Nursing Journal, 14,* p. 79. Copyright 1985 by the Graduate Programs of Maternity Nursing and Nursing Care of Children at the University of Pittsburgh. Reprinted by permission.

Table A–5
STUDIES OF MULTIMODAL STIMULATION OF PRETERM INFANTS

Investigator	Subjects	Type of Stimulation	Results
Hasselmeyer, 1964	30 E, 30 C 1501–2000 g	Held during feeds; stroking, rocking for 10 min every 8 h	E quieter and had more rapid weight gain
Scarr-Salapatek & Williams, 1973	15 E, 15 C; 1300–1800 g 28- to 36-wk gestation	Visual (mobile), tactile and vestibular stimulation during feedings and when awake, starting when admitted to nursery and continued during hospital stay (N 6 wk); weekly home visits to teach infant stimulation for 10 mo	E's had higher Cattell scores at 1 y
Kramer & Pierpont, 1976	11 E, 9 C; less than 34 wk gestational age	Stimulation from age 2 to 7 d including: placement on rocking water bed for 1 h prior to each feeding and tapes of heart-beat sound and woman's voice during rocking	E's ate better and were more active; had increased weight gain and head growth
Rice, 1977	15 E, 15 C; 1420–2245 g 32- to 37-wk gestation	Cephalocaudal stroking, massage, and rocking 20 min qid for 30 d beginning day after hospital discharge	E's had better weight gain, increased Bayley scores at 4 mo, and better reflex maturity
White & Labarba, 1976	6 E, 6 C; 1588–2041 g 32- to 36-wk gestation	Rubbing body and passive flexion of arms and legs 15 min each hour for 4 h between 2 and 11 d of age	E's had increased weight gain and increased formula ingestion and "seemed" more responsive and alert
Chapman, 1979	Total N = 35, randomly divided into E and C; 26- to 33-wk gestational age at birth	5- to 10-min tapes of mother's voice, alternating with Brahm's lullaby, played midway between feeds, starting at age 5 d until hospital discharge; 10 mo home program to teach infant stimulation to parents after discharge	E's have increased Bayley scores at 9 and 18 mo and increased Standford-Binet scores at 36 mo

Leib, Benfield, & Guidubaldi, 1980	14 C, 14 E; 1200–1800 g Mean gestational age: C = 32.5 wk E = 32.79 wk	Starting when infant reached 1700 g and intermediate care status; visual stimulation (mobile), rubbing, talking, rocking during/after feedings; 5-min music box song after feedings.	E's had increased Bayley scores at 6 mo past EDC; no difference in weight gain, but E's received fewer calories
Naqvi & Hyatt, 1980	15 E, 15 C; less than 36 wk gestational age	30-min stimulation, 5 d/wk starting with admission to intermediate care and continuing until discharge: tactile stimulation of chin and mouth, visual stimulation with toys, and auditory stimulation with music box and parent's voices	E's had stronger sucks, increased weight gain, and shorter hospital stay
Rausch, 1981	20 E, 20 C 1000–2000 g Not requiring intubation	Gentle body rubbing and limb exercises 15 min/d	E's had increased fluid intake and fewer abnormal stooling patterns
Barnard & Bee, 1983	26 E_1, 23 E_2, 10 E_3, 28C Mean gestational age: E_1 = 31.21 wk E_2 = 31.02 wk E_3 = 30.48 wk C = 31.09 wk Mean birthweight ranged from 1277 to 1420 g in the four groups	E_1—15 min rocking and heart-beat sound per hour; E_2—15 min rocking and heart-beat stimulation after each 90 s of inactivity; E_3—same as E_2 but would repeat only once per hour; all starting at age 3–15 d and continuing an average of 21 d	In hospital, all E's had decreased rates of activity for first 8 d and then increased rates; fewer abnormal reflexes and better orienting responses; higher Bayley scores at 24 mo; E_3 had most favorable response

Source: L. Harrison (1985). Effects of early supplemental stimulation programs for preterm infants. *Maternal Child Nursing Journal, 14,* pp. 81–84.

REFERENCES

Barnard, K. E., & Bee, H. L. (1983). The impact of temporally patterned stimulation on the development of preterm infants. *Child Development, 54,* 1156–1167.

Chapman, J. S. (1978). The effect of pre-term infants' decreasing mortality on their future morbidity: Preliminary examination of long-term outcomes of stimulation programs for pre-term infants. *Nursing Papers, 10*(2–3), 31–54.

Chapman, J. S. (1979). Influence of varied stimuli on development of motor patterns in the premature infant. In G. Anderson & B. Raff (Eds.), *Newborn behavioral organization: Nursing research and implications.* New York: Alan R. Liss.

Hasselmeyer, E. C. (1964). Handling and premature infant behavior: An experimental study of the relationship between handling and selected physiological, pathological, and behavioral indices related to body functioning among a group of prematurely born infants who weighed between 1501 and 2000 grams at birth and were between the ages of seven and 28 days of life (Doctoral dissertation, New York University, 1963). *Dissertation Abstracts International, 24B,* 2874B–2875B. (University Microfilms No. 64-257)

Jay, S. S. (1982). Effects of gentle human touch on mechanically ventilated very-short-gestation infants. *Maternal-Child Nursing Journal, 11*(4), 199–256.

Jones, D. A. (1981). Controlled trail of a regularly cycled oscillating waterbed and a non-oscillating waterbed in the prevention of apnea in the preterm infant. *Archives of Disease in Childhood, 56,* 889–891.

Kattwinkel, J., Nearman, H. S., Fanaroff, A. A., Katona, P. G., & Klaus, M. H. (1975). Apnea of prematurity: Comparative therapeutic effects of cutaneous stimulation and nasal continuous positive airway pressure. *The Journal of Pediatrics, 86*(4), 588–592.

Katz, V. (1971). Auditory stimulation and developmental behavior of the premature infant. *Nursing Research, 20,* 196–201.

Korner, A. F. (1981). What we don't know about water beds and apneic preterm infants. *Pediatrics, 68,* 306–307.

Korner, A. F., Guilleminault, C., Van den Hoed, J., & Baldwin, R. B. (1978). Reduction of sleep apnea and bradycardia in preterm infants on oscillating waterbeds: A controlled polygraphic study. *Pediatrics, 61,* 528–533.

Korner, A. F., Kraemer, H. C., Haffner, M. E., & Cosper, L. M. (1975). Effects of waterbed flotation on premature infants: A pilot study. *Pediatrics, 56,* 361–366.

Korner, A. F., & Schneider, P. (1983). Effects of vestibular-proprioceptive stimulation on the neurobehavioral development of preterm infants: A pilot study. *Neuropediatrics, 14,* 170–175.

Kramer, L. I., & Pierpont, M. E. (1976). Rocking waterbeds and auditory stimuli to enhance growth of preterm infants. *The Journal of Pediatrics, 88,* 297–299.

Kramer, M., Chamorro, I., Green, D., & Knudtson, F. (1975). Extra tactile stimulation of the premature infant. *Nursing Research, 24,* 324–334.

Leib, S. A., Benfield, G., & Guidubaldi, J. (1980). Effects of early intervention and stimulation of the preterm infant. *Pediatrics, 66,* 83–89.

Malloy, G. B. (1979). The relationship between maternal and musical auditory stimulation and the developmental behavior of premature infants. In G. Anderson & B. Raff (Eds.), *Newborn behavioral organization: Nursing research and implications.* New York: Alan R. Liss.

Measel, C. P., & Anderson, G. C. (1979). Nonnutritive sucking during tube feedings: Effect on clinical course in premature infants. *Journal of Obstetric, Gynecologic, and Neonatal Nursing, 8,* 265–272.

Naqvi, M., & Hyatt, K. (1980). Neonatal stimulation program reduces hospital time and cost. *Pediatric Research, 14,* 436.

Neal, M. V. (1969). The relationship between a regimen of vestibular stimulation and developmental behavior of the small premature infant. In American Nurses Association (Ed.), *Fifth Nursing Research Conference.* New Orleans, March 3–5, 1969.

Powell, L. F. (1974). The effect of extra stimulation and maternal involvement on the development of low-birth-weight infants and on maternal behavior. *Child Development, 45,* 106–113.

Rausch, P. B. (1981). Effects of tactile and kinesthetic stimulation on preterm infants. *Journal of Obstetric, Gynecologic, and Neonatal Nursing, 10,* 34–37.

Rice, R. D. (1977). Neurophysiological development in premature infants following stimulation. *Developmental Psychology, 13,* 69–76.

Scarr-Salapatek, S., & Williams, M. L. (1973). The effects of early stimulation on low-birth-weight infants. *Child Development, 44,* 94–101.

Segall, M. (1971). Relationship between auditory stimulation and heart rate response of the premature infant. In American Nurses' Association *Nursing Research Conference,* Vol. 7, 119–129. Kansas City: American Nurses' Association.

Solkoff, N., Yaffe, S., Weintraub, D., & Blase, B. (1969). Effects of handling on the subsequent developments of premature infants. *Developmental Psychology, 1,* 765–768.

Tuck, S. J., Monin, P., Duvivier, C., May, T., & Vert, P. (1982). Effect of a rocking bed on apnea of prematurity. *Archives of Disease in Childhood, 57,* 475–476.

White, J. L., & Labarba, R. C. (1976). The effects of tactile and kinesthetic stimulation on neonatal development in the premature infant. *Developmental Psychobiology, 9,* 569–577.

Author Index

See also general index, p. 437

General Index

Numbers in *italics* indicate figures; numbers followed by a "t" indicate tabular material.

See also author index, p. 417